AF801063

Published by Dr Joe Cheung, Sydney, Australia

First published in 2025

Copyright © Dr Joannes C W Cheung 2025

Purchasers of the book may wish to photocopy portions of the text or figures for use with their patients or for educational purposes. Such copies should not be for sale. This is acceptable to the publisher, who, nevertheless, disclaims any responsibility for the consequences of any such use of this material in clinical practice. It is not necessary to write to Dr Joannes C W Cheung for permission to make such photocopies. This permission does not extend to making multiple copies of the book for use by the purchaser, for use by others, or for resale.
Individuals or clinics requiring copies may purchase them through **www.joecheung.com.au**

Printed in Sydney, Australia

Common Pain Syndromes: A NEW APPROACH
Includes bibliographical references.

ISBN 978-0-646-73418-7 Paperback

Common Pain Syndromes:
A NEW APPROACH

Dr Joe Cheung MB BS

ACKNOWLEDGEMENTS

To Dr Janet G Travell and Dr David G Simons, their tireless work on the concept of trigger points and pain.

To Dr Toshikatsu Yamamoto, the ingenious innovator and the discoverer of YNSA.

To Dr Emily Teo, the eternally enthusiastic, generous healer and teacher, who taught me YNSA.

To my colleagues from different specialities, Dr Ali Gursel, MBBS (Hons), FRACS (Ortho), Associate Professor Jonathon S Mulford, MBBS (Hons), FRACS (Ortho), Diploma Clinical Trial, and others who have reviewed and contributed to the four common musculoskeletal regions, in their diagnostic features and conventional treatments.

The innumerable teachers and colleagues I learnt from.

My medical students, together we clarified numerous ideas and concepts.

To Catriona Murdie, who proofread and made the book immensely more readable.

To Peter Mackie, whose design skills and unwavering patience, gave the content balance and brought the book to life.

To Jesse Cheung, the 170 odd drawings, many of which had been re-worked multiple times, would not be in the book without his IT skills and patience.

My family, who helped me in all aspects in writing this book, and

Most of all, to all my patients, who taught me something in every encounter.

PREFACE

I have worked in primary healthcare as a general practitioner for over 35 years. My special interests include musculoskeletal (MSK) medicine and teaching, and I wish to share some knowledge on pain syndromes and treatment methods learnt during my career. This book has been written with medical graduates interested in MSK medicine and acupuncture practitioners in mind, but I hope that others in the healthcare profession may find this useful as well.

MSK problems are common, comprising about 20% of all primary care presentations.[1] With recent technological advancements, when presented with MSK problems there appears to be an over-reliance on imaging findings. Imaging results are not always reliable in making a diagnosis, and a false positive result can often mislead the clinician. For example, in one study 65.3% of sampled patients with rotator cuff tears were asymptomatic.[2] In anyone over 40, imaging of any joint can show varying degrees of osteoarthritis (OA), but this does not mean that the presenting pain is due to OA. While imaging has an important role in the diagnostic process, it should not replace a thorough history, detailed examination and palpation.

Another trend involves our eagerness to resort to various medications or invasive interventions to treat MSK problems too early on. In literature review of pain syndromes, strains and sprains are often listed as the most common causes. Manual treatments, mechanical interventions and exercises to address these muscular dysfunctions are usually recommended as a first-line approach. Logically, the aim should be a curative approach with these modalities rather than pain management with medications, but in practice this is not the case. Furthermore, in order to address our ever-rising opioid overuse problem, we need to treat pain syndromes better and aim to cure or improve each condition instead of just treating the pain caused by it.

Over the years, the more I worked with MSK problems, the more I became convinced that muscles and their **myofascial trigger points (TrPs) account for a lot of the pain in any pain syndrome.** TrPs are increasingly being recognised by physiotherapists and other manual therapy practitioners, but often overlooked by medical practitioners as a source of pain. One of the main reasons for this is that **TrPs can only be diagnosed by careful targeted palpation and cannot be diagnosed by imaging.** It is for these reasons that I embark on writing this book. The book will cover the four most common regions of MSK pain presentations, namely lower back, knee, shoulder and neck. We will look at how TrPs can cause pain in these regions. As there are hundreds of muscles in the body, this book focuses on the most common TrPs and ones that are more difficult to palpate.

Having discussed the importance of TrPs in many pain syndromes, this book then describes a relatively new but, from my experience, very effective way of treating them – Yamamoto New Scalp Acupuncture (YNSA), which I have been practising for about 17 years. Throughout the book, I outline 35 case studies to examine the diagnostic process, the relevance of TrPs in each of these cases, and how to treat these TrPs using YNSA and other conventional methods.

It is my hope that this book will prompt readers to rethink how pain is conceptualised and treated, and that for any pain syndrome they are presented with, **it is very useful to consider TrPs of all the muscles and their attachment sites close to the pain.** TrPs may well be part of – if not the sole cause of – the pain. Over millenniums, doctors and healers have known about myofascial TrPs and treated them with various methods. I have tried many techniques myself – some conventional Western medicine and some more traditional – and have found YNSA to be a very useful modality.

In summary, **this book contains firstly a revision of pain syndromes,** their diagnostic features and conventional Western medical management. **Secondly, an emphasis will be made on the important role myofascial TrPs play in any pain syndromes and how to palpate for them. Lastly, I will introduce a relatively new, 50-year-old modality – YNSA – to treat TrPs.** While many treatment methods exist for TrPs, I hope readers will give this modality a try. This book will give precise instructions for trained acupuncturists to treat TrPs with some YNSA techniques. **For the readers who are not interested in the modality of acupuncture, the section on acupuncture can be omitted.**

For any health practitioners who want to try YNSA, they should check with their professional governing bodies the necessary qualification requirements before they can practise acupuncture, as different states and countries may have different regulatory requirements. For others who do not want to go down the path of learning acupuncture themselves, they can refer to acupuncturists that are familiar with YNSA.

DISCLAIMER

The published content is not to be relied upon by anyone using it as being in the manner of a medical consultation or advice. All medical information is general in nature and in no way provides individual clinical advice. Readers should be advised to contact their own doctor or other health professional in relation to any specific clinical concern they may have.

MYOFASCIAL TRIGGER POINTS

A trigger point (TrP) can be defined as a focus of hyperirritability in a tissue, palpable as a nodule or a cord that, when compressed, is locally tender and can give rise to referred pain. Types of TrPs include myofascial, cutaneous, fascial, ligamentous and periosteal.[3] This book focuses on myofascial TrPs.

Myofascial TrPs were brought to medical attention by the late Dr Janet Travell, the personal physician to the late US President John F Kennedy. Dr Travell had a diverse background; she worked as a cardiologist and also served as a professor in pharmacology. She co-authored a two-volume book with Dr David Simons, **Myofascial Pain and Dysfunction: The Trigger Point Manual.[4]** Dr Travell observed that palpable tender muscular knots/cords/nodules or TrPs can cause pain at the site and refer to adjacent regions, often mimicking other conditions. For example, TrPs in the left latissimus dorsi can mimic angina, or TrPs in the piriformis and gluteus minimus can mimic lumbar radiculopathy. Travell and Simons painstakingly listed, studied and mapped the pain distribution of every trigger point for all the muscles in the body.

Basically, I believe that TrPs can result from:

1. **traumatic injury to a muscle e.g. a fall or misstep straining some thigh muscles.**
2. **constant contraction of a muscle due to repetitive strain e.g. an antalgic gait of a patient walking with a severe knee OA or a heel pain, thereby straining the lumbosacral muscles.**
3. **constant activation of a muscle in order to protect a nearby painful joint or structure e.g. constant activation of the gracilis and quadriceps to protect the pain of an osteoarthritic knee joint, or constant activation of multiple shoulder muscles to protect the pain of a supraspinatus tear.**

It is thought that this strain in the muscle causes a neuromuscular dysfunction (an abnormal depolarisation) of the motor endplate and excessive release of acetylcholine, leading to a sustained sarcomere shortening. This sustained contraction leads to the compression of local blood vessels, causing a reduction of oxygen and nutrients as well as the release of sensitising chemicals. These events activate muscle nociceptors, thereby causing central and peripheral sensitisation.[5] As every muscle is enclosed by fascia, and fascia microscopically is filled with blood vessels, lymphatics and nervous tissues, it is possible that fascia may well be a system of communication by itself. The theory is that adjacent muscles are not separated but linked by fascias, which can affect and influence each other. This concept is useful in both diagnosis and in treatment.[6,7]

TrPs can be minor, for example, a strained neck muscle from a bad night's sleep or painful shoulder muscles from playing a game of tennis. These will settle spontaneously over time, or with some stretches and gentle manual therapies. TrPs can also be severe and chronic, for example, a serious whiplash injury to the neck muscles from a severe motor vehicle accident, or a strained back muscle with fractured vertebrae from a significant fall down a flight of stairs. These TrPs are much harder to treat and eradicate.

Since the pioneering work of Dr Janet Travell and Dr David Simons, more and more doctors and other health practitioners have recognised the importance of TrPs in pain syndromes and undertaken research. It is difficult to carry out research on TrPs, as there is a lack of standardised diagnostic criteria. At present, TrPs are not diagnosed by imaging. This may explain why more physical therapy practitioners than medical practitioners recogonise the importance of TrPs in pain syndromes. A systemic review on diagnosing TrPs by imaging showed that ultrasound techniques using vibration sonoelastography and shear wave elastography appeared to have some reliable results, with MRI able to detect some TrPs when using MRE and T2 mapping, and work is also being done on thermography.[8] At present, TrPs are diagnosed by palpation and, therefore, subjected to examiners' expertise, making accuracy in research difficult.

I believe that doctors and healers across different cultures, over hundreds, potentially thousands of years, have observed that these TrPs are the cause of many pain syndromes. Numerous methods have been created and evolved to eliminate them, with manual therapies and physical treatments remaining the mainstay of treatment. Most cultures have developed their own styles of massage, muscle release techniques, mobilisation and manipulation methods over time. Other modalities include acupuncture, moxibustion (heat treatment generated by burning the moxa plant powder), cupping (glass suction cups to suck/disperse the muscle knots, found in Eastern and Middle Eastern cultures), heat packs, hot spas and Japanese onsens have been invented and practised. Different types of stretching and strengthening exercises have also been created to treat these TrPs, such as yoga and Tai Chi.

Nowadays, there are some positive research findings for treating TrPs with manual therapies and 'dry needling'. A meta-analysis on 37 randomised controlled trials (RCTs) with 1,574 participants found that a combination of different types of manual therapies are more effective than the control group. However, the improvement of Visual Analogue Scale (VAS) was only at 1.75.[9] A systemic review and meta-analysis on the effectiveness of 'dry needling' on TrPs showed low to moderate evidence of improvement as compared to sham needling.[10] Other types of physical therapeutic modalities are also used, from the McKenzie method, osteopathy, Feldenkrais method and Alexander technique, to more modern physiotherapy-based programs and neuromuscular exercises.

Modern technological advances such as mechanical massage gadgets, transcutaneous electrical nerve stimulation (TENS) machine, interferentials and photobiomodulation (PBM) therapy (low-level laser light treatments) have also been used. Pharmacological therapies such as analgesics, non-steroidal anti-inflammatory drugs (NSAIDs), muscle relaxants, antidepressants, anticonvulsants and opioids are widely used. In recent years, calcitonin gene-related peptide (CGRP) monoclonal antibodies have been used to target an inflammatory peptide to treat migraines. Doctors have tried injecting TrPs with saline, hypertonic dextrose solutions, local anaesthetics, corticosteroid and Botox (the PREEMPT protocol for migraines). In-depth patient education and psychological approaches are used for chronic pain as well. Unfortunately, none have been consistently successful.

If an illness is easily cured by one or two very effective treatment methods – for example, penicillin for follicular tonsillitis, or appendectomy for appendicitis – there would be no need to search for additional methods. There exists so many different methods to treat TrPs, implying that probably none has consistent success.

From my experience, in many chronic and severe pain syndromes, TrPs are a very important part, and at times the main cause of the pain. Notably, some of these palpable tender muscular nodules can persist for many years, resistant to many different treatments.

Research and reviews of the efficacies of different treatment modalities, such as different manual therapies, massage techniques and acupuncture, often yield conflicting results. It is easy to dismiss a 'non-Western medicine' modality by looking at just one or a few negative reviews. For example, some would dismiss the efficacy of acupuncture after reading a few negative reviews despite its continued practice over 4,500 years and the existence of positive reviews.[11,12]

Acupuncture is also recommended as a treatment for 43 diseases by the World Health Organisation.[13] Interestingly, modern 'mainstream' therapists are revisiting some of these old methods, whether it be physiotherapists using dry needling, or cupping used on Olympic swimmers.

It is true many of these modalities cannot be easily standardised and therefore cannot be accurately measured. They are more of an art, with individual practitioner variations and success dependent on individual therapists. For example, two physiotherapists using similar treatment techniques can have completely different results.

Logically, we should try to eradicate these TrPs using various physical therapies first before invasive interventions or long-term drug treatments. Our objective is to cure or improve the MSK condition rather than a pain management approach.

It is my hope that this book, with its many drawings of muscle palpation, will invite the reader to palpate muscles more readily and **to palpate for TrPs in all the muscles close to the pain of any pain syndromes,** even in muscles not mentioned in this book. Having located the TrPs, to consider them as part of, if not the main cause of the pain.

NB. Three short videos on TrP palpation techniques for the knee, lower back, neck/ shoulder regions are available on YouTube under joecheungYNSA, or visit http://www.joecheung.com.au

YAMAMOTO NEW SCALP ACUPUNCTURE (YNSA)

This section of the book is only intended for readers who are interested in, or practise the modality of, acupuncture.

YNSA is a 'microsystem' of acupuncture. A microsystem, or somatotope, is a small area or a miniature topographic map of the body located somewhere on the body, which can be utilised to treat the different anatomical parts it represents. The concept of a somatotope is not new. For example, maps of the body have long been used in various ancient traditions. In Egypt, India and China, reflexology treatments focused on a map of the body on the feet. Korean acupuncture uses a similar map on the hand, while French acupuncturists are known for their proficiency in treating the body through a map on the ear. The ear microsystem was discovered in the 1950s when a French MD Dr Paul Nogier from Lyon observed the Algerian practice of charring a spot on the ear to treat sciatic pain, and from that he developed a whole system of auricular acupuncture.

Dr Toshikatsu Yamamoto, MD, PhD, is a Western medical doctor in Japan who discovered a scalp microsystem by chance about 50 years ago.[14] Again, quite accidentally he discovered that a spot on the forehead was effective in treating shoulder pain, and from that he mapped out somatotopes on the scalp representing the whole body. YNSA is a new map, one that does not follow the traditional Chinese acupuncture meridian system. It is particularly effective in treating MSK and neurological problems. Dr Yamamoto's books have been translated into more than ten languages, including Chinese and Russian. He has established a rehabilitation hospital in Miyazaki, Japan, which draws patients from all over the world who suffer neurological and MSK problems resistant to other treatments.

From my experience, YNSA is particularly effective in treating TrPs. During the treatment, one would:

1. Identify the problem – for example, a TRP in the levator scapulae in a patient with cervicogenic headache.

2. Find an active point representing the levator scapulae TRP on the scalp somatotope/map. (An active point is usually a tiny, very tender area on the skin specific to that TRP. When there is no problem, there would not be any active points and, interestingly, the area would normalise when the condition subsides.)

3. An acupuncture needle is then inserted about 5mm deep and activated by twirling the needle clockwise several times. From my experience, if the needle is inserted accurately, the TRP in the levator scapulae would soften immediately. An average of six needles are used for one condition, treating different TrPs involved. If the treatment is successful, there would be 10 – 15% progressive improvement after each treatment. For minor problems, only several treatments are required. For severe or chronic cases, it would take

more treatments, with progressive improvements. Like any other modalities, treatments can continue until improvements have plateaued.

The single most significant feature of this modality is that, for each and every one of the treatments that is successful, the evidence of improvement is instant (by retesting the range of movement, repalpating the TrPs and patient feedback). If there is no improvement on the TrPs, then it is likely that either the point location is wrong, or the insertion has missed the point.

From my experience, another unique feature of YNSA is it can often resolve and eradicate TrPs that may be significant in size, have been in existence for many years and are resistant to many modalities of treatments.

Having practised YNSA for 17 years, I have found that once these TrPs are treated successfully by YNSA, they do not return unless the muscle is reinjured.

Acupuncture in general is quite well accepted and practised not just in Asian countries, but also in many European countries. This is most likely due to the missionaries spreading Christianity in China and merchants from the trade routes bringing the practice from China back to their own countries from the sixteenth century onwards.

In the last 50 years, YNSA has been embraced by many countries in Asia and Europe. Interestingly in Brazil, their health system has included YNSA in their medical training and it is practised in their hospitals. These countries have recognised the efficacy of YNSA and the fact that it is very safe to practise (the scalp does not have many vulnerable structures), easy to learn and does not require the very complex traditional Chinese medicine theoretical knowledge as a prerequisite.

There is emerging international research regarding YNSA treatment,[15,16] with some key articles summarised as follows. Dr Thomas Schockert, a Western-trained medical doctor from Germany, learned YNSA from Dr Yamamoto in 1995 and has been running YNSA courses in Europe for many years.[17] Schockert undertook a study of 17 stroke patients who were treated with YNSA and assessed, aided by functional MRIs. The treated sample showed premotor and motor activities in the functional MRIs and some improvement of movement and spasticity.[18]

A prospective randomised control of stroke patients treated by YNSA was undertaken by the University of Pécs in Hungary.[19] In the study, 520 post-stroke patients were given rehabilitation and YNSA acupuncture, while the control group was treated with rehabilitation only. The acupuncture group was given a small absorbable thread (instead of acupuncture needles) into YNSA points. The outcome was measured by the Barthel Index, Rivermead Mobility Index, SF-36 questionnaire and Visual Analogue Scale (VAS) The outcome was very favourable, with the quality-of-life SF-36 showing significant improvement (P:0.005) and VAS showing significant improvement (P: 0.001).

A small sample study of 20 patients in Brazil with head and neck pain showed an average VAS improvement from 7.9 to 0.8 with YNSA treatment.[20] Another study on 80 patients with non-specific lower back pain (LBP) from Brazil showed significant improvement.[21] A study of 46 patients with neck and shoulder pain in Italy's San Luca Hospital also showed significant improvement.[22]

A systemic review on painful conditions using YNSA treatment was undertaken by Derrick Patrick Artioli et al.[23] Using PubMed, PEDro, SciELO and LILACS databases, the treated group was found to be superior to the control group ($P<0.05$). In considering the research evidence of the efficacy of YNSA, there are an increasing number of studies being done. However, further research is still required. In these small number of studies, YNSA appeared to show promising results.

Now, why and how can this microsystem work? How can some highly resistant TrPs the size of half a squash ball, that have 'existed' for 20 years, be tamed by a few tiny needles on the scalp, never to return? Noting that one of the current treatments of chronic cervicogenic headaches is a session of 30 or so Botox injections every three months (the PREEMPT Protocol), and that this is not curative either. I am afraid that no one really knows the answer at this point in time.

I once asked a professor in anatomy and embryology that question. He offered that, 'As the embryo develops, the ball of cells unrolls itself and migrates, it is possible that some cells that are destined to be the lower limbs, for example, can leave a trail of such cells all the way to the scalp.' It is an interesting theory, but it probably would not hold up in the scientific world.

When I set out to write this book, I originally intended to separate the conventional medical aspects of MSK problem from the YNSA treatment content. However, from my experience, YNSA has been so effective in treating myofascial trigger points, as indicated in many of the case studies, it would be logical to discuss these together.

How do we find out more about YNSA or even learn to practise it?

I believe that every medical graduate is well suited to learn and practise YNSA, as:

1. They are trained to diagnose and rule out red-flag conditions that need urgent intervention and to use conventional treatment for the condition if it is deemed to be more appropriate.
2. YNSA does not require the full understanding of the complicated traditional Chinese medicine theories and meridians.
3. It is completely safe as most of the YNSA acupuncture points are on the scalp, free of vital blood vessels and nerves, and the depth of needle insertion is only about 5mm.
4. Acupuncture needle insertion is easy to learn (Fig. 27).
5. YNSA can also be practised by directing a laser beam from a dedicated acupuncture laser gun or even a laser pointer – instead of acupuncture needles – on the active points, making the application even simpler (Fig. 30).

In order to practise acupuncture (including laser acupuncture) in Australia and charge a Medicare item with rebates, a medical graduate is required to complete an acupuncture training course from the Australian Medical Acupuncture College (AMAC) or a university applied science bachelor or master degree on acupuncture.

For any health practitioners who want to try YNSA, they should check the necessary qualification requirements with their professional governing bodies before they can practise acupuncture as different states and countries may have different regulatory requirements. For others who do not want to go down the path of learning acupuncture themselves, they can refer to acupuncturists that are familiar with YNSA.

There are many other conventional modalities that can successfully treat MSK problems and TrPs, many of which are described in this book. Introducing a relatively new modality of treatment can often be met with resistance from more established systems. However, I believe this is a treatment worth seriously considering. Having tried most of the conventional MSK treatment modalities and experienced firsthand the results YNSA can bring, I am constantly impressed by the treatment's effectiveness especially for patients suffering from chronic and daily pain.

The YNSA system is quite complex; it is made up of a number of points, somatotopes and diagnostic methods. There are A, B, C, D, E, F, G, H and I points, also sensory points, brain points, cranial nerves and Ypsilon points. There are also the J, K, I and chest somatotopes. It is not the intention of this book to describe the whole YNSA treatment system – there are other published books written for that purpose.[24,25] In order to simplify the YNSA system, this book focuses mainly on the J and K somatotopes to treat the TrPs. They are very easy to learn and I believe sufficient by themselves in treating most TrPs.

1. HISTORY-TAKING AND DIAGNOSIS

HISTORY, HISTORY, HISTORY

Experienced clinicians often say that, if we cannot narrow the differential diagnoses down to two to three conditions through history-taking, doing a routine general examination and casting a net of numerous imaging and tests would likely cause further confusion. A good history, reasoning out the cause of the pain, and a targeted examination should yield the correct diagnosis, where imaging should play a more supportive role. **Spending more time to take a thorough history will actually save time in the long run.**

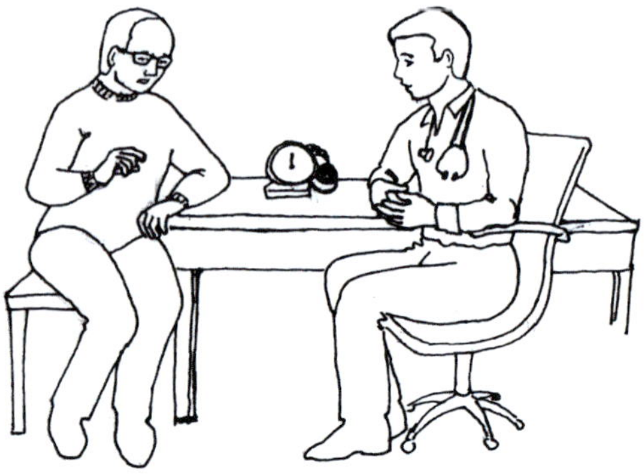

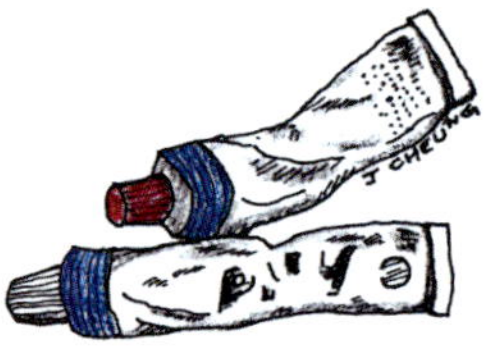

My suggested approach is to **superglue ourselves to our chairs** and not get up to examine the patient until we have asked all the possible questions. If we think all the questions have been asked, ask some more! Set aside our provisional diagnosis, and ask more questions on our differential diagnoses. I have a habit of retelling the history back to the patient, to ensure that all the details are correct, while also collecting my thoughts on the case. I always challenge myself to make the diagnosis by just using the history, before getting up from my chair to examine the patient.

Dr Arthur Doyle, the creator and author of the Sherlock Holmes series of books, was actually a practicing physician. Surely, when challenged with a clinical problem, like Dr Doyle, we must all have a bit of Sherlock Holmes in us?

FRAMEWORK OF QUESTIONING IN PAIN SYNDROMES

A **framework of questions is useful** when approaching pain syndromes. With practice, a mental framework of questioning will become automatic.

1. Are there any **red flags**? e.g. unstable fractures, urgent neurological presentations (cauda equina), urgent vascular presentations (aortic aneurysm, subarachnoid haemorrhage), acute/serious infections and undiagnosed malignancies.
2. Any history of **trauma or sporting injuries?** *Causing possible fractures, joint injuries, muscle and ligament injuries. Bear in mind that injuries can occur without any trauma in the older age group.*
3. Could the patient's **employment, sports and activities** have contributed to the presenting problem? *e.g. a handyman building a stone retaining wall.*
4. **Is it infective?** *Unexplained pain with fever, abscess, septic arthritis, osteomyelitis.*
5. **Is it osteoarthritis?** *e.g. insidious in onset, 'I have had this knee pain for years', morning stiffness less than 30 minutes, pain worse with activities, improves with rest.*
6. Is it an **inflammatory joint disease?** *Typically, prolonged morning stiffness of greater than 30 minutes, pain worse with rest, improves with activities, other joint involvement.*
7. **Is it gout?** *Can affect joints and ligaments, thought to be underdiagnosed.*[26,27]
8. Is it a **radiculopathy?** *Pain fits the corresponding dermatomes, possible sensory and motor changes.*
9. Is the pain from **muscle strain/myofascial trigger points?** *This can give rise to referred pain.*
10. **Is it a neuralgia?** *e.g. neuralgia in the occipital nerves, sciatic nerve, pudendal nerve, genitofemoral nerve, post herpetic neuralgias.*
11. **Is it a tumour (benign or malignant) or a cyst**? *e.g. primary or metastatic cancer, synovial cysts.*
12. Is the pain coming from **neighbouring structures?** *e.g. neck strain causing headaches, soleus TrPs causing plantar heel pain, hip joint problems referring pain to the knee or lower back, abdominal pathologies referring pain to the lower back.*
13. Is the pain coming from **distal pathologies?** *e.g. antalgic gait from chronic knee or heel problems causing lower back pain, liver pathologies giving right shoulder pain, renal colic causing pain in the back.*

DIFFERENTIATING NEUROMUSCULAR PAIN SYNDROMES

While OA, radiculopathy, trigger points and neuralgias share some common features, they can be differentiated (see Table 1).

Table 1: Different Neuromuscular Pains

	Nerve root impingement	**Peripheral nerve entrapment***	**Facet joint arthropathy**	**Muscular myofascial trigger points**
Distribution of pain	Fits the dermatomes, tends to include the extremities in distribution	Area innervated by the nerve, can radiate along the course of the nerve	Fits the facet joint pain distributions, tends to be more axial in distribution, rarely passes the elbow or knees	The affected muscles, their attachment sites and adjacent areas (these can overlap with other causes of pain e.g. TrPs in Latissimus dorsi overlapping with C8 radiculopathy)
Nature of pain	Tends to be more constant, tends to be severe	Tends to be more constant, tends to be severe	Worse on movements, especially in extension and rotation (when the facet joints are loaded)	Tends to be intermittent, tends to be less severe, pain can be aggravated by certain movements when the affected muscles are activated
Numbness	Possible	Possible	Usually not	Possible
Muscle weakness and associated clumsy movements	Possible	Possible	Nil	Nil
Reflex changes	Possible	Rarely	Nil	Nil
Tenderness on palpation on the painful area	Nil	Can be tender at the site of impingement	Can be tender on the facet joint and the overlying intervertebral muscles	Tender trigger points of the relevant muscles
Useful clinical examination/tests	Reflexes, power, sensation	Reflexes, power, sensation	Localised tenderness on palpating over the facet joints, extension – rotation test	Palpation of all the muscles in the painful area and adjacent muscles

Dr Joe Cheung

*Peripheral nerve entrapment can occur, for example, at the occiptal nerves, median sciatic nerve, pudendal nerve etc.

NB. The pain distribution of intervertebral joints/discs degeneration and injury is thought to be similar to that of facet joint arthropathy.

ASSESSMENT OF THE PATIENT'S STATUS AFTER DIAGNOSIS

After making the diagnosis of a pain syndrome, we need to **record** the patient's status and **review** them regularly as the treatment progresses.

1. **Duration of pain**
2. **The nature of the pain, how severe and how constant** is the pain. An easy way to quantify it is by using Visual Analogue Scale (VAS).
3. **Range of movement (ROM)** e.g. record ROM in a neck, shoulder or lower back condition.
4. Specific **activities that could have affected or been aggravated by the pain** e.g. lying on one side in bed, fastening a bra, getting in and out of a car.
5. Effect on **activities of daily living (ADL) and employment** (mobility, household duties, shopping) e.g. a shoulder bursitis in a plasterer with a young family and a mortgage, chronic neck pain and headache in a bus driver.
6. Quality of **sleep.**
7. **State of mind and psychological status** e.g. patient's outlook on the condition, motivation and resistance in the healing process, presence of depression, status of relationships.
8. Efficacies of **previous treatment modalities and medications.**

2. THE KNEE REGION

Briefly, this chapter will cover the following aspects:

Knee problems are common. If 20% of general practitioner (GP) presentation are musculoskeletal problems,[28] with knee problems being the second most common after lower back, a GP would probably see at least one case each day.

The knee joint is the largest and most complex joint in the body. As knees are weight-bearing joints, osteoarthritis (OA) naturally develops over time, more so for patients with prior injuries or high participation in sport. **There are far too many instances when patients are given a diagnosis of OA for their knee pain simply due to the imaging findings.** Most clinicians would agree that the pain and dysfunction of an arthritic joint deteriorates very gradually. Consequently, if a patient presents with a relatively sudden onset of pain or a sudden increase of pre-existing pain – with or without a history of injury – we cannot assume it is purely just from the OA. Muscle and ligamentous injury and strain must be considered as well. Imaging of the knee in anyone over the age of 40 would likely show some evidence of OA, but it may not necessarily be the cause of pain. As doctors, we need to diligently screen and look for other causes of knee pain besides OA, especially muscular/ligamentous strains (trigger points), which can be treated successfully and cured.

Unless you work in the area of sports medicine or trauma, a clinician is unlikely to see too many anterior cruciate ligament (ACL), posterior cruciate ligament (PCL) or collateral ligament rupture. Listed here are some relatively rare conditions which are useful to keep in mind when making a diagnosis.

There are causes of knee pain which are intra-articular and there are causes which are extra-articular or peri-articular. There are more than 20 muscles and tendons attached close to the knee joint. Dysfunction in these muscles and ligaments is very common and can certainly cause pain in the knee area. Unfortunately, these causes are often overlooked. Conditions that can cause knee muscle and tendon dysfunction and pain are trauma (e.g. sporting injuries, falls, misstepping), repetitive strain (e.g. walking with a chronic heel pain) and constant muscle activation in order to protect a nearby painful structure (e.g. constant activation of the gracilis and quadriceps to protect a painful arthritic knee joint). Other factors are obesity and poor core muscle strength, muscle imbalance, faulty walking dynamics and de-conditioning due to a sedentary lifestyle. Often, this muscle and tendon dysfunction are secondary to coexisting lower back pain, hip and foot problems. For example, someone with chronic heel pain can end up straining the thigh adductors, or someone with hip OA straining the iliotibial band (ITB) and the soleus.

It is also important to note that dysfunction or osteoarthritis in the hip joint can refer pain to the knee. A knee pain from any cause can lead to straining of the surrounding muscles, which then become painful themselves. Often, such muscular pain can become the dominant pain, over and above the original cause of pain. Therefore, it is always worthwhile palpating for tightness and tenderness **(TrPs)** in all the nearby muscles and their attachments, and to treat them first, before embarking on invasive treatments or continuing medications.

Trigger point (TrP) can be defined as a focus of hyperirritability in a tissue, palpable as a nodule or a cord, that when compressed, is locally tender and can give rise to referred pain. Types include myofascial, cutaneous, fascial, ligamentous and periosteal.

FRAMEWORK OF QUESTIONING IN KNEE PAIN SYNDROMES

A **framework of questions is useful** when approaching pain syndromes. With practice, a mental framework of questioning will become automatic.

1. Are there any **red flags?** e.g. unstable fractures, urgent neurological presentations, urgent vascular presentations, acute/serious infection and undiagnosed malignancies.

2. Any history of **trauma or sporting injuries?** Causing possible fractures, joint injuries, muscle and ligament injuries. Bear in mind that injuries can occur without any trauma in the older age group e.g. ACL and collateral ligament ruptures.

3. Could the patient's **employment, sports and activities** have contributed to the presenting problem? e.g. a tiler or a netball player.

4. Is it **infective?** Unexplained pain with fever, abscess, septic arthritis, osteomyelitis.

5. Is it **osteoarthritis?** e.g. insidious in onset, 'I have had this knee pain for years', morning stiffness less than 30 minutes, pain worse with activities, improves with rest.

6. Is it an **inflammatory joint disease?** Typically, prolonged morning stiffness of greater than 30 minutes, pain worse with rest, improves with activities, other joint involvement.

7. Is it **gout?** Can affect joints and ligaments, thought to be underdiagnosed.[29,30]

8. Is it a **radiculopathy?** Pain fits the corresponding dermatomes, possible sensory and motor changes.

9. Is the pain from **muscle strain/myofascial trigger points?** This can give rise to referred pain.

10. Is it a **neuralgia?** e.g. peroneal nerve neuralgia.

11. Is it a **tumour (benign or malignant) or a cyst?** e.g. primary or metastatic cancer, synovial cysts.

12. Is the pain coming from **neighbouring structures?** e.g. hip joint problems referring pain to the knee.

13. Is the pain coming from **distal pathologies?** e.g. antalgic gait from a chronic lower back pain or a chronic heel pain can strain the gracilis, thus causing knee pain.

ELEMENTS IN THE HISTORY THAT CAN HELP THE DIAGNOSIS

Age of patient

- Young – septic arthritis or osteomyelitis
- Teenagers to young adults – patellofemoral pain syndrome, osteochondritis dissecans, Osgood-Schlatter Disease, sporting injuries and trauma
- Middle-aged – spontaneous osteonecrosis of the knee (SONK), degenerative meniscal tear
- Older – arthritis
- Any age – referred pain from trigger points, tendinosis and bursitis can affect any age group

Trauma – the mechanism of injury can give a good idea as to what has happened

- ACL – pivot and twist (while playing in a sport) – immediate swelling and cannot keep playing
- Meniscal tear or chondral lesion – twist but can keep playing – swelling the next day
- PCL – dashboard motor vehicle accident (MVA) injury or tackled front-on below the knee (in contact sports)
- Varus or valgus force can result in collateral ligament injury or plateau fracture

Arthritis

- Inflammatory joint diseases – family history, coexisting polyarthritis, inflammatory bowel disease; rheumatoid arthritis (RA) often commences with symmetrical polyarthritis in the metacarpalphalangeal joints (MCPJs), metatarsophalangeal joints (MTPJs) and/or proximal interphalangeal joints of the hands and feet; history of psoriasis in psoriatic arthritis; history of a preceding genital chlamydia or digestive infection in reactive arthritis/Reiter's syndrome
- Gout – rapid onset of severe joint pain, swelling and erythema; absence of trauma
- Osteoarthritis – gradual onset, 'I have this knee pain for years but it has been gradually worsening in the last six months'
- Patellofemoral joint OA – worse going up stairs
- Tibiofemoral joint OA – worse going down stairs

Table 2: Comparison Between RA and OA

Rheumatoid Arthritis (RA)	Osteoarthritis (OA)
• Early morning stiffness • >30 minutes duration • Stiffness and pain are worse after a period of inactivity • Pain improves with use of the joint	• Morning stiffness <30 minutes and often <15 minutes • Pain improves on resting • Pain is worse with use

DIAGRAMMATIC REPRESENTATION OF KNEE CONDITIONS

The causes of knee pains are highly positional, so the site of the pain is very useful in the history-taking.

RIGHT LEG

Anterior Knee Pain

1. Patellofemoral Pain Syndrome
2. Patellofemoral OA
3. Patellar Bursitis
4. Patellar Tendinopathy
5. Osgood-Schlatter Disease
6. Hoffa's Disease
7. Synovial Plica Syndrome
8. Osteochondritis Dissecans
9. Rectus Femoris TrPs
10. Vastus Medialis TrPs
11. Fracture of Patella

Lateral Knee Pain

12. Lat. Collateral Ligament Injury
13. Lat. Meniscal Tear
14. ITB TrPs, Tendinosis, Bursitis
15. Vastus lateralis TrPs

TrPs = trigger points

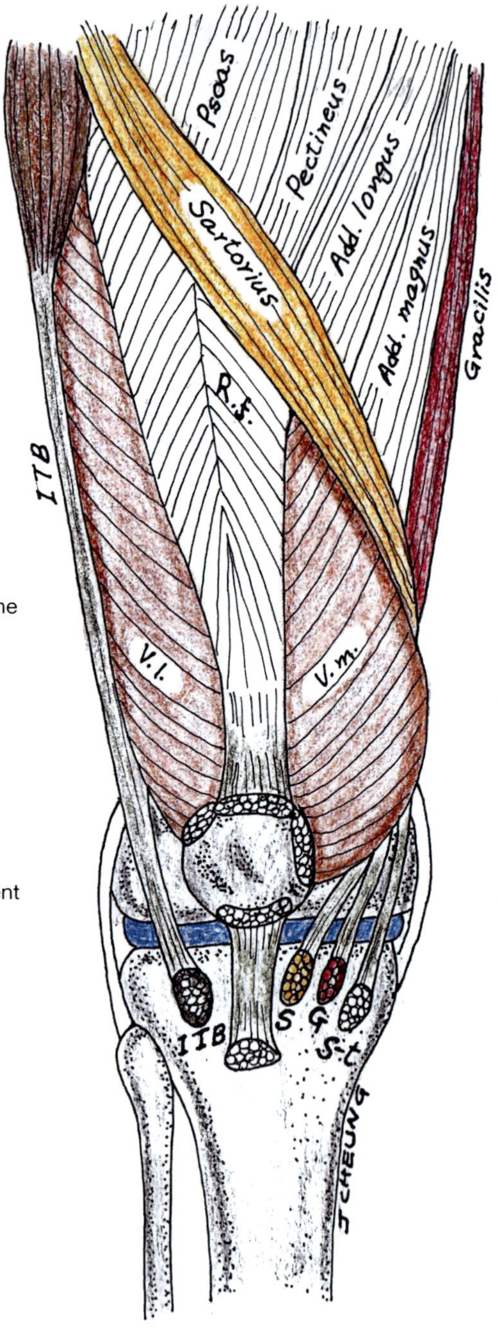

Antero-Medial Knee Pain

16. Spontaneous Osteonecrosis of the Knee
17. Med. Collateral Ligament Injury
18. Med. Meniscal Tear
19. Sartorius TrPs, Tendinosis, Bursitis
20. Gracilis TrPs, Tendinosis, Bursitis
21. Semi-tendonosis TrPs, Tendinosis, Bursitis
22. Add. longus & Brevis TrPs
23. Vastus medialis TrPs
24. Rectus femoris TrPs, Tendinosis

General Knee Pain

25. Tibiofemoral OA
26. Inflammatory Joint Disease
27. Gout
28. Septic Arthritis
29. ACL Rupture
30. Tumour, Cysts, Malignancies
31. Fracture of Tibial Plateau

Figure 1: Front view of knee pain sites

RIGHT LEG

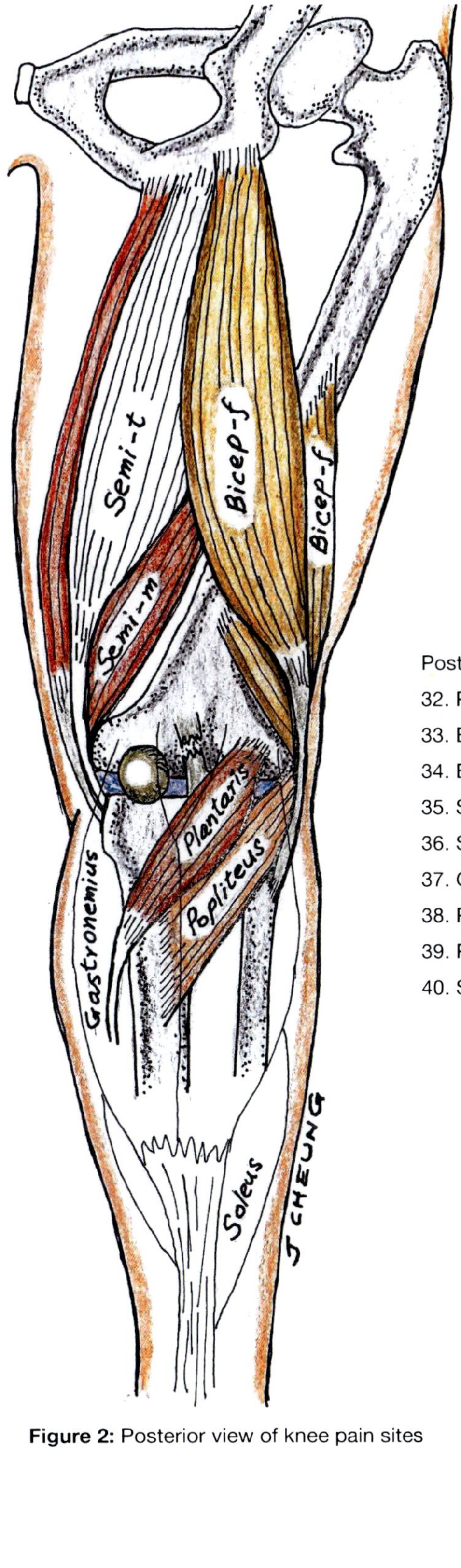

Posterior Knee Pain

32. PCL Rupture
33. Baker's Cyst
34. Bicep femoris TrPs
35. Semi-tendinosis TrPs
36. Semi-membranosis TrPs
37. Gastrocnemius TrPs
38. Popliteus TrPs
39. Plantaris TrPs
40. Soleus TrPs

Figure 2: Posterior view of knee pain sites

PAIN SYNDROMES OF THE KNEE REGION

This section outlines 16 pain syndromes affecting the knee region, ranging from Patellofemoral Pain Syndrome to Baker's cyst.

PATELLOFEMORAL PAIN SYNDROME (PFPS) (no.1 in Figure 1)

PFPS is also known as anterior knee pain syndrome, patella instability syndrome, patellar maltracking, chondromalacia (sick cartilage) of the knee or runner's knee. As the names imply, it is a knee pain caused by malaligned patellar frictional movements. It is important to diagnose and treat PFPS as it is not a simple, self-limiting condition, with more than 50% of individuals describing chronic pain. Incidence is reported to be between 3–6% of the population and **accounts for 25–40% of all knee problems.** It is more common in women.[31]

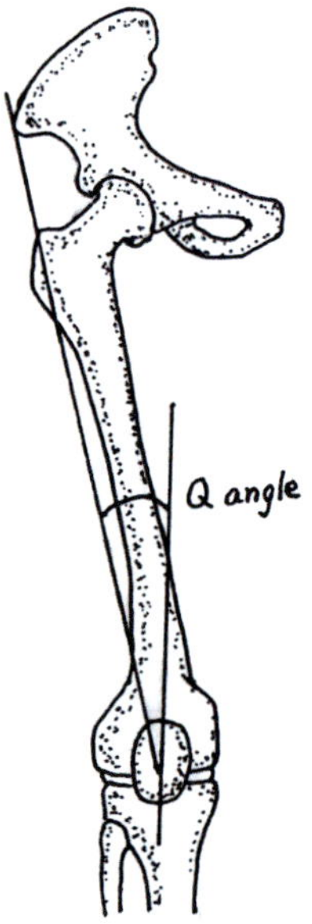

Figure 3: Q angle

The symptom of PFPS is anterior knee pain, which increases when the knee is in flexion during weight-bearing activities. For example, going up and down stairs, squatting, prolonged sitting and running.

The Q angle is the angle formed between a line from the anterior superior iliac spine to the centre of the patella and the line drawn between the centre of the patella and the tibial tubercle. Normal is 14 degrees in men and 17 degrees in women; and an increase in the Q angle is considered a significant risk in PFPS. In a metanalysis, the presence of pain on squatting is the most sensitive examination finding for PFPS, with a positive Tilt test having the highest positive likelihood ratio of 5.4.[32]

Like a lot of MSK conditions, a cluster of positive tests rather than one test would be needed to make a diagnosis. Some useful tests are tenderness on applying pressure on the patellar facets, J-sign on knee extension, the Clarke's test, and pain during squatting and climbing stairs.

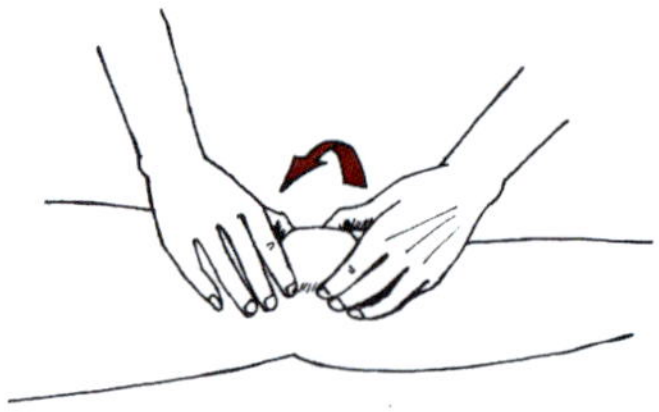

Figure 4: Tilt Test – The lateral edge of the patella lifting >15 degrees is positive.

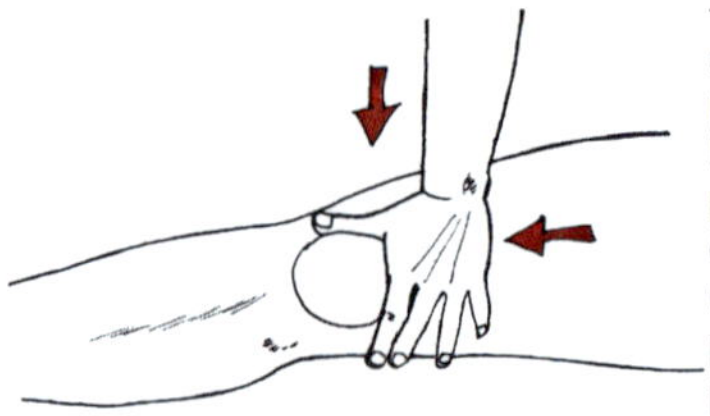

Figure 6: Clarke's Test – Push downwards above the patella and push on the patella laterally, then ask patient to contract the quads. If they are unable to do so or it is painful, the test is positive.

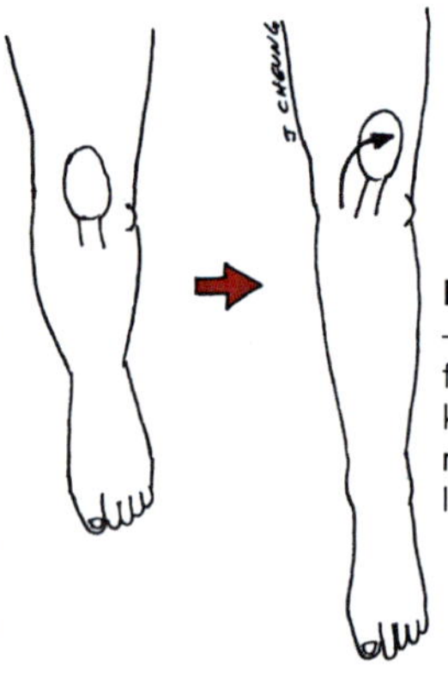

Figure 5: J-sign – On extension from a flexed knee, the patella moves like the letter J.

Essentially, PFPS is a clinical diagnosis for which imaging only helps to exclude other conditions. With this condition the initial approach is to avoid aggravating activities. Common in PFPS is the imbalance between the vastus medialis and the vastus lateralis. As the vastus medialis is the weaker of the two, the main goal is to build up the vastus medialis.[33] This can be done with exercises such as lunges, monosquats and lateral step-ups, with or without patellar taping (like the McConnell taping, which can be done quite easily). Weakness in the hip external rotators and abductors (gluteus medius and gluteus minimus) can also play a part.[34]

A study by Peterson et al showed that a patient's inability to stand on one leg for one minute is a sign of weakness in the hip muscles. It is a useful secondary test in the assessment of PFPS.[35] Tightness in the hamstring and the ITB also needs to be addressed, and a stretching regime is important as studies have shown a significant association between PFPS and hamstring tightness.[36] It is important to address patellar instability and early patellofemoral (PF) osteoarthritis in order to prevent and deter the development of severe PF osteoarthritis, as it is difficult to treat.

OSTEOARTHRITIS OF THE KNEE (no.2 and 25 in Figure 1)

Osteoarthritis (OA) can be defined as a degenerative disease characterised by joint tissue damage that fails to repair. Knee OA is common, affecting 37% of the population older than 60 years old.[37] It increases with age, with the incidence peaking at 70–79 years of age. The ratio of prevalence female to male is 1.69, commonly occurring with women in their 50s and men in their 40s.[38] Knee OA can be classified as primary/idiopathic or secondary. It occurs more and earlier in athletes participating in certain sports (e.g. netball, basketball and various contact sports) in which injuries are common. Previous structural injuries and surgery (meniscectomy, ACL and PCL repair) would also predispose the onset of OA. Other common causative factors are malalignment, muscle weakness, muscle imbalance, dysfunctional walking dynamics, coexisting lower back, hip and foot problems and obesity.

Symptoms

The symptoms are pain, stiffness, reduction in range of movement (ROM) and muscular weakness. The pain is usually dull, localised or involving the whole knee. It increases with use and abates with rest. Morning stiffness can occur but usually lasts <30 minutes and more often <15 minutes (>30 minutes in inflammatory joint diseases).

Examination

Examination may show bony enlargement, mild erythema, warmth and swelling. There may be a reduction in ROM.

Diagnosis

The diagnosis can be radiological or clinical/subjective. Radiological OA can be graded 0 to 4 (the Kellgren-Lawrence scale) according to the presence and severity of osteophytes, joint space loss, sclerosis and cysts. Knee OA can affect the tibiofemoral compartment and/or the patellofemoral joint.

It is important to note that individuals with early painful OA may be free from radiographic changes and, conversely, those with severe radiographic changes may be entirely asymptomatic. There is a correlation between the severity of radiographic disease and symptoms, however, the association is not strong.[39]

Treatments

Weight Loss First and foremost, **the most important treatment is to lose weight** in an overweight patient with knee OA, whether the OA is mild, moderate or severe. Logically, extra weight would put more pressure on the knee joint and causes OA; statistically, the numbers are staggering. In Australia, over 35% of total knee replacements (TKRs) are attributed to patients with BMIs >25. In the 18- to 54-year-old age group, the incidence of TKRs in the population with Obese class I (BMI 30-35) and class II (BMI 35–40) was 15 times that of the population in the same age group. With Obese class III (BMI >40), it was 30 times. It is postulated that the proportion of TKRs being attributed to being overweight and obese in the community could be reduced by over 20% if this population were to all move down one BMI category.[40] In another analysis for overweight patients, for every 1% reduction in weight, there is a 2% reduction in the risk of TKR.[41] In the Australian National Health Survey 2017-2018, two-thirds of the population is overweight (BMI 25-30), and one-third is obese (BMI >30).[42]

To address this grave problem of widespread and increasing obesity, there is only so much a clinician can do on a one-to-one basis. Excessive refined sugar in our diets has contributed immensely to the obesity epidemic we face. Action on a national scale with legislation to reduce the amount of sugar in food products and accompanying public awareness campaigns would be far more effective. In 2018, the UK decided to instigate a sugar tax and, as a result, the food and beverage industry cut 300,000 tonnes of sugar from their products compared to the year prior.

The Australian Medical Association's (AMA) submission in 2023 to a parliamentary inquiry found that, if a sugar tax were to be introduced, we could save $3.1 billion in Australia's health system from mitigating the impact of diabetes alone. The submission also found that preventable disease resulting from people being overweight and/or obese accounts for 18% of health spending ($4.3 billion).[43]

However, in Australia the sugar and food and beverage industry lobbying are so effective that we lack even a discussion or debate about a sugar tax in our parliament. In the meantime, 26 countries in the world have adopted a sugar tax.

TrP Treatment and Preventative Exercises The pain from a knee joint with OA can be from the synovium or from the adjacent muscle TrPs that have developed from the continuing muscle activation to protect the painful knee. Often it is impossible to determine whether the pain is coming from the synovium or from the muscle TrPs. It is worthwhile palpating for TrPs and treating them first. Often the pain can improve significantly. Modalities such as regular stretching exercises, heat and manual therapies (soft tissue massage, mobilisation, etc.) can be trialled.

Treatment in mild and asymptomatic cases should be directed at preventing its progression. Exercises to strengthen the knee extensors (Fig. 65) and hip external rotators and abductors (gluteus minimus and gluteus medius); exercises to improve balance; to lose excessive weight; and general level of fitness. There is strong evidence that various dedicated exercise programs can improve pain and function in arthritic knees, such as the GLA:D® Program (Good Life with osteoArthritis: Denmark), aquatic exercises, yoga and tai chi.[44] I believe that, as clinicians, we should familiarise ourselves with these exercise regimes. While GPs do not have the training to supervise complicated rehabilitations, they should be able to make definitive diagnoses and plan appropriate management. In mild to moderate cases, GPs should be able to prescribe an exercise program for patients and monitor them.

Pharmaceutical Treatments For moderate cases, pharmaceutical treatments can be introduced in addition to exercise programs. There is evidence that topical non-steroidal anti-inflammatory drugs (NSAIDS) diclofenac cream can be effective.[45,46] It should be trialled first before oral NSAIDs. Oral NSAIDs can be used if not contraindicated in patients with gastrointestinal or cardiovascular conditions. Different NSAIDs can be trialled, as one may work while another does not, but the lowest doses should be used and in short pulses rather than continuously to avoid side effects. Paracetamol has a lower efficacy than NSAIDs but is certainly worth trying. Opioids also have a lower efficacy than NSAIDs but, given their side effects outweigh their usefulness, they should be avoided in the treatment of osteoarthritis. In meta-analysis, glucosamine or chondroitin did not lead to reduction in pain from osteoarthritis.[47]

Unloader Braces In mild and moderate knee OA, unloader braces are worth trying. The braces redistribute loads away from either the medial or lateral compartments of the knee on extension, thus reducing the friction and pain. There even exists tri-compartment unloader knee braces, which ease the pressure on the patellofemoral joint. In young patients, unloader braces and osteotomy should be considered. Unloader braces can be fitted by a trained physiotherapist. They are expensive – at about $1,000 – but private fund rebates and assistance may be available.

Different Intra-Articular Injections Intra-articular corticosteroid injections (CSIs) can be effective for short-term relief, usually lasting only a few weeks. However, caution must be exercised as recent studies have shown that intra-articular CSIs used three months prior to knee arthroscopies, meniscectomies and hip replacements increase the post-operative infection significantly.[48] Recent studies suggest that dose-dependent repeated CSIs may have a chondrotoxicity effect and may be associated with the development of osteoarthritis, leading to an increased rate of TKRs.[49]

Looking at the efficacy of intra-articular platelet-rich plasma (PRP) injection, there was a double-blind, randomised placebo-controlled trial comparing PRP and saline injections on 102 patients with early knee OA. The patients were followed up at six weeks, 12 weeks, six months and 12 months. The conclusion was that there was no difference between the two.[50] The efficacies of intra-articular hyaluronic acid have not been substantiated.

Surgery In isolated disease, partial knee replacement can be very effective. In severe cases, knee replacement is the treatment of choice. The success rate in pain relief and restoring function is 80–85% with proven cost-effectiveness.[51] However, the timing of surgery is important. Usually, the pain and disability would be the deciding factor for the patient, as the pain may become unbearable. In patients with very severe knee OA, the GP should have periodic earnest discussions about the timing of knee replacement with the patient. Surgery must be done before the patient's other comorbidities and frailty have developed to the stage that a knee replacement is prohibited. It is a sad situation when faced with an elderly patient with crippling OA knee pain, but is medically unfit to have the operation. However, if possible, surgery should not be done *too early,* as a 65-year-old patient has a 7% lifetime risk of requiring revision surgery following a knee replacement, and this risk increases substantially with younger age groups.[52]

In formulating a treatment plan for knee OA, the knee should not be assessed in isolation as comorbidities that can aggravate the knee OA – such as problems in the lower back, hip, foot, obesity, sedentary lifestyle and general de-conditioning – should be addressed at the same time. For example treating a coexisting severe lower back pain can often improve the knee pain, and vice versa.

PATELLAR BURSITIS (no.3 in Figure 1)

Patella bursitis can include suprapatellar, prepatellar or infrapatellar bursitis, and can be classified as septic and aseptic. Septic bursitis needs to be treated with drainage and antibiotics. While aseptic prepatellar bursitis is usually caused by repetitive trauma, it can also be caused by various inflammatory conditions e.g. rheumatoid arthritis, sarcoid, etc. Symptoms include an obvious swelling, which is usually painless. Aseptic bursitis usually subsides spontaneously with conservative measures such as compression bandaging or needle aspiration, and at times requiring corticosteroid injections. On rare occasions drainage tube insertion or bursectomy is required.

PATELLAR TENDINOPATHY (no.4 in Figure 1)

Patellar tendinosis, sometimes called jumper's knee, is a degenerative condition which usually results from overuse in sports, particularly in those that require jumping and quick changes in direction e.g. netball, basketball, soccer and rugby. Inflammatory tendonitis, avulsion injuries and rupture must also be considered.

Patellar tendinosis can occur at the superior pole and inferior pole of the patella, and at the insertion of the patellar ligament to the tibial tubercle, the most common being at the proximal attachment of the patellar ligament. Usual symptoms include pain at the site, with pain worse during loading activities or getting up after prolonged flexion of the knee. Examination shows localised patellar tenderness. Basset's sign may be positive; when the most tender part of the ligament is palpated and located in the fully extended position, subsequent 90-degree flexion reduces the tenderness markedly. Treatment includes rest, massage, stretching and strengthening;[53] surgical excision is rare but necessary for severe recalcitrant cases.

OSGOOD-SCHLATTER'S DISEASE (OSD) (no.5 in Figure 1)

OSD is a traction apophysitis of the tibial tubercle. Symptoms include anterior knee pain of the patellar ligament at its insertion site. The mean incidence in one study was 3.8 per 1000 person in the 8- to 18-year-old age group, peaking in the 12- to 15-year-old age group.[54] Examination shows mildly swollen, tender and thickened patellar tendon. Diagnosis is usually clinical but an X-ray would exclude bony injuries, tumors and infection.

There is limited literature evaluating the efficacies of different treatments for OSD. A consensus approach includes physical activity modifications, taping/patellar strapping, stretching and strengthening of the quadriceps, and stretching of the hamstrings.[55]

HOFFA'S DISEASE (no.6 in Figure 1)

Hoffa's Disease is the impingement of the inflamed and hypertrophied infrapatellar fat pad (Hoffa's fat pad) between the articular surfaces of the knee, which measures about 21 cm^3 in females and 29.7cm^3 in males. The hypertrophy is thought to be in response to repetitive trauma and sports. Symptoms include sharp anterior knee pain, often aggravated by sporting activities and walking up and down stairs.

Incidence is rare. Hoffa's Test can be used for diagnosis, while MRI can provide a definitive diagnosis. Treatments include activity modifications, NSAIDs, steroid injections and resection.[56]

SYNOVIAL PLICA SYNDROME (SPS) (no.7 in Figure 1)

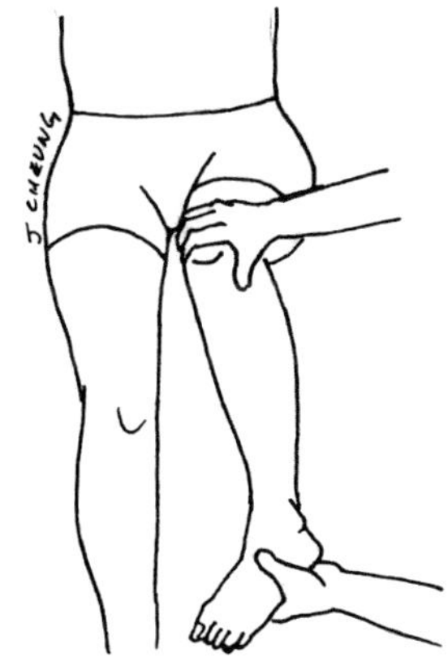

Figure 7: Hoffa's Test - The knee should be flexed at 90 degrees, with the examiner holding the patella with the thumb exerting pressure laterally at the level of the patellar tendon, then passively extending the knee.

Severe pain during the last 10 degrees of extension indicates presence of the disease.

Plicae are inward folds of synovial lining which can become inflamed and fibrotic through overuse and trauma, and may bowstring across the femoral trochlea, leading to impingement. It can be supra, medial or lateral patellar, with medial being the most common. The prevalence is thought to be around 10%.[57] Symptoms include a sharp anterior or anteromedial knee pain with a clicking, clunking or a popping sensation during activities such as walking up and down stairs, squatting or arising after sitting for a long time.

Clinical examination includes:

1. Palpating for the plicae over the anterior joint line,
2. Hughston's plica test - The examiner stands on the affected side, places one hand around the heel while the palm of the other hand is positioned over the lateral border of the patella with the fingers over the medial femoral condyle.

The examiner flexes and extends the patient's knee while rotating the tibia and pushing the patella medially. Pain and popping in the knee are a positive test. It is typically at 30–60 degrees of extension.

3. Plica Stutter Test: The patient is positioned sitting on the side of the bed with knee flexed to 90 degrees. The examiner crouches down to knee level, placing the index and middle fingers on the centre of the patella. Action: the examiner asks the patient to extend the knee slowly while keeping their fingers on the patella and watching its movement. Positive finding: if the patella stutters or jumps during the course of movement, it is indicative of a plica. It is typically in the range of 45–70 degrees towards extension. Crepitus of the patella may also be felt. Imaging including US or MRI are not conclusive. The diagnosis is made more from clinical findings.

Treatments include activity modifications, building up limb strength, NSAIDs, steroid injections and resection. A Cochrane Review of 31 studies with 1690 participants found consistent evidence supporting conservative treatment. SPS of the knee is a commonly overlooked cause of anterior knee pain.[58]

OSTEOCHONDRITIS DISSECANS OF THE KNEE (no.8 in Figure 1)

This is defined as osteochondral loose bodies within a joint, affecting the knee, elbow or ankle joints. It occurs more in active paediatric and young adult populations, rarely in patients under 10 and over 50 years of age. It affects males four times more than females. In the age group between six to 19, the incidence is 9.5 of 100,000 knees.[59] Trauma can cause the condition but it may be idiopathic as well. Symptoms differ between stable and unstable cases. Stable ones have non-specific and intermittent knee pain. Unstable ones present with catching/locking mechanical symptoms. Examination may show joint effusion and reduced range of movements. For diagnosis, MRI has excellent sensitivity and specificity. Treatment includes conservative activity modifications and surgery in unstable cases.

LATERAL COLLATERAL LIGAMENT INJURIES (no.12 in Figure 1)

Isolated lateral collateral ligament injuries are rare and often associated with more serious combined ruptures of ACL and/or PCL. It usually occurs in MVA and sporting injuries.

MENISCAL TEAR (MT) (no.13 and 18 in Figure 1)

The main function of the meniscus is load sharing and shock absorbing in the tibiofemoral joint. Meniscal tears are common. They can be traumatic (in the younger age group) or degenerative. The incidence of acute MT is 60/100,000, usually occurring in sporting injuries such as netball, basketball, rugby, soccer and skiing, and causative factors include lack of warming up before sports and excessive loading. MT is often associated with ACL ruptures. Male to female ratio is 2-4/1. Ratio of medial to lateral MT is 3/1.[60] Degenerative MT is more common for those over 40 years old, where significant trauma may be absent, and incidence increases with age.

Symptoms of acute MT are sharp pain on injury, swelling and stiffness. In degenerative cases, symptoms may be minor or even absent. After the initial injury, the pain and swelling usually settle down after several days. Subsequently, there may be recurrent dislodgement of the torn but attached tear causing periodic swelling, pain and 'locking' (the inability to fully flex or fully extend), which settles until the next episode. Examination usually shows an effusion. For diagnosis, useful tests are localised mid medial knee joint tenderness, a positive McMurray Test and Apley Test, and MRI provides a definitive diagnosis.

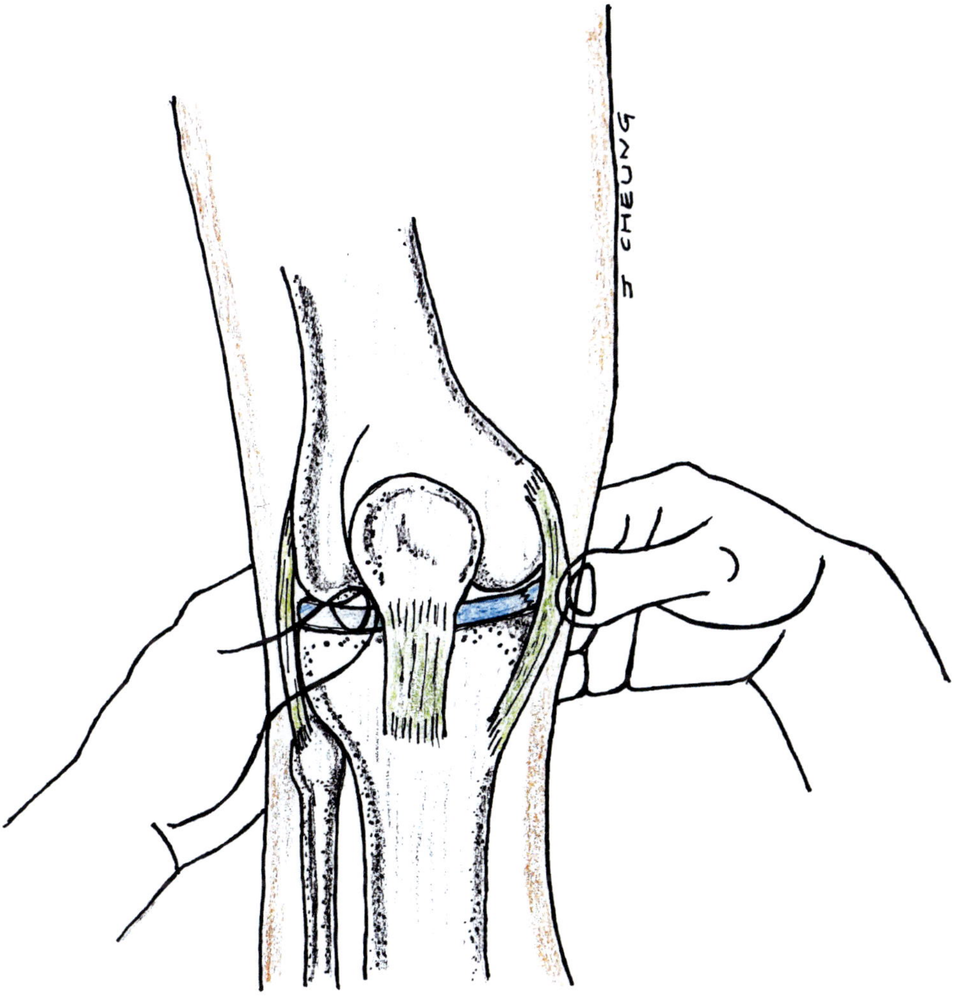

Figure 8: Medial Meniscal Tear

Localised mid medial line joint tenderness points to medial meniscal tear.

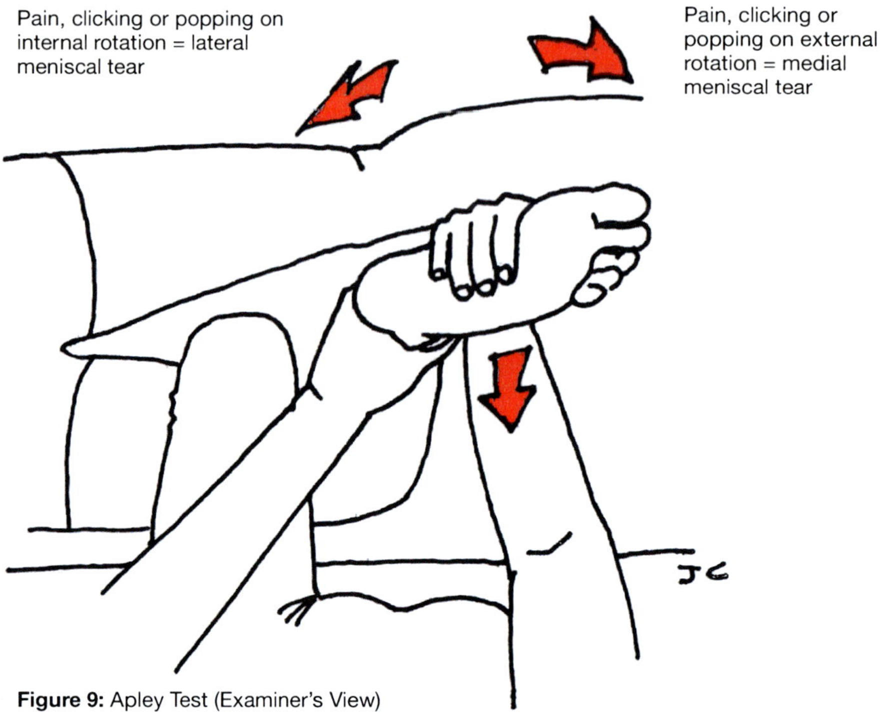

Figure 9: Apley Test (Examiner's View)

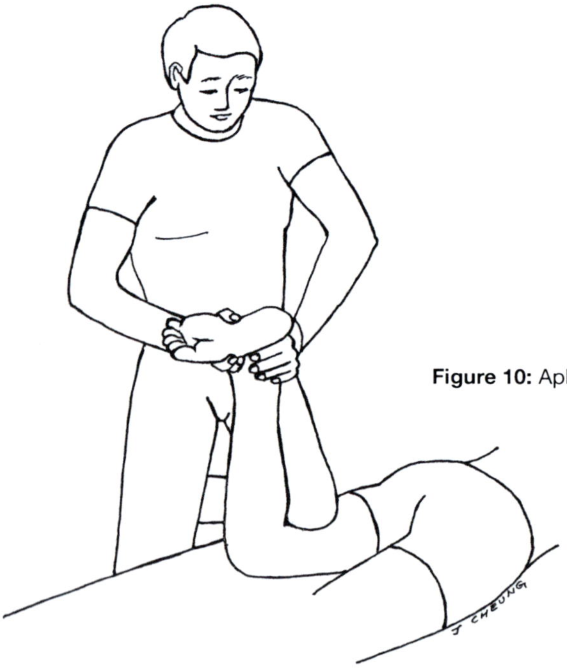

Figure 10: Apley Test

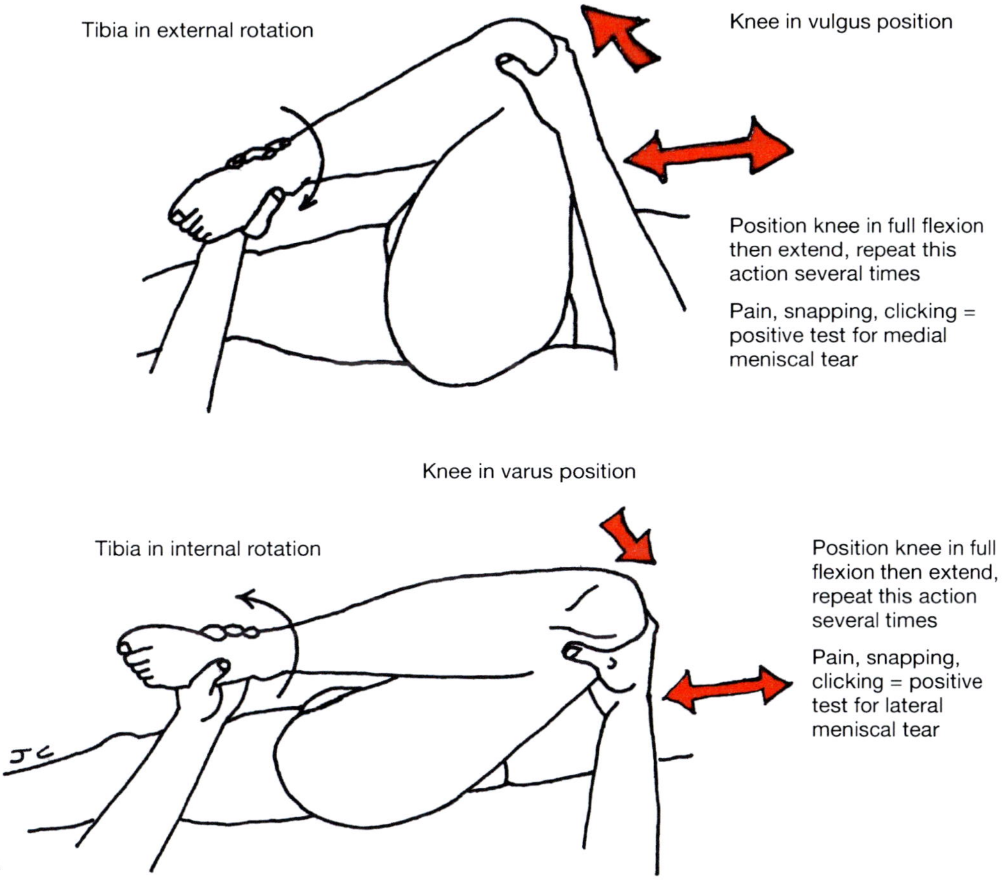

Figure 11: McMurray Test (Examiner's View)

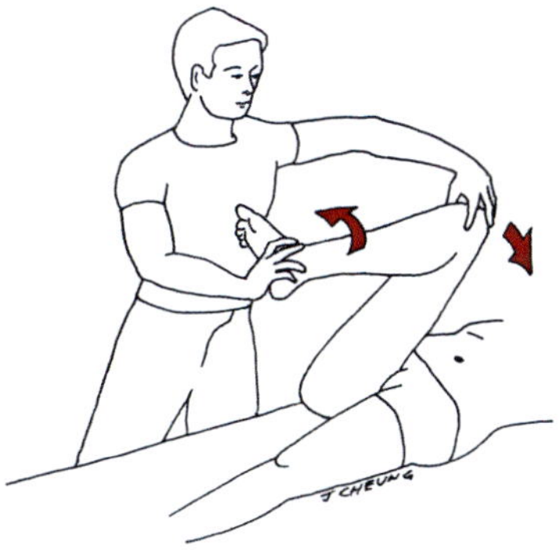

Figure 12: McMurray Test

Treatment tends to be limited to conservative monitoring, moving away from a previous high rate of meniscectomy, given the evidence of development of OA associated with meniscectomy.[61] Surgery can involve suturing and other repairing techniques besides meniscectomy, which is reserved for unstable severe cases. Surgical treatment of meniscal injuries depends on the age of patient, type of tear and degree of existing degenerative disease. The treatment of a meniscal tear of a 20-year-old would be quite different to the degenerative tear in someone over 40; the latter would be treated more conservatively.

SPONTANEOUS OSTEONECROSIS OF THE KNEE (SONK) (no.16 in Figure 1)

SONK is a relatively common idiopathic condition, with one study estimating the prevalence to be 3.4% of the population.[62] It is described as a focal, subchondral lesion, which may lead to an end-stage osteoarthritis of the knee, or as a subchondral insufficiency fracture. It is usually unilateral, affecting the medial femoral condyle 94% of the time.[63] SONK primarily affects the middle-aged and elderly, and more in females than males. Patients usually report symptoms including sudden onset of anteromedial knee pain upon weight bearing; however, pain can also occur when the knee is not loaded and at night. Initially, an X-ray may not show the crescent-shaped lesion, whereas MRI would after more than six weeks of its onset. Treatment includes crutches-assisted, non-weight-bearing ambulation for the first six weeks and stick-assisted walking for the next six weeks, together with NSAIDs and bisphosphonates. For the more severe cases, joint arthroplasty is the treatment of choice.[64]

MEDIAL COLLATERAL LIGAMENT INJURIES (no.17 in Figure 1)

The medial collateral ligament is a major stabiliser of the knee and the most common ligament injured during knee trauma, usually during sports such as netball, skiing, soccer and rugby. It can be presented in isolation or combined with ACL rupture. Examination shows localised tenderness and medial laxity of the knee at 30-degree flexion while abducted by a valgus force. Treatment is usually conservative as extra-articular ligamentous injuries usually heal well, but surgery is indicated in severe and unstable cases.[65]

INFLAMMATORY DISEASE (no.26 in Figure 1)

Inflammatory disease in the knee includes rheumatoid arthritis, psoriatic arthritis and reactive arthritis (Reiter's syndrome). They have the usual features of prolonged morning pain and stiffness of more than 30 minutes.

GOUT (no.27 in Figure 1)

Gout can affect any joints in the body. In acute gout, patients present with rapid onset of severe pain, swelling and erythema of the affected joint, tendon or bursa. Knee joints are a common site for gouty arthritis. Definitive diagnosis is by the presence of monosodium urate crystals in joint aspirations.

ANTERIOR CRUCIATE LIGAMENT (ACL) RUPTURE (no.29 in Figure 1)

ACL rupture is a common sports injury, occurring more in females. Symptoms include acute, painful swelling and haemarthrosis. The ACL normally stops the tibia from sliding out in front of the femur. Clinical tests for diagnosis include the Lachman test and anterior drawer test; an MRI is a definitive diagnostic test.

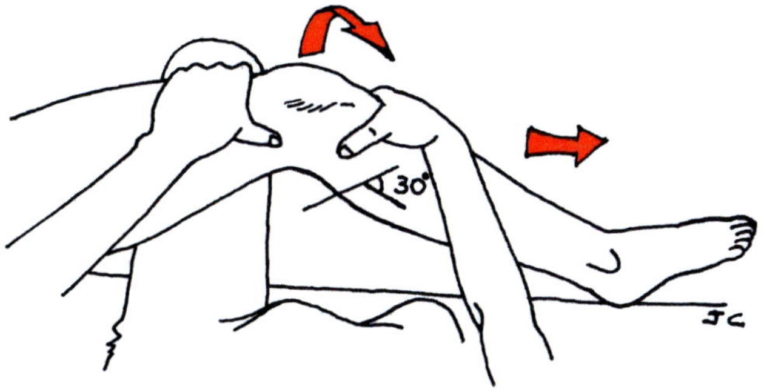

Figure 13: The Lachman Test (Examiner's View) – Rest patient's knee at 30° flexion onto examiner's knee. Fix the femur with one hand, externally rotate the tibia then try to move the tibia anteriorly. Laxity and no end point = ACL tear.

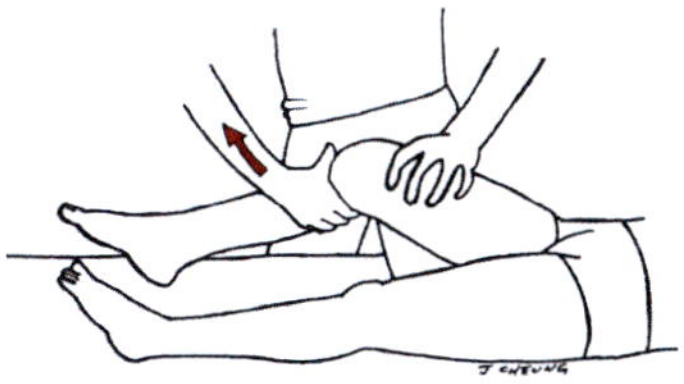

Figure 14: The Lachman Test

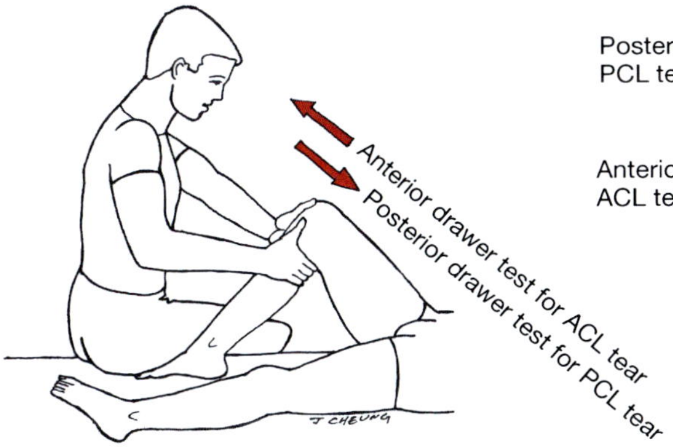

Figure 15: Anterior and posterior drawer tests for ACL tears

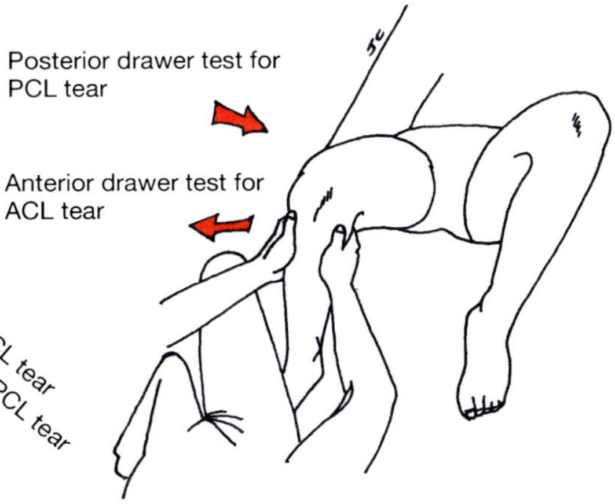

Figure 16: Anterior and posterior drawer tests for ACL tears (Examiner's View)

TIBIAL PLATEAU FRACTURE (no.31 in Figure 1)

A tibial plateau fracture is usually sustained in high-impact injuries such as motor vehicle or motor bike accidents, or trauma with a varus or vulgus force. In the older age group where osteoporosis is common, a much lesser impact incident, such as a fall with the knee extended, can cause it.

POSTERIOR CRUCIATE LIGAMENT (PCL) RUPTURE (no.32 in Figure 2)

Isolated PCL rupture is uncommon; causes include a dashboard direct anterior blow in MVAs and hyperflexion injuries. Clinical test for diagnosis includes posterior drawer test, and MRI provides a definitive diagnostic test.

BAKER'S CYST (no.33 in Figure 2)

Baker's cyst, sometimes called popliteal cyst, is a fluid-filled sac in the posterior knee that is, typically, in the medial aspect, between the semimembranosus tendon and the gastrocnemius insertion. It occurs more frequently in adults with a history of trauma (e.g. cartilage or meniscal tear) in association with degeneration and joint disease (e.g. OA or RA). In children, it arises from a herniated knee joint capsule. Baker's cysts do not usually cause severe pain and treatment is usually not necessary. If symptoms are more significant, ultrasound-guided aspiration and steroid injection are used. Rupture of the Baker's cyst is rare, and the resulting swelling and bleeding can resemble deep vein thrombosis or acute thrombophlebitis.

GRACILIS (AND OTHER MUSCLES) TRIGGER POINTS, TENDINOSIS & BURSITIS (Figures 1 and 2)

Many muscles have attachments near the knee joints and, when these muscles are injured or strained, trigger points (TrPs) can develop. Dysfunction in these muscles and their ligamentous attachments can cause pain in the knee area.

Basically, TrPs can result from either a traumatic injury to the muscle, constant contraction of the muscle due to repetitive activities, or continuing activation to protect a nearby painful joint or structure.

Examination may elicit wasting of the relevant muscles. Careful, purposeful and targeted palpation can detect tender muscular knots/cords/nodules or TrPs. Patients often exclaim, 'Ouch! That's it! That's the pain I was telling you about! That's the centre of my pain.' As outlined earlier, an osteoarthritic joint can cause adjacent muscle dysfunction and the resulting pain can actually become the dominant pain experienced by the patient. It is therefore very important to treat it first. Modalities such as regular stretching exercises, heat and manual therapies (e.g. mobilisation and soft tissue massage) can be utilised.

Pain in the sartorius, gracilis and semitendinosus distal attachment on the tibia (at 5 o'clock of the patella for the right knee and 7 o'clock for the left knee) is often referred to as bursitis, which may be a misnomer, as it can be a tendinosis as well as a bursitis. Together, the pain in the three distal attachments is sometimes called pes anserine bursitis. Bursitis and tendinosis in these can cause anteromedial knee pain. Tendinosis of the distal attachment of the ITB is common as well and can cause anterolateral knee pain. Similarly, TrPs in the quadriceps can cause anterior knee pain, and TrPs in the popliteus and plantaris can cause posterior knee pain.

It is of interest that, while the TrPs are palpable on the muscles, the pain is often not felt at the TrPs but at the insertion sites (Fig. 20). At times, the pain at the attachment sites of the ITB, sartorius, gracilis or semitendinosus is so intense that a single targeted corticosteroid injection can be very effective. However, frequent repeated corticosteroid injections are not advisable as this can weaken the ligamentous structures. The causes of the tendinosis need to be addressed otherwise recurrences are common. Treatments include manual therapies (e.g. soft tissue massage and mobilisation), a stretching regime and acupuncture.

POSITION OF THE PATIENT AND EXAMINER WHEN PALPATING FOR TRIGGER POINTS IN THE KNEE REGION

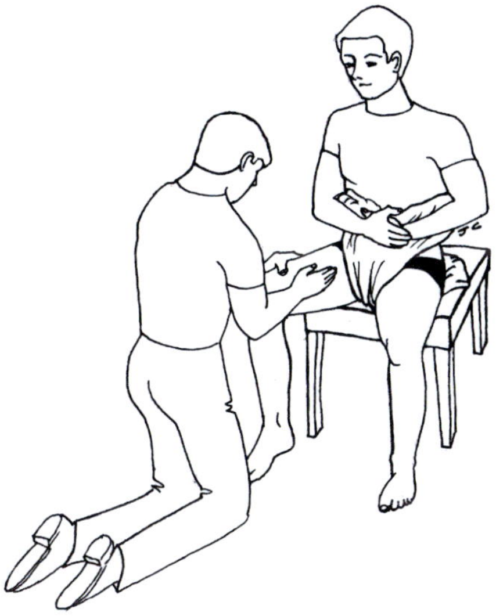

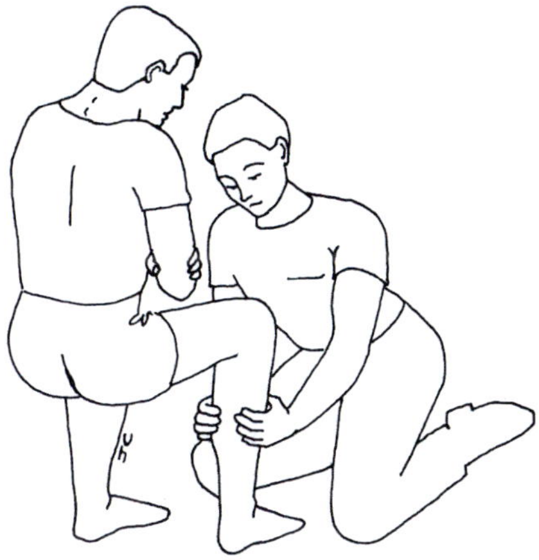

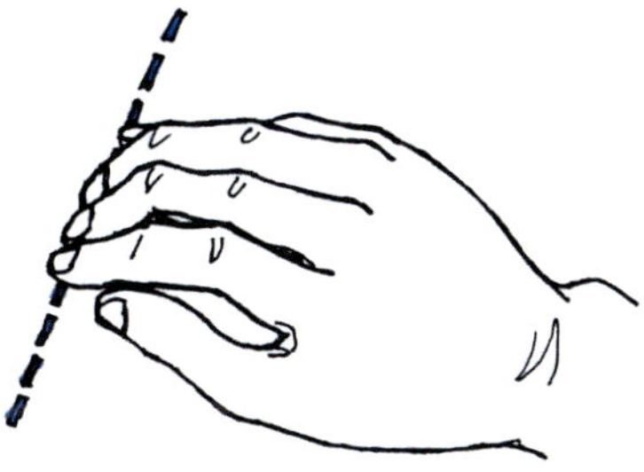

Place the pulp of four fingers in a line to cover more area. A small amount of soluble bath oil increases the sensitivity.

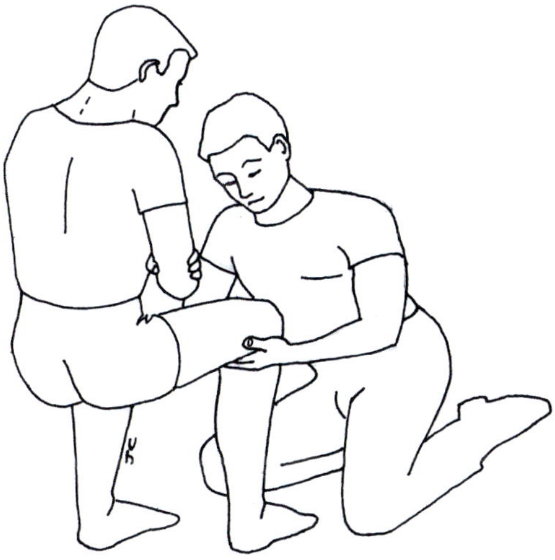

Figure 17: Palpation diagrams for examining the lower limb

NB. Three short videos on TrP palpation techniques for the knee, lower back, neck/ shoulder regions are available on YouTube under joecheungYNSA, or visit http://www.joecheung.com.au

The causes of knee pains are highly positional

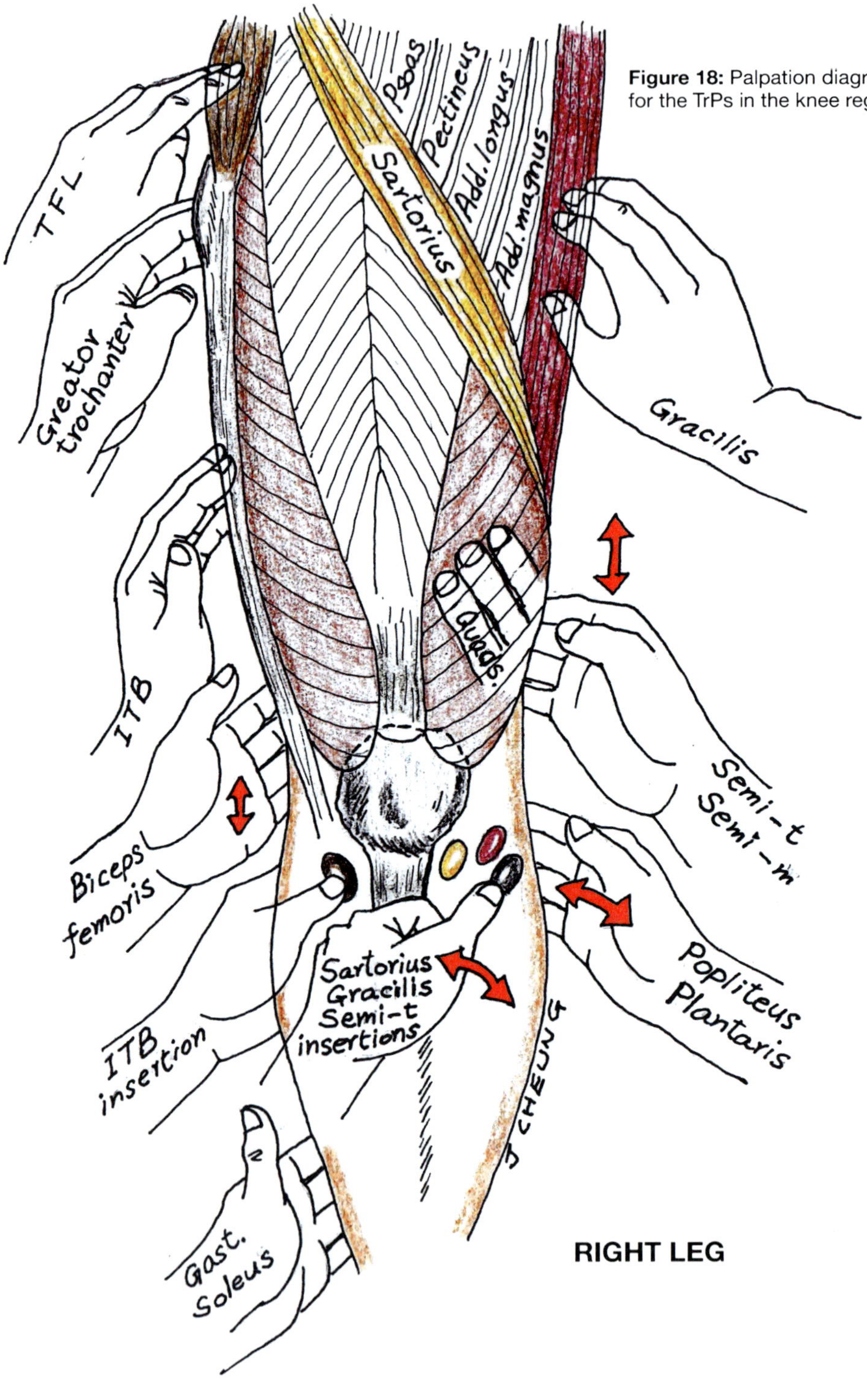

Figure 18: Palpation diagram for the TrPs in the knee region

THE GRACILIS MUSCLE AND ITS TrPs

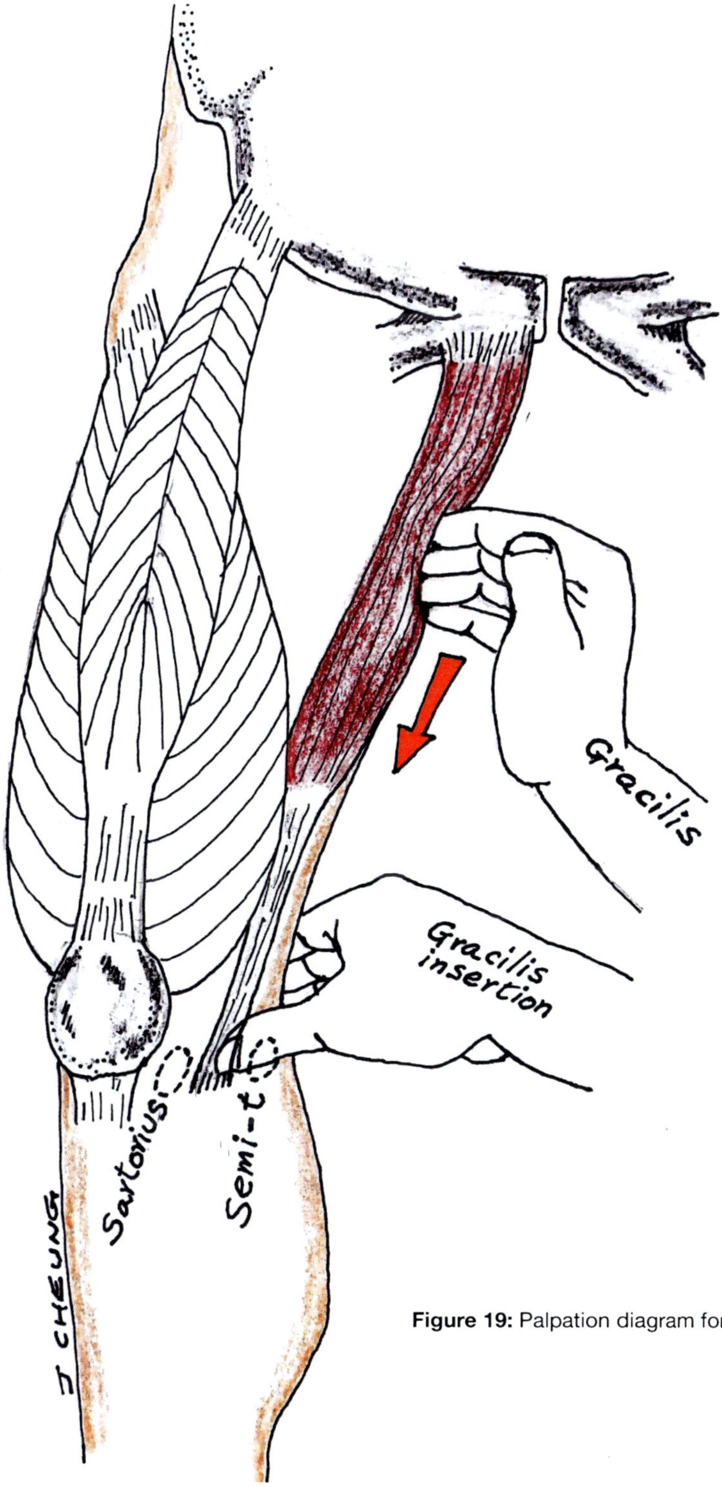

Figure 19: Palpation diagram for the gracilis TrPs

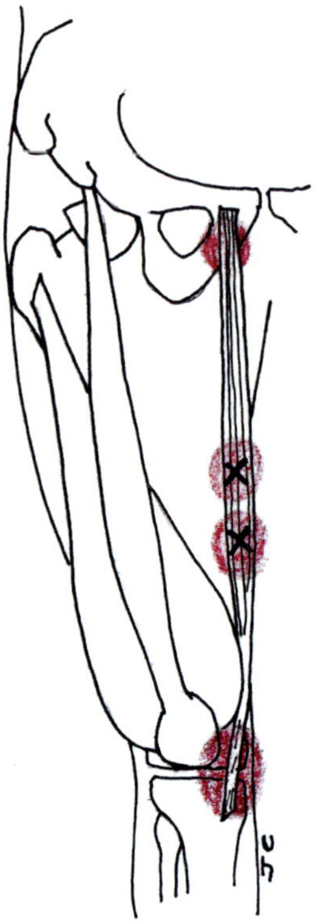

Figure 20: Gracilis TrPs and their referred pain pattern

X = TrPs
Red area = the referred pain

One of the most common causes of anteromedial knee pain are gracilis TrPs, especially in patients with OA of the tibiofemoral joint. A likely explanation is as follows – OA is more common in the medial compartment of the tibiofemoral joint. Given the gracilis helps to adduct the knee joint from a valgus position, its contraction would lessen the contact pressure in the medial compartment when in a weight-bearing position. Therefore, in patients with tibiofemoral OA, the gracilis is in constant contraction to ease the OA pain thereby creating the TrPs. While the TrPs may be along the length of the muscle and usually in the distal third area, the pain is usually felt in the distal insertion near the patella. Often, the TrP pain at the distal insertion site can become the dominant pain, over and above the original OA pain. It is therefore worthwhile treating the gracilis TrPs whenever they are present.

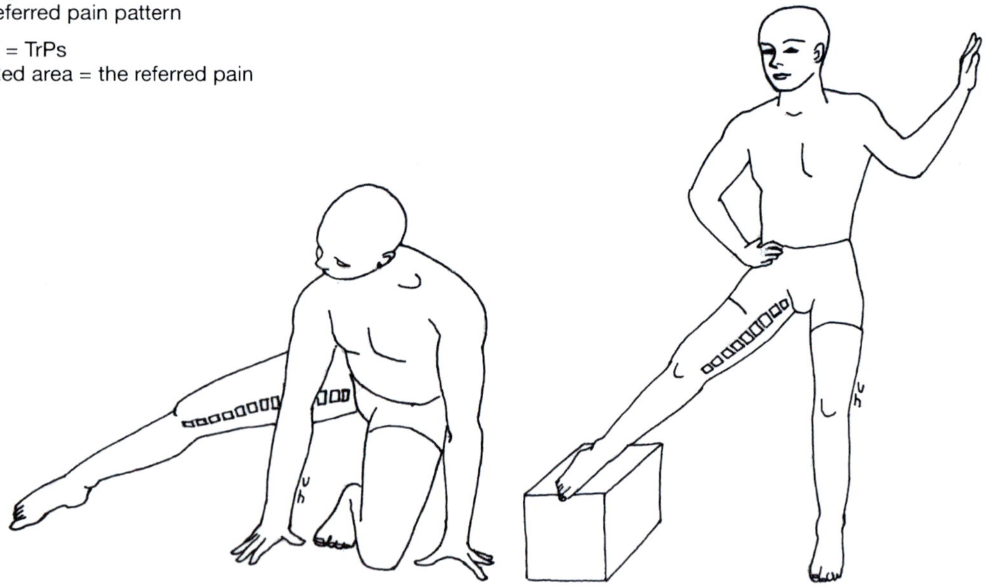

Figure 21: Useful stretches for the gracilis

TREATMENT OF TRIGGER POINTS WITH YNSA (USING THE KNEE AS AN EXAMPLE)

This section of the book is only intended for readers who are interested in or practise the modality of acupuncture.

It is not the intention of this book to describe the whole YNSA treatment system as there are other published books written for that purpose.[66,67] The YNSA system is quite complex; it is made up of a number of points, somatotopes and diagnostic methods. Including A, B, C, D, E, F, G, H and I points, sensory points, brain points, cranial nerves and Ypsilon points. There are also the J, K, I and chest somatotopes. (A somatotope is a small area or a miniature topographic map of the body located somewhere else on the body.)

This book mainly focuses on the J and K somatotopes to treat the TrPs. I believe they are very easy to learn and sufficient on their own in treating TrPs.

In this section the gracilis is used as an example of how to use YNSA to treat the TrPs of a muscle. The described treatment methods apply to other muscles as well and therefore won't be repeated again.

To find the J and K somatotopes, we first need to locate the 'centre point' of the scalp, which demarcates the border between the J and K somatotopes. It is located one to two centimeters behind the intersection between the sagittal suture and a line drawn between the tips of the ears. It is characterised by a consistently small depression on the skull, it is present in everyone. In Chinese acupuncture, this centre point is an important acupuncture point called **'Baihui'** or governing vessel channel point number 20 (GV 20). Once the GV 20 point has been identified, the J somatotope is located just anterior to it, representing a miniature topographic map of the body lying supine. The head is next to the GV 20 (Fig. 22) and the K somatotope is just posterior to the GV 20, representing the body lying prone, with the head next to the GV 20. From my experience, the J and K somatotopes are quite small, each measuring about 6 cm in length.

As an example, for an active point representing a right gracilis TrP, it would be located on the J somatotope, some estimated distance below and to the right of the GV 20 (Fig. 22). An active acupuncture point on the scalp for a left trapezius TrP would be located on the K somatotope, some estimated distance below and to the left of the GV 20 point. **From my experience, the location of the active points on the J and K somatotopes are highly proportional to the anatomical sites of the TrPs.**

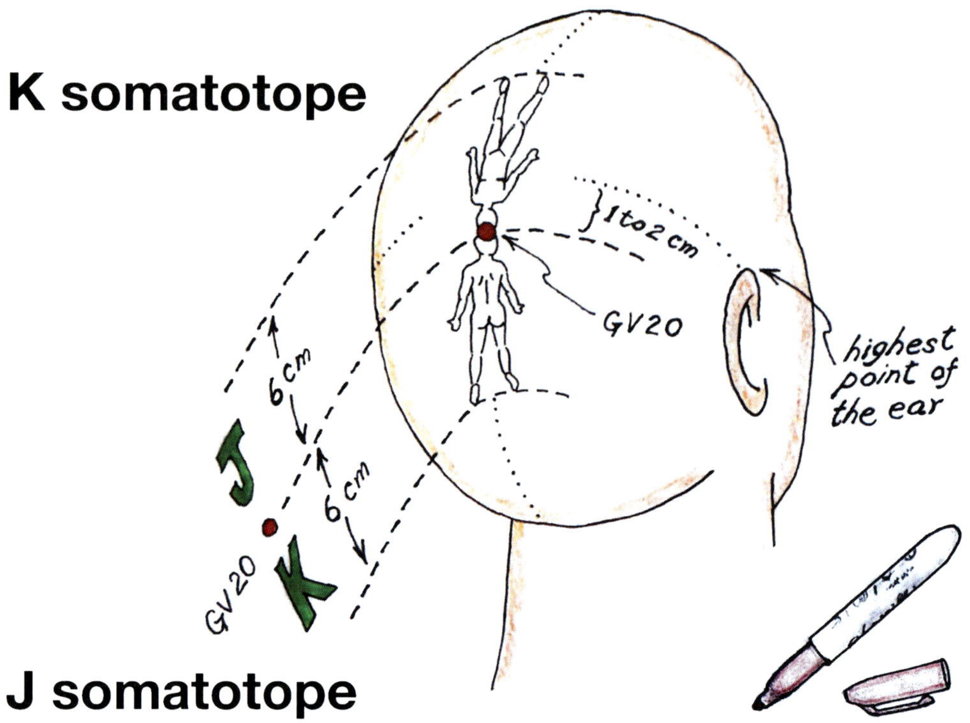

Figure 22: Locating the GV 20 point, K and J somatotope

HOW TO LOCATE GV 20: If you draw a line between the highest points of the ears, where it crosses the sagittal suture, about 1 to 2 cm behind that intersection is a small depressed spot on the skull bone, an acupuncture point called 'Baihui' or the GV 20 point. GV 20 demarcates the J and K somatotopes. After you locate the GV 20, I find it useful to landmark it with a small dot with a coloured permanent marker, to avoid looking for it repeatedly during a treatment session.

NB. From my experience, **the J and K somatotopes are quite small**. According to my estimation, **each measures about 6 cm from head to toe.** As the somatotopes are so small, it follows that the location of active points has to be very accurate. After the needle insertion, one must repalpate the TrPs to confirm a 15–20% improvement. If there is no improvement to the TrPs, then either the point location is wrong, or the needle has missed the point. The point then has to be repalpated and the needle reinserted. Often, I have to re-locate the needle quite a few times. When a treatment is unsuccessful in improving the Trp, it is almost always due to inaccuracy of the point location.

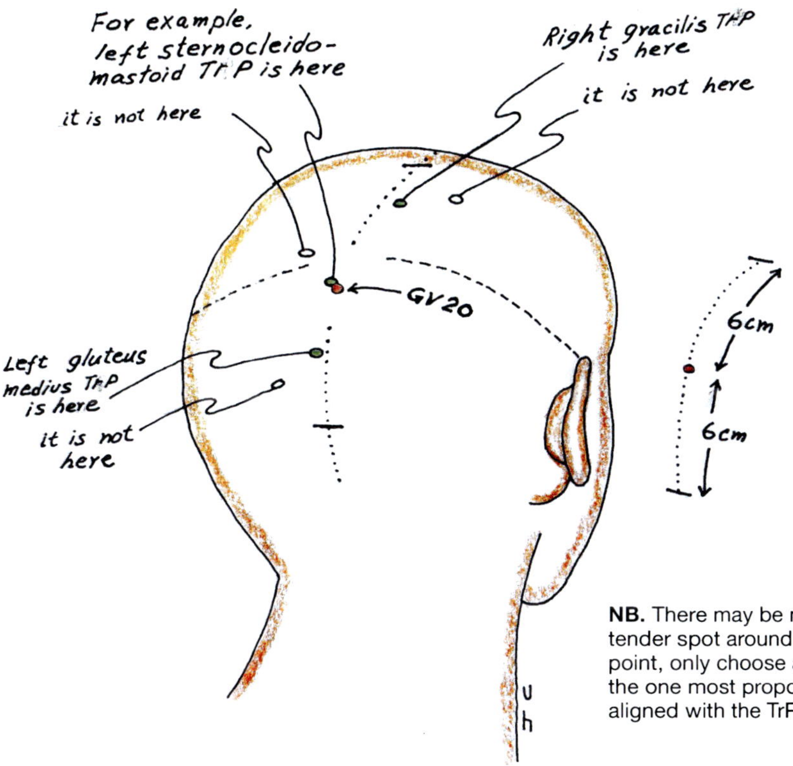

NB. There may be more than one tender spot around the true active point, only choose and acupuncture the one most proportionately aligned with the TrP.

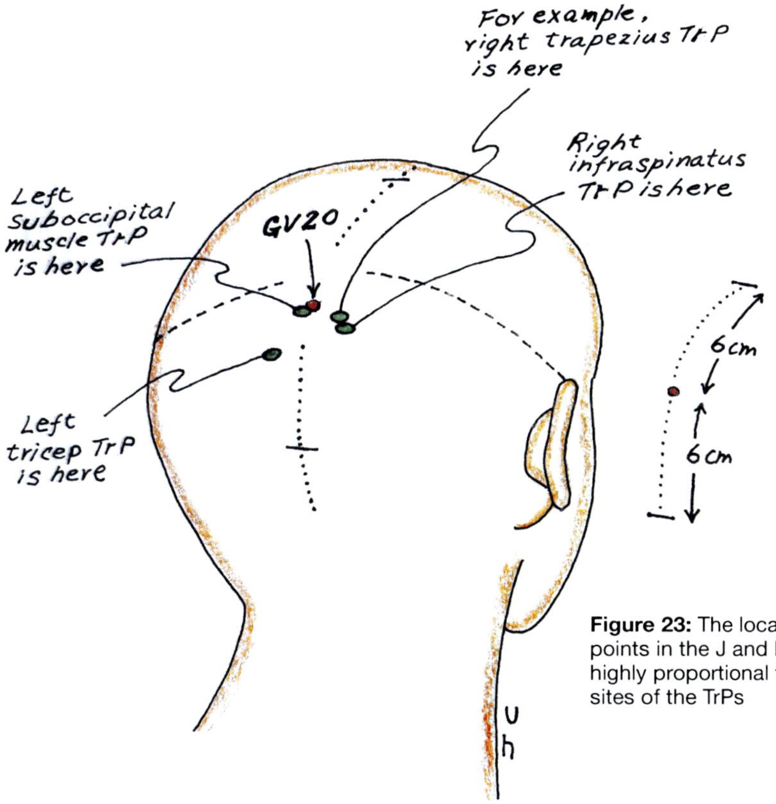

Figure 23: The location of active points in the J and K somatotopes are highly proportional to the anatomical sites of the TrPs

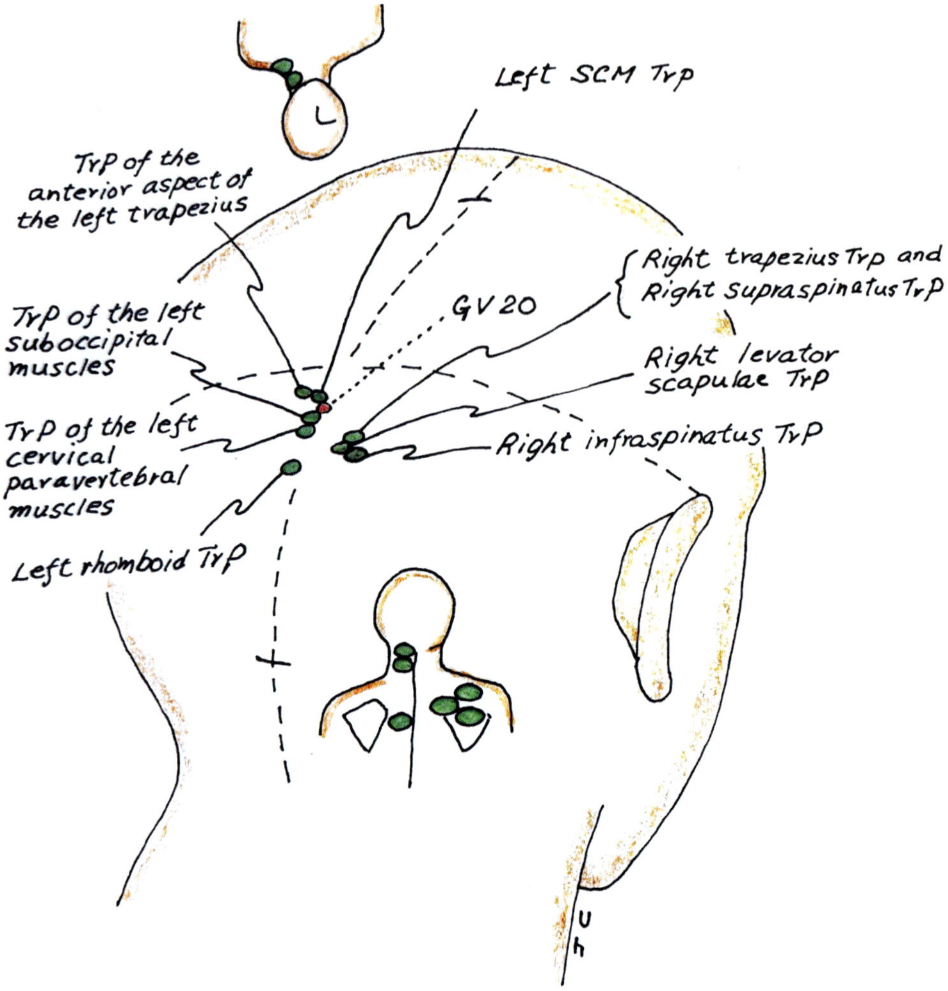

Figure 24: Some active acupuncture points are located **very close** together, sometimes within 3 mm of each other.

Once you have inserted a needle into one point, it would be difficult to palpate for another active point close-by.

You can:

1. treat each active point one by one, if time permits, or
2. mark multiple active points with a fine tip permanent marker; acupuncture them all, without palpating between each insertion, or
3. use laser instead of needles.

NB. Three short videos on TrP palpation techniques for the knee, lower back, neck/ shoulder regions are available on YouTube under joecheungYNSA, or visit http://www.joecheung.com.au

The location of each active acupuncture point on the J and K somatotopes, is highly proportional to the TrP you want to treat in the full-sized body.

An active point is a tiny, very tender spot on the skin specific to that TrP. It is usually located within a softer, depressed area that feels like a tiny bruise on an apple.

While this softer, depressed area is about 1 cm in diameter, the challenge is to find the 2 mm active point that is located within it. (On rare occasions, the active point can be a tiny raised lump.)

The consistent characteristic of an active point is that **it is always, always intensely tender on FIRM palpation.** If a patient has no problems, there will be no active points. Interestingly, the area normalises when the condition subsides.

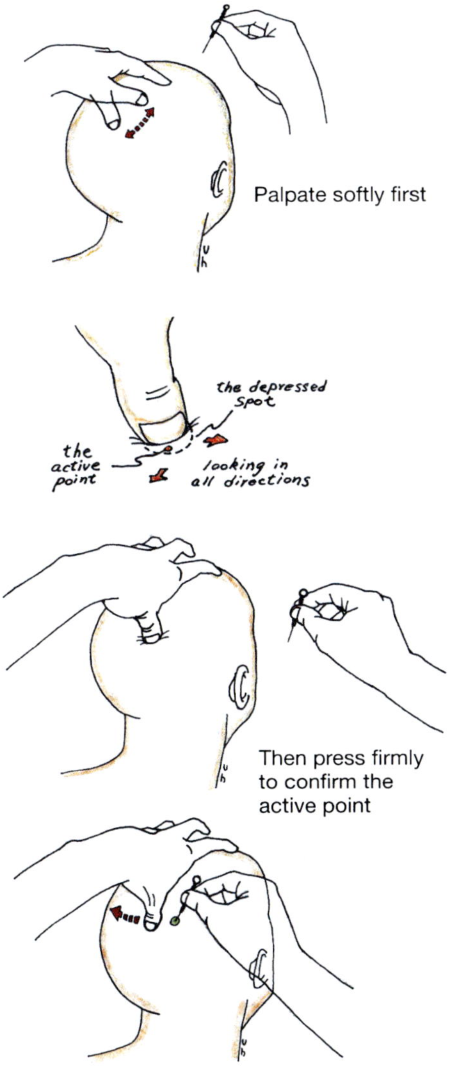

Figure 25: Needle insertion without the use of guide tubes

1. Palpate for the active point with the thumb or index finger of your non-dominant hand. **Search for the softer depressed area gently and softly first** (for sensitivity).
2. To locate the active acupuncture point within this softer area, **press FIRMLY in all directions** to illicit its characteristic sharp tenderness. The palpating fingertip should be pointing almost perpendicularly, for accuracy and precision of location.Meanwhile, the dominant hand is holding the needle ready for insertion.
3. Move the palpating finger slightly away from the point in order to insert the acupuncture needle into the designated point at 15-degree angle, then activate it by twirling the needle clockwise several times. The accuracy of insertion is very important as the active point is often only 2 mm in diameter and can be easily missed. If the insertion is accurate there would be an immediate 10 to 20 % improvement when you **re-palpate the TrP,** which you **must do for confirmation.** When there is absence of improvement, you have probably missed the point. I often have to reinsert the needle several times before succeeding.

HOW TO INSERT AN ACUPUNCTURE NEEDLE WITH A GUIDE TUBE

I prefer using a guide tube, as I feel that it allows for a more precise needle insertion.

1. If there is a safety peg that locks the needle in the tube, remove it to free up the needle.

2. First, hold the needle and the guide tube together with the thumb and index finger of your dominant hand in readiness. Make sure the sharp end of the needle tip is not protruding from the guide tube.

3. Locate the acupuncture point with your non-dominant thumb or index fingertip, almost perpendicularly to be more precise; your dominant hand is holding the needle, ready for insertion.

4. Slide the guide tube with the needle inside under your palpating fingertip, precisely onto the acupuncture point (the active point is 2–3 mm in diameter).

5. Hold and secure the position of the guide tube with the thumb and index finger of your palpating hand, then gently tap the rear end of the acupuncture needle into the active point at an angle of about 15 degrees and about 5mm deep.

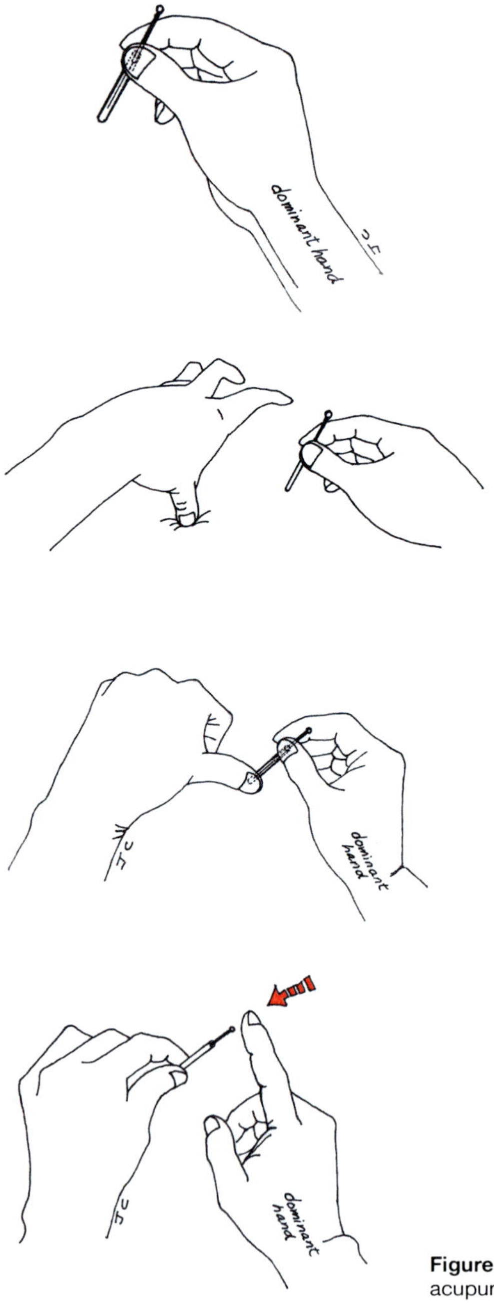

Figure 26: Method for inserting acupuncture needle with a guide tube

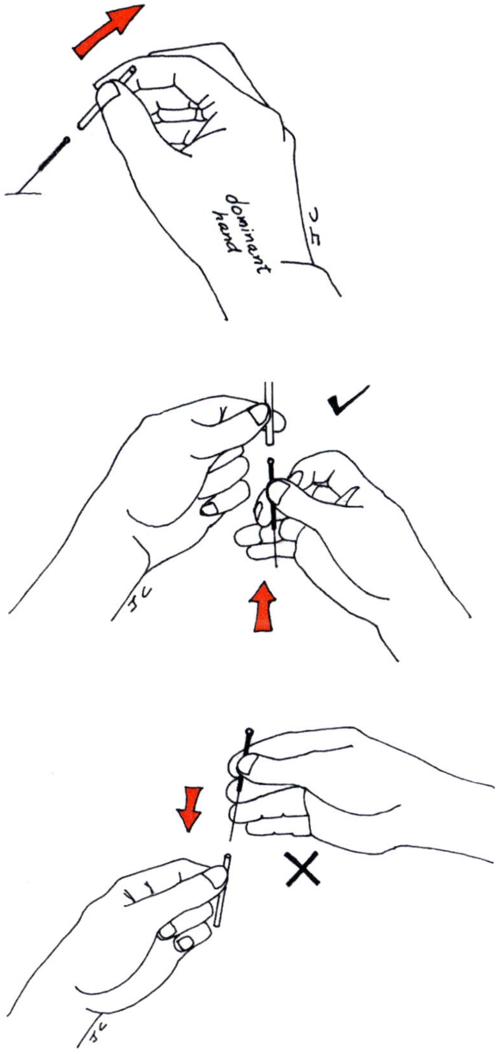

Figure 27: Method for reinserting acupuncture needle into a guide tube

6. With the needle securely in situ, remove the guide tube and gently stimulate the needle by twirling it a few times clockwise.

7. Leave the needles in for 20 minutes before removal. At the time of removal, have some cottonwool balls ready in case some minor bleeding occurs.

8. If you need to remove the needle and re-locate it, reinsert the needle back into the guide tube. This is done by entering the guide tube with the blunt end of the needle rather than the sharp end, as you may miss and puncture yourself.

NB. Most of the time, there is only minor discomfort when the needle is inserted; on rare occasions, the pain is sharp and significant. It is then advisable to remove the needle and wait for the pain to subside before reinsertion. Otherwise, the pain can persist or even cause a headache that can linger for hours afterwards. However, this complication is infrequent and it is worthwhile persevering with the treatment given its effectiveness.

PROCESS: FROM DIAGNOSIS TO COMPLETION OF TREATMENT

1. Diagnosis – the gracilis TrPs are identified as the possible cause or partial cause of the patient's knee pain and the **TrPs located.**

2. **Locate the active points on the J somatotope on the scalp** corresponding to the gracilis TrPs. It is located anatomically as shown in the diagram below. An active point is usually a tiny, very tender area on the skin specific to that problem. **It is usually a softer, depressed spot that feels like a tiny bruised area on an apple. On some occasions, it can be a tiny raised lump.** The consistent characteristic of an active point is that it is always intensely tender. If a patient has no problems, there will be no active points. Interestingly, the area normalises when the condition subsides.

3. **Needle insertion:** Gently insert a small-gauge acupuncture needle (e.g. 0.22 gauge) at a 15-degree angle, to a depth of about 5 mm, then twirl it clockwise several times.

4. **Assess the result of the treatment:** Go back and palpate the gracilis TrPs to ensure a minimum of 15% improvement, or you may ask the patient to walk and see if the pain has improved. (In other cases, for example, the ROM of a restricted shoulder abduction may have improved, or a reduced neck rotation to the left may have improved.) If there is no difference, twirl the needle anticlockwise a few times. If there is still no improvement, reinsert the needle as it may have missed the active point. The active points are as tiny as 2–3 mm and easily missed. **It is important to note that, if the diagnosis is correct and the needle is inserted accurately, the improvement will occur immediately.** Sometimes I have to reinsert the needle three or four times before succeeding! Note that it is important to treat ALL the TrPs along the length of the muscle, including the attachment sites.

5. **Leave needles in for 20 minutes** and then remove – have a cotton ball or gauze ready in case of a small amount of bleeding.

6. **Continuing treatment regime:** Repeat the session once or twice a week until the pain is cleared or improvement has plateaued. For chronic conditions, it usually averages between six to eight treatments.

7. **After all the TrPs are eradicated, reassess the patient.**

8. **Review the diagnosis.**

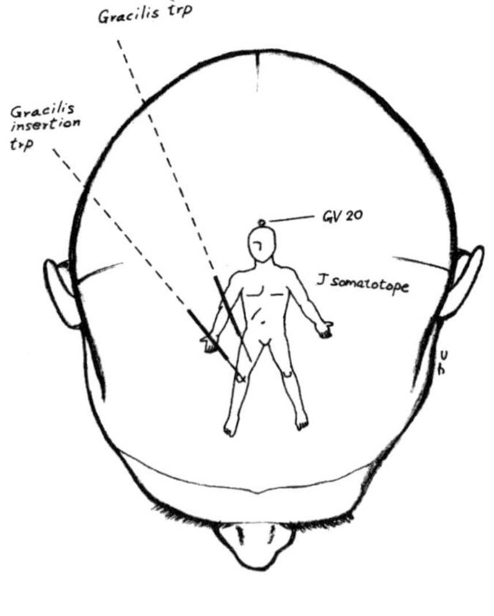

Figure 28: Example of treating gracilis TrPs

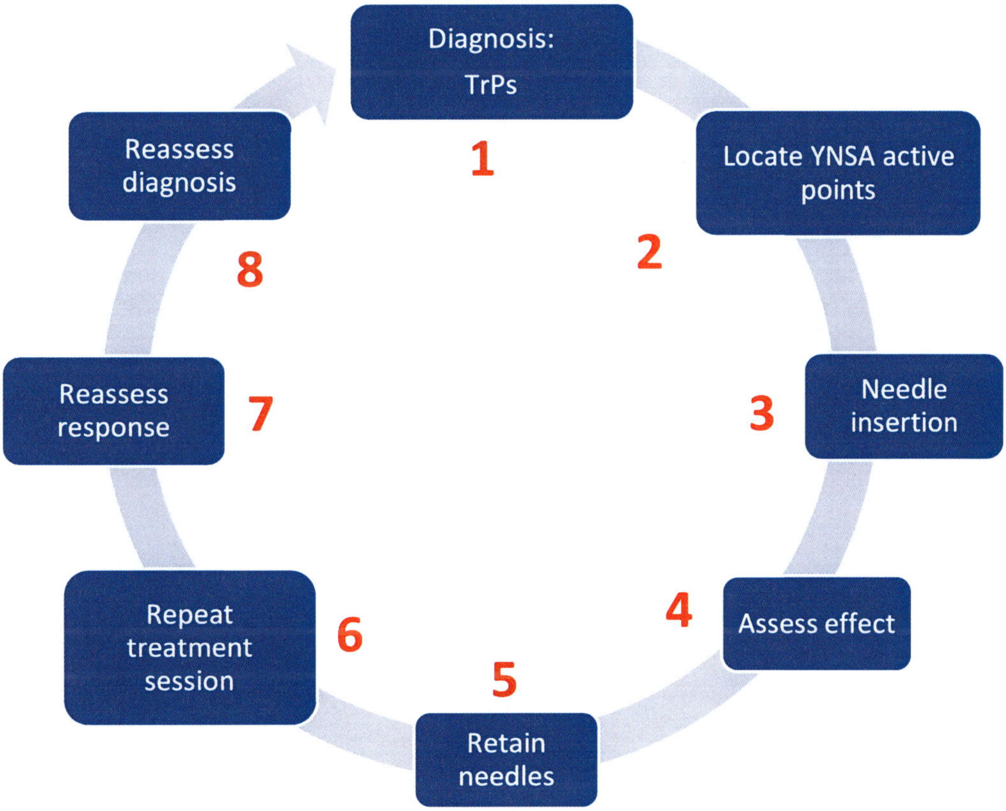

Figure 29: Flow chart of TrP treatment in pain syndromes

ACUPUNCTURE USING LASER INSTEAD OF NEEDLES

The world's first laser (light amplification by stimulated emission of radiation) was developed about 60 years ago and its usage has expanded ever since. Laser acupuncture has been used since the 1970s and increasingly so now due to its easy application, the potential of fewer adverse side effects, the lack of needling discomfort and quicker treatment time. International research on laser acupuncture is still trying to clarify its efficacy and whether there is any difference in effect compared to needle acupuncture.[68]

The emission wavelength of laser acupuncture commonly used in YNSA ranges from 685 nm (in the red spectrum) to 885 nm (in the infrared spectrum). As to the amount of laser energy (joules or watt-seconds) applied to each point, no unified consensus has been made and the research on this continues.[69,70] It is advisable to adjust the treatment dose depending on the patient's response, starting from low to high. Laser pointers with similar wavelengths and varying emission power have also been used, although their efficacy requires more research.

Laser is particularly useful in patients whose active points are very sensitive and painful for needling. Another advantage is that the laser beam covers a larger target area than the point of a needle, therefore requiring less precision. **Care should be taken not to look at the laser beam directly, and protective glasses should be worn by the practitioner and patient to avoid eye damage.** While the initial outlay for a laser machine appears high compared to acupuncture needles, it is a one-off purchase.

From my experience, I have found acupuncture needles, dedicated acupuncture lasers and laser pointers to be all effective in practising YNSA.

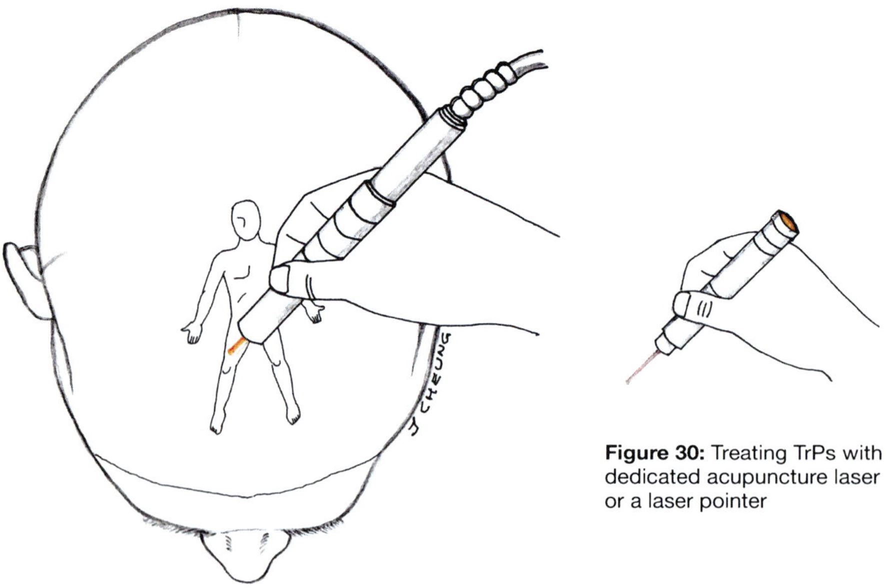

Figure 30: Treating TrPs with dedicated acupuncture laser or a laser pointer

CASE STUDIES ON KNEE PAIN

Most of the case studies (with a few exceptions) use the modality of YNSA for treatment. This is only intended for readers who are interested in or practise the modality of acupuncture.

CASE STUDY 1: Right medial knee pain – gracilis, vastus medius TrPs, treated with YNSA

HISTORY: A 60-year-old male presented with a ten-day history of 6/10 pain in his right knee. The pain was in the medial aspect of the knee and severe on walking and on getting up from a seated position. There were no previous knee pain or injuries to the knee. He reported no swelling or locking and he had no constitutional symptoms. He had no prolonged morning stiffness and no other joint problems. The patient did have a very severe left heel pain in the preceding month, which had settled with some orthotic inserts. He had regular annual check-ups and cancer screenings with his GP. A plain X-ray showed moderate OA in the tibiofemoral joint and a trial of a NSAID had failed.

REASONING: As there was no previous history of knee pain and the onset was sudden, it would unlikely be due to OA. There was no history to support a diagnosis of ligamentous rupture or meniscal tear. There were no symptoms of inflammatory joint diseases. It was likely to be related to muscular strains, as the pain was directly related to movement.

EXAMINATION: The patient was limping with pain, he was afebrile and there was no knee effusion. The range of movement was normal and tests for meniscal or ligament tears were negative. On careful palpation, there were very tender TrPs on his right gracilis, at a point about a third from its distal end and also at the insertion of the distal end of the muscle. The patient confirmed the latter was the centre of his pain. Minor TrPs were found in his vastus medialis as well.

INVESTIGATIONS: No further tests planned.

DIAGNOSIS: It was postulated that his antalgic gait from the left heel pain had strained his right gracilis and vastus medialis.

TREATMENT: He was treated with YNSA, with three needles used on the J somatotope targeting the right gracilis, gracilis insertion and vastus medialis TrPs. Immediately after the insertion of the needle in the correct position (it had to be reinserted three times before an improvement was

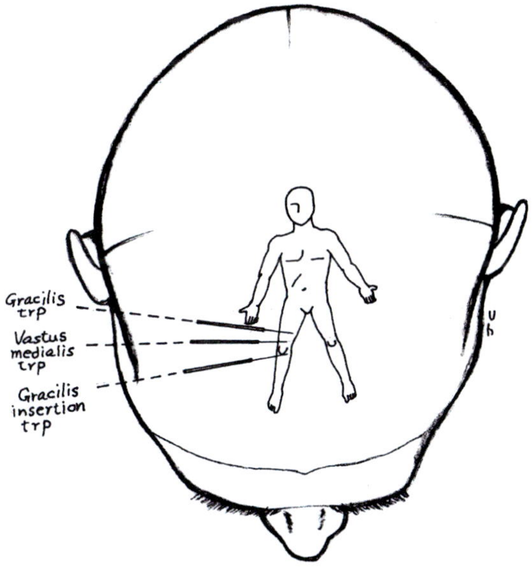

Figure 31: TRP treatment for Case Study 1

achieved), there was a significant reduction of tenderness at the TrPs. The patient was asked to walk while the needles were still in. He was pleasantly surprised by how much less pain he felt.

OUTCOME: After three treatments at weekly intervals, he was pain-free. From my experience, once the TrPs are cleared, they do not usually return unless the muscles are reinjured. In this case, for example, if the patient's left heel pain were to recur, it may strain the gracilis again.

THE QUADRICEPS AND ITS TrPs

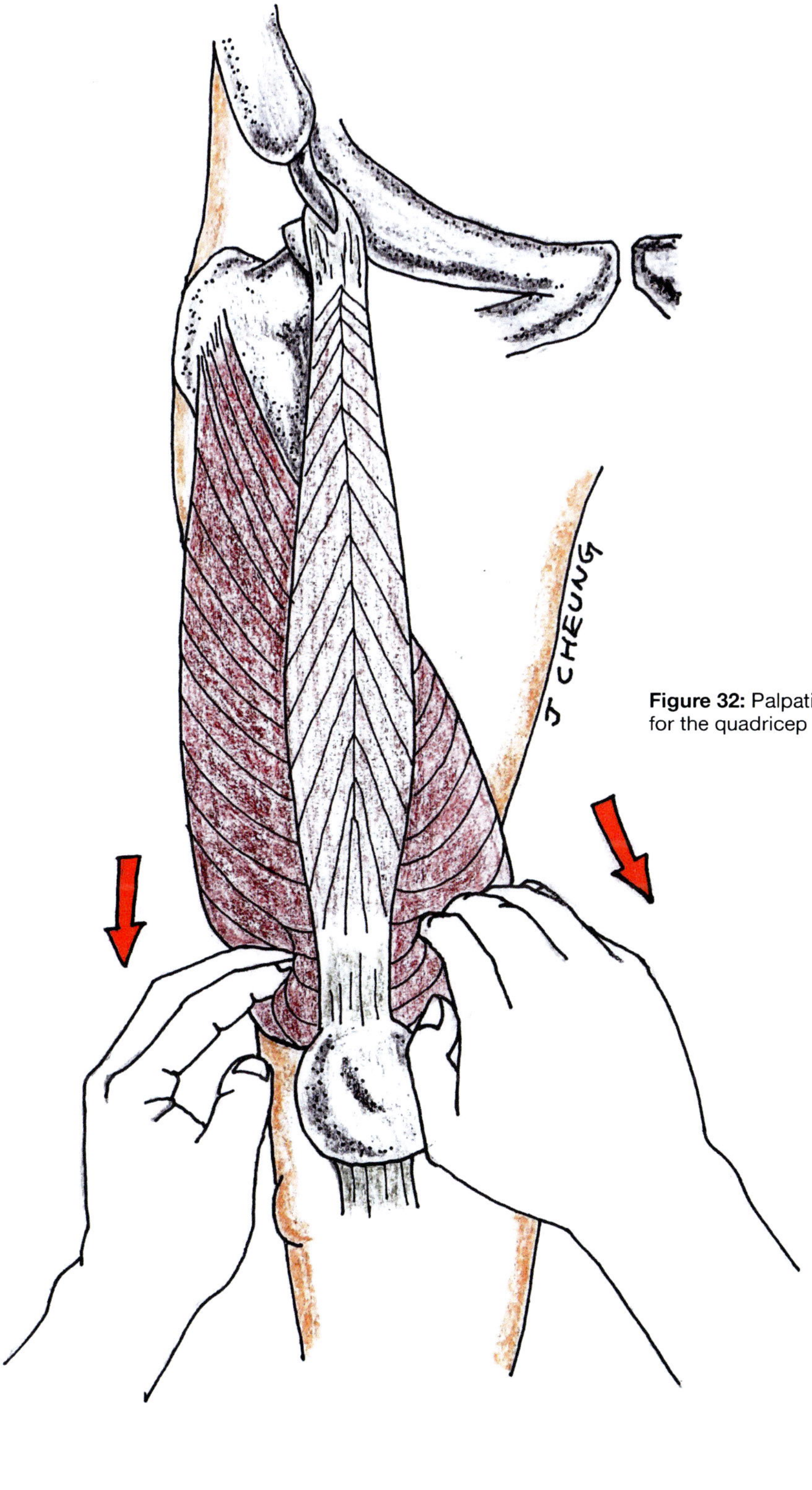

Figure 32: Palpation diagram for the quadricep TrPs

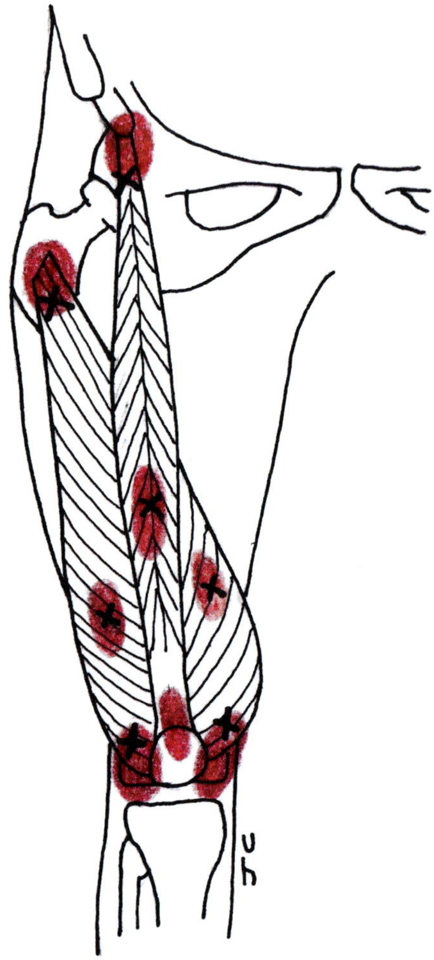

Figure 33: Quadricep TrPs and their referred pain pattern

X = TrPs

Red area = the referred pain

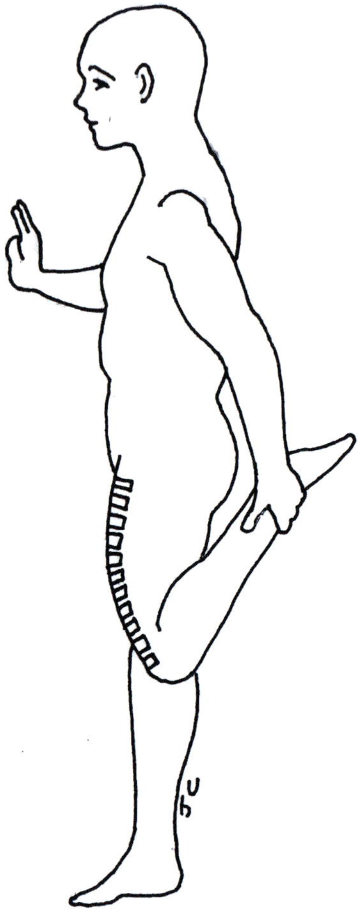

Figure 34: A useful stretch for the quadricep

CASE STUDY 2: Left knee pain – gracilis, quadriceps, ITB and semitendinosus TrPs, treated with YNSA

HISTORY: A 45-year-old female, a full-time office worker, presented with a two-year history of severe left knee pain. She has X-ray and MRI evidence of a medial meniscal tear and very severe OA in the left knee, having played a lot of sports all her life – netball, soccer, running, etc. Interestingly, her right knee OA was relatively mild. Two orthopaedic surgeons had said her left knee was 'bone on bone' and would eventually require a total knee replacement (TKR), however, were reluctant to do so due to her relatively young age. The patient's pain was so severe she found it difficult to walk even 100m. She said that her left knee locking or swelling was rare. She heard positive reviews of acupuncture and hoped it would help the pain and buy her some time before knee replacement surgery.

REASONING: The main diagnosis was a known severe OA and there were no recent sudden exacerbations to point to other additional diagnoses. Her recent MRI had excluded lytic and sclerotic lesions.

EXAMINATION: The patient limped in. Examination reviewed a surprisingly normal-looking left knee with no effusion. There was localised mid medial joint line tenderness, confirming the known meniscal tear. Tender TrPs were found on the left gracilis, distal quads, ITB and distal semitendinosus.

INVESTIGATIONS: None necessary.

DIAGNOSIS: Severe knee OA, with coexisting TrPs.

TREATMENT: YNSA was given on TrPs of the left gracilis, distal quads, ITB on the J somatotope and semitendinosus on the K somatotope. The YNSA treatment was unlikely to affect the end-staged OA but may buy her some time before the eventual TKR.

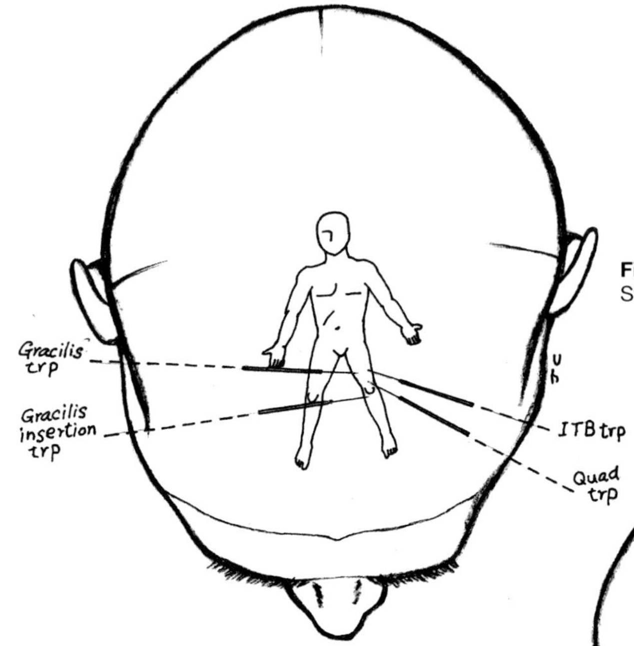

Figure 35: TrP treatment for Case Study 2 (J somatotope)

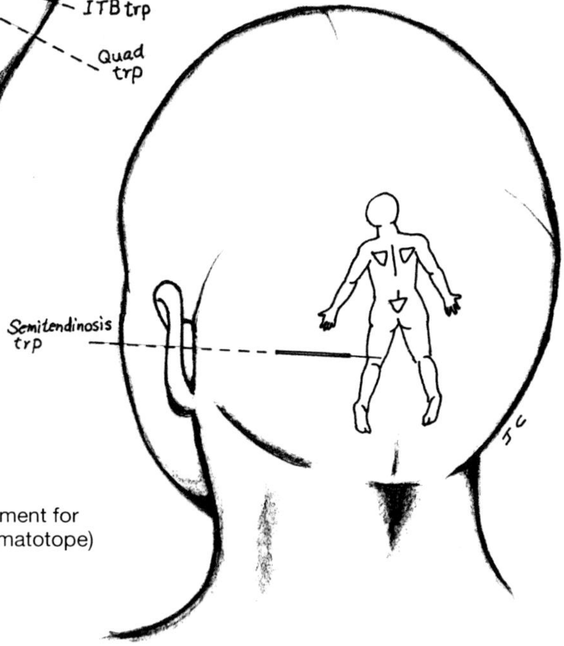

Figure 36: TrP treatment for Case Study 2 (K somatotope)

OUTCOME: Surprisingly, the results of the first two treatments were amazing. She reported pain in the left knee went from a VAS of 8/10 to 4/10 and she was able to go for a 15-minute walk after the first treatment without much pain. The tender TrPs were also normalising. Unfortunately, her pain returned after the second treatment and the subsequent three treatments yielded no improvement at all, with the pain back to a VAS of 8/10. A decision was made to return to the surgeon to discuss the possibility of a trial of an unloader brace or an osteotomy prior to a TKR.

DISCUSSION: In hindsight, it was still worthwhile to try to eradicate the TrPs that were found. It is important to note that individuals with painful OA may be free from radiographic changes and, conversely, those with severe radiographic changes may be entirely asymptomatic. There is a correlation between the severity of radiographic disease and symptoms, however, the association is not strong.[71]

CASE STUDY 3: Right medial knee pain – gracilis TrPs treated with massage and stretching

HISTORY: A 12-year-old boy presented with a ten-day history of constant 6/10 right knee pain. He indicated that the pain was more on the medial aspect of the knee. There were no specific injuries, but he played soccer at least twice a week and trained twice a week as well. Unfortunately, post-game stretching was not always reinforced. He had no previous knee problems, there was no joint swelling or 'locking' of the knee and there were no other joint problems.

REASONING: There was no specific injury pointing to fractures or ligamentous ruptures. Rather, it pointed more to muscular TrPs as the cause.

EXAMINATION: He was afebrile and there was no knee effusion. The range of movement of the knee was normal, but external rotation of the hip exacerbated the knee pain. Tests for collateral, patellar ligaments and meniscal injuries were negative. On palpation, it was very tender at the distal insertion of the gracilis. The patient confirmed this was the 'centre' of his pain. Tracing back along the gracilis, there were TrPs along it, mostly at the lower third of the muscle.

DIAGNOSIS: Gracilis TrPs were diagnosed as the cause of his pain.

INVESTIGATIONS: None planned.

TREATMENT: The patient had a moderate degree of needle phobia and the decision was made not to use acupuncture but to instead use manual therapy/massage (Fig. 37) and stretching (Fig. 21) as treatment.

OUTCOME: He was pain-free after the second treatment, and some gracilis stretches were also prescribed.

MANUAL TREATMENT AND MASSAGE FOR THE GRACILIS

Apply some massage oil or soluble bath oil to the area, then massage the muscle firmly along its length in a downwards motion, with the four fingertips in line, for two minutes. Then rhythmically strike along the muscle with the edge of your palms (like hitting a drum) for two minutes. Alternate the two methods five times. It can be quite painful, but the condition should settle after two or three treatments at a weekly interval.

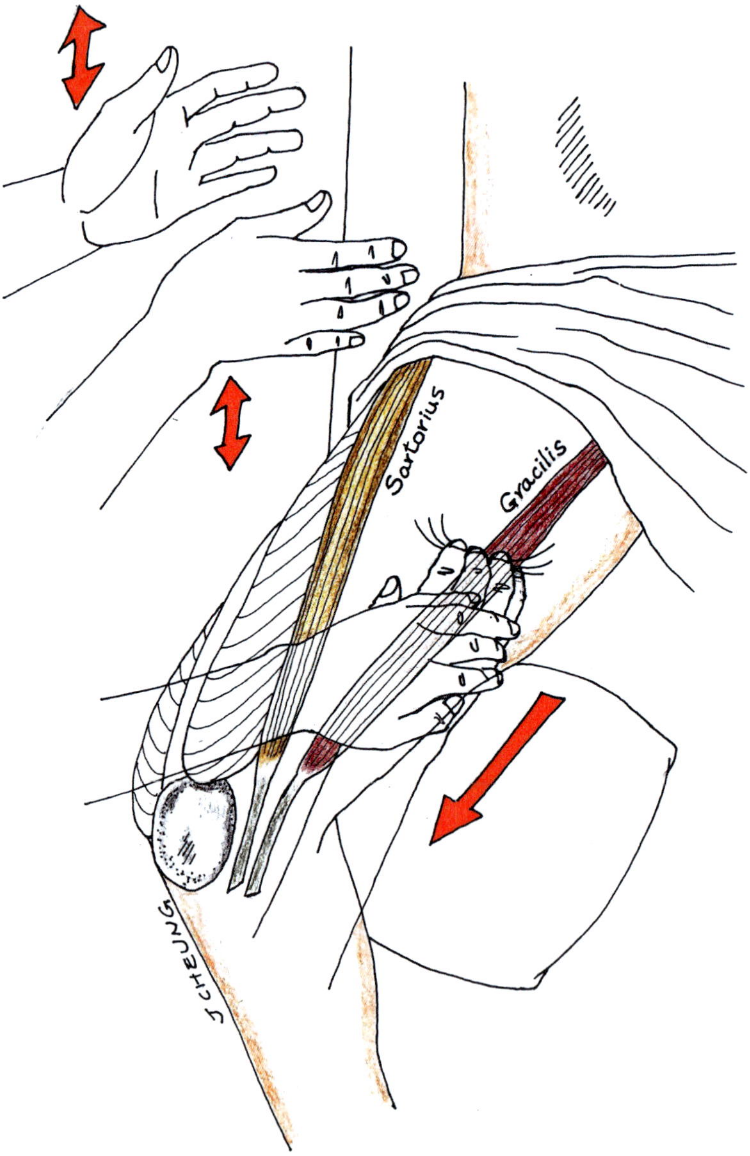

Figure 37: A method of massage for the gracilis in Case Study 3

CASE STUDY 4: Left medial knee pain – gracilis, vastus medialis, rectus femoris and ITB TrPs, treated with YNSA

HISTORY: A 35-year-old female part-time office worker presented with a two-month history of moderate left knee pain. She used to play a fair bit of soccer and remembered several notable knee injuries. The patient described a low-grade pain, VAS at 1/10 to 2/10 for the last eight years and had to stop playing soccer. She avoided long walks or running. Pain was present on stairs, worse going up than going down; squatting was also painful. The patient denied any locking or joint swelling. Previous imaging showed moderate osteoarthritis (OA) but no meniscal tears. While she did not recall any recent injuries, the left knee pain had increased to 5/10 in the last two months and seemed to be located more on the medial aspect of the knee. She had no other joint problems and no prolonged morning stiffness.

REASONING: Inflammatory joint disease was unlikely from the history. Her sporting history, long-term knee pain and previous imaging results pointed to a degree of OA but the relatively sudden increase in pain meant that it may not be the cause of the increased pain. Even though there was no locking, a medial meniscal tear was still possible. With painful squatting and a long history of knee pain and inactivity, patellofemoral pain syndrome (PFPS), a very common condition, needed to be considered. TrPs or meniscal tear were also high on the list, while lytic and sclerotic lesions were still possible.

EXAMINATION: This patient was afebrile and there was no joint effusion. Her left vastus medialis was noticeably thinner than the right side. Clinical tests for meniscal tears were negative. However, on the left side, the Tilt test and Clarke's Tests were positive for PFPS. All the muscles in the knee area were palpated and a comparison made to the contralateral side. Very tender TrPs were found on the left gracilis at the lower third of the muscle and at the distal insertion site, at which point she exclaimed, 'That's it! That's the pain I was telling you about!' There were milder TrPs at the vastus medialis, rectus femoris and iliotibial band as well. The diagnosis made was that the knee TrPs were causing the increase in pain, on the background of OA and PFPS. It is likely that she had strained her gracilis when protecting her painful arthritic knee in the last two months, which caused the increased pain, and the gracilis TRP pain had overshadowed the original OA pain.

INVESTIGATIONS: An X-ray was ordered for a baseline assessment of her OA and to rule out lytic and sclerotic lesions. The X-ray confirmed moderate OA in both the tibiofemoral joint and the patellofemoral joint.

DIAGNOSIS: PFPS as well as TrPs in the gracilis, vastus medialis, rectus femoris and ITB.

TREATMENT: She was treated with YNSA (points on the left gracilis, vastus medialis, rectus femoris and ITB were needled in the J somatotope).

DISCUSSION: In this case study, the real cause of the patient's increased pain was addressed - the TrPs rather than OA – then treated and she began an exercise program to prevent further progression of her problem. Patients with chronic low-grade OA knee pain do not usually consult their GPs as many have tried numerous treatment modalities without success and have accepted the disability. However, an exercise program can often slow down the progression of OA. **In many cases, even when exercises are the correct approach, the patients are unable to continue due to the pain. Therefore, the pain has to be addressed first. Worse still, patients are often told that their pain is due to OA, and long-term medications are then prescribed.**

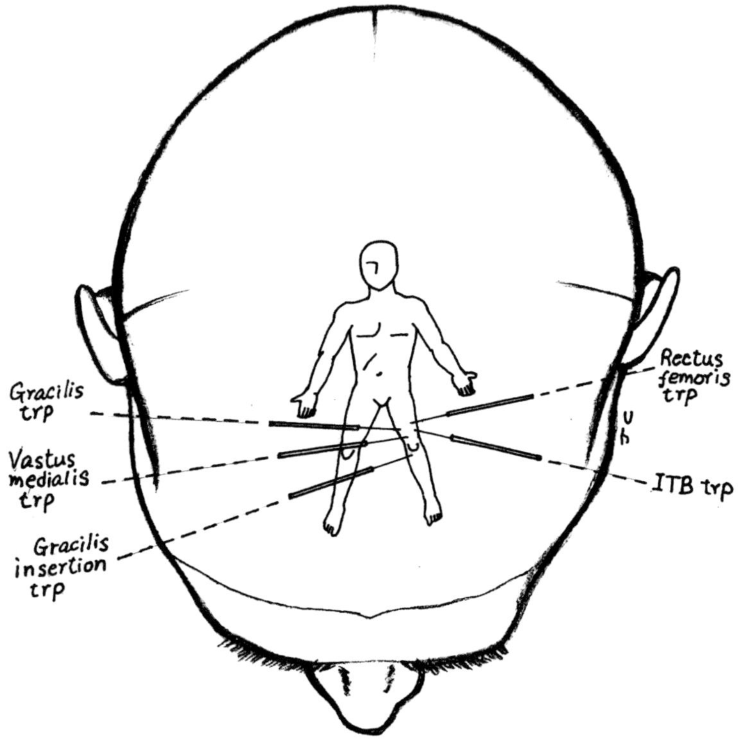

Figure 38: TRP treatment for Case Study 4

Tips: At times, when a few TrPs are close to each other, the acupuncture active points on the scalp would be <10mm next to each other. Once the first needle has been inserted, it would be difficult to palpate the other active points close by. Instead, you should first palpate for all the clustered active points in the scalp, memorise these locations and then insert all the needles.

OUTCOME: She had 15% improvement with each treatment and, after six treatments, her pain improvement plateaued and returned to mild. Treatment was ceased, but the patient was strongly advised to begin an exercise program of strengthening and stretching for her PFPS and OA, in order to slow their progression and prevent a premature knee replacement. Neuromuscular exercise programs such as the GLA:D® (Good Life with osteoArthritis: Denmark) program are increasingly being used by orthopaedic surgeons to do just that.

CASE STUDY 5: Right medial knee pain – gracilis TrPs, treated with a corticosteroid injection

HISTORY: A 68-year-old retired female presented with sudden onset of severe 8/10 medial right knee pain with the background of known moderate OA (usually 2/10 to 3/10 pain). She denied any trauma or misstepping. There was no history of locking, no pain when seated or lying, and no night pain. The pain was only present with movement and weight-bearing activity, and it was worst when getting up from sitting and she struggled to even walk. The patient was obese with a BMI of 38. Past history included atrial fibrillation (on Warfarin), poor renal function, type 2 diabetes and osteoporosis (treated). She was extremely poorly motivated and only compliant in very dire situations.

REASONING: As the onset of severe pain was sudden, we could not assume it was from OA. Muscle and ligamentous injury and strain also had to be considered. The patient was diabetic, so septic arthritis had to be ruled out. Degenerative medial meniscal tear, spontaneous osteonecrosis of the knee and lytic lesions had to be considered. The examination was to help confirm or exclude muscle TrPs or tears.

EXAMINATION: She limped into the room precariously with her husband's help. She was afebrile, which was comforting for a diabetic. Both knee joints were enlarged from the knee OA, there was no redness or obvious effusion (bulge sign was negative), and knee passive flexion and extension were painless and full. Her medial mid joint line was not tender. There was, however, very localised tenderness at 5 o'clock below the patella – at the site of the gracilis insertion. The patient confirmed this was the centre of her pain. There was also marked tenderness along the length of the gracilis.

DIAGNOSIS: The diagnosis was pretty certain to be a gracilis strain resulting in a tendinosis at the site of its distal insertion.

INVESTIGATIONS: If the pain persisted, a CT scan would be ordered to rule out lytic and sclerotic lesions and spontaneous osteonecrosis of the knee.

TREATMENT: The first thought was that an imminent fall was highly likely, resulting in a neck of femur fracture. Ideally, she would be admitted to hospital to be assessed and treated but she declined. The patient also preferred not to have manual therapies or acupuncture. A decision was therefore made to inject her insertion site with corticosteroid and local anaesthetic, which was performed in the office. The most tender spot was located precisely by careful palpation and injected.

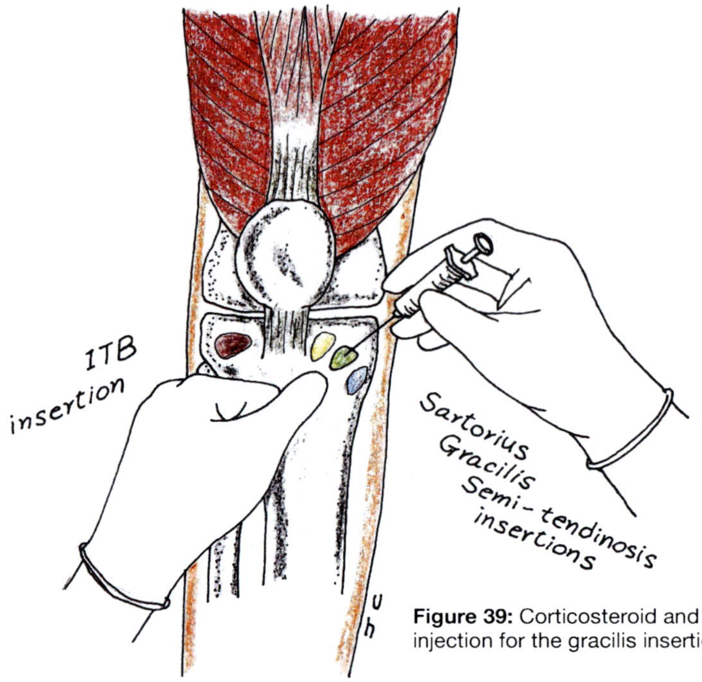

Figure 39: Corticosteroid and local anaesthetics (LA) injection for the gracilis insertion site in Case Study 5

OUTCOME: Ten minutes after the injection, her pain had improved by 80% and she could get up without trouble. I reviewed her an hour after the injection and the pain came back somewhat after the local anaesthetic had worn off, but it was still about 50% better than when she first presented. Caution must be exercised with corticosteroid injections as repeated injections would weaken the injected muscle and ligamentous structures.

I asked her to get a walking frame and not leave home for the next three weeks. I was expecting the pain to recur but, surprisingly, it did not. Some manual therapies and massage on her gracilis were refused, as was attending falls prevention classes (refused on numerous occasions). However, she did agree to keep the walking frame and use it to walk at home regularly, three times a day when her pain settled. As she left, I asked her to organise a plain knee X-ray to rule out lytic and sclerotic lesions.

THE TENSOR FASCIAE LATAE (TFL), THE ILIOTIBIAL BAND (ITB) AND THEIR TrPs

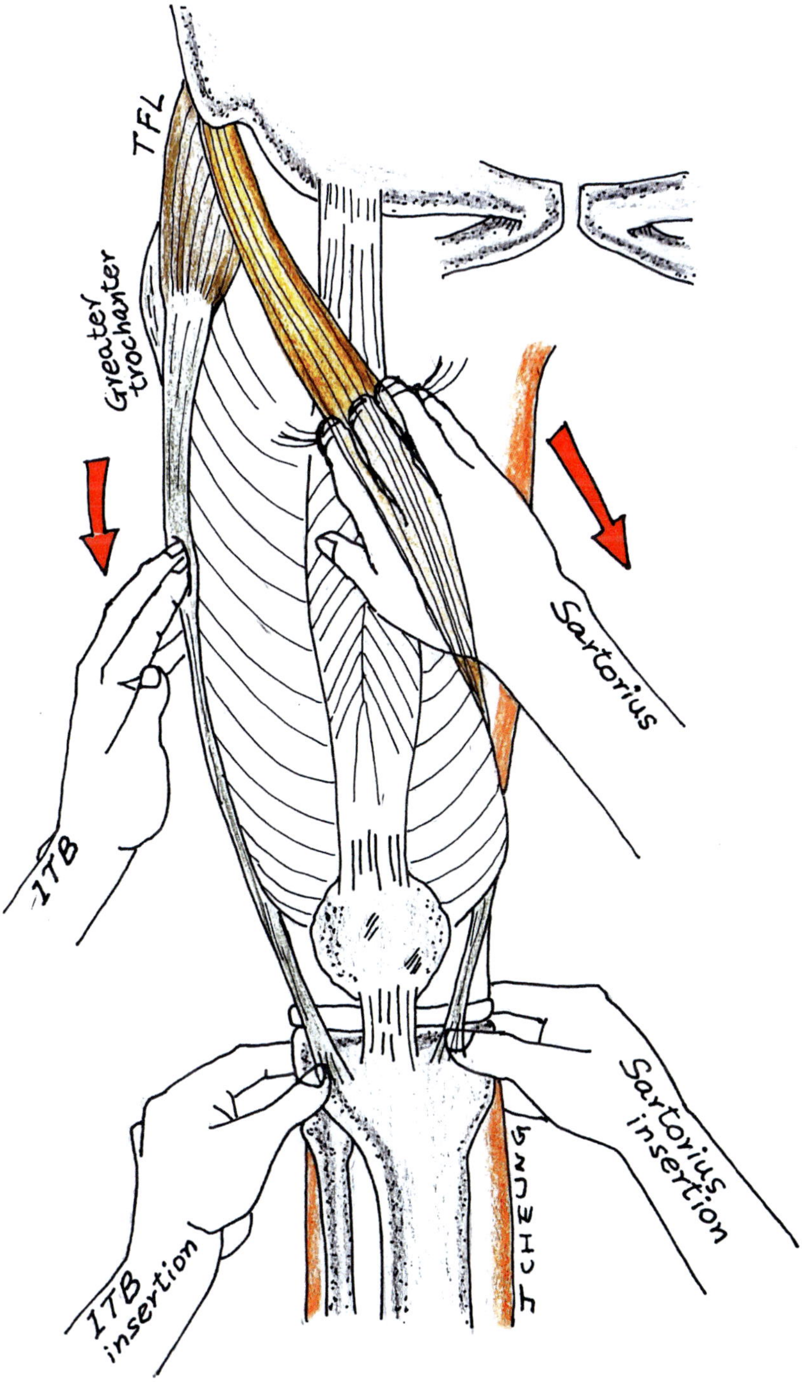

Figure 40: Palpation diagram for the TFL and ITB TrPs

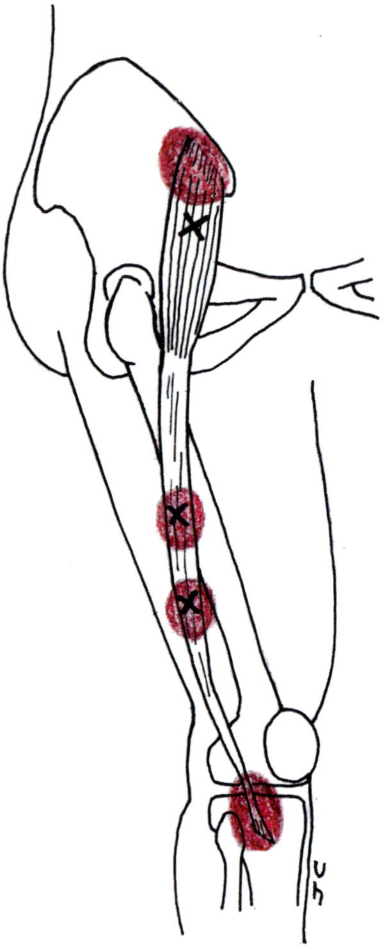

Figure 41: TFL and ITB TrPs and their referred pain pattern

X = TrPs

Red area = the referred pain

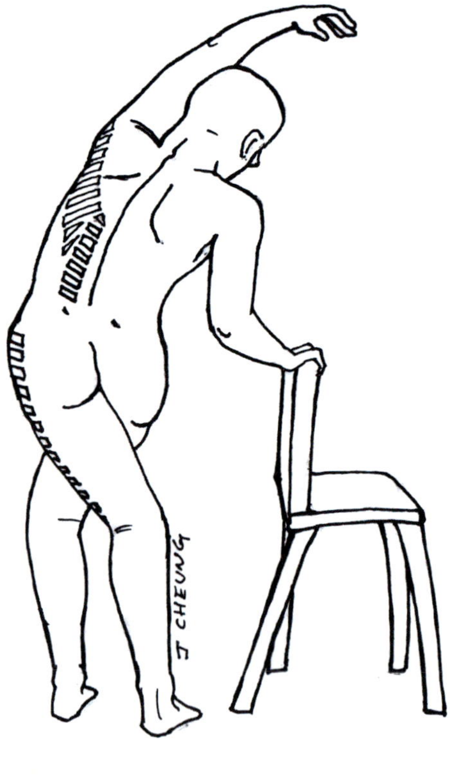

Figure 42: A useful stretch for the TFL and ITB

CASE STUDY 6: Right knee pain – ITB TrPs, treated with YNSA

HISTORY: A 65-year-old man presented with a two-month history of right lateral knee pain with VAS of 5/10. The pain was sharp and aggravated by walking and squatting. He recalled misstepping into a small pothole on one of his usual daily walks. He didn't notice any swelling or locking of the knee, there was no pain at rest and no prolonged morning stiffness. The patient had no previous knee or other joint issues. He had no significant medical problems. Other aspects of his history that are useful in assessing older patients with pain syndromes – such as prostate cancer and bowel cancer screening, bone density, vitamin D and calcium levels – were normal. His usual GP examined him and ordered an X-ray, which showed mild OA. He was diagnosed with OA of the knee and NSAID prescribed. As the pain continued, he presented for a second opinion.

REASONING: As there was no previous knee problem and the pain started relatively suddenly, it was highly unlikely OA was the cause. In the older age group, it was reassuring that he had regular screening for common malignancies and osteoporosis. There were no symptoms supporting the diagnosis of inflammatory joint disease. It was likely to be caused by TrPs resulting from the misstepping. However, a lateral meniscal tear and lateral collateral ligament strain had to be considered.

EXAMINATION: A normal-looking knee joint with full ROM. Lateral collateral ligament was not tender and tests for lateral meniscal tear (McMurray Test and Apley Test) were normal. TrPs were found at the insertion of the ITB, medial to the proximal fibular head, at which point the patient's face lit up. 'That's the pain!' he exclaimed. Palpating up the length of the ITB, more TrPs were found along it.

DIAGNOSIS: TrPs of the ITB.

INVESTIGATIONS: None needed.

TREATMENT: The patient was treated with YNSA (active points of the right ITB on the J somatotope were needled) and was given stretching exercises for the ITB. While YNSA was chosen, the patient could also have been treated with massages to the ITB with similar success.

OUTCOME: After three treatments, he was pain-free.

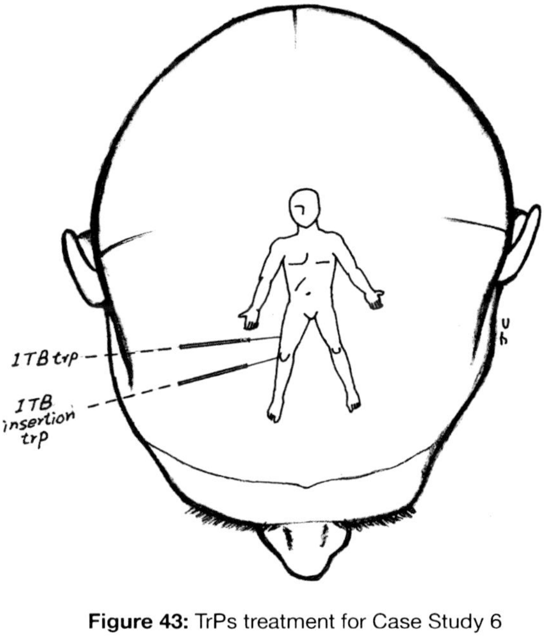

Figure 43: TrPs treatment for Case Study 6

THE HAMSTRING AND ITS TrPs

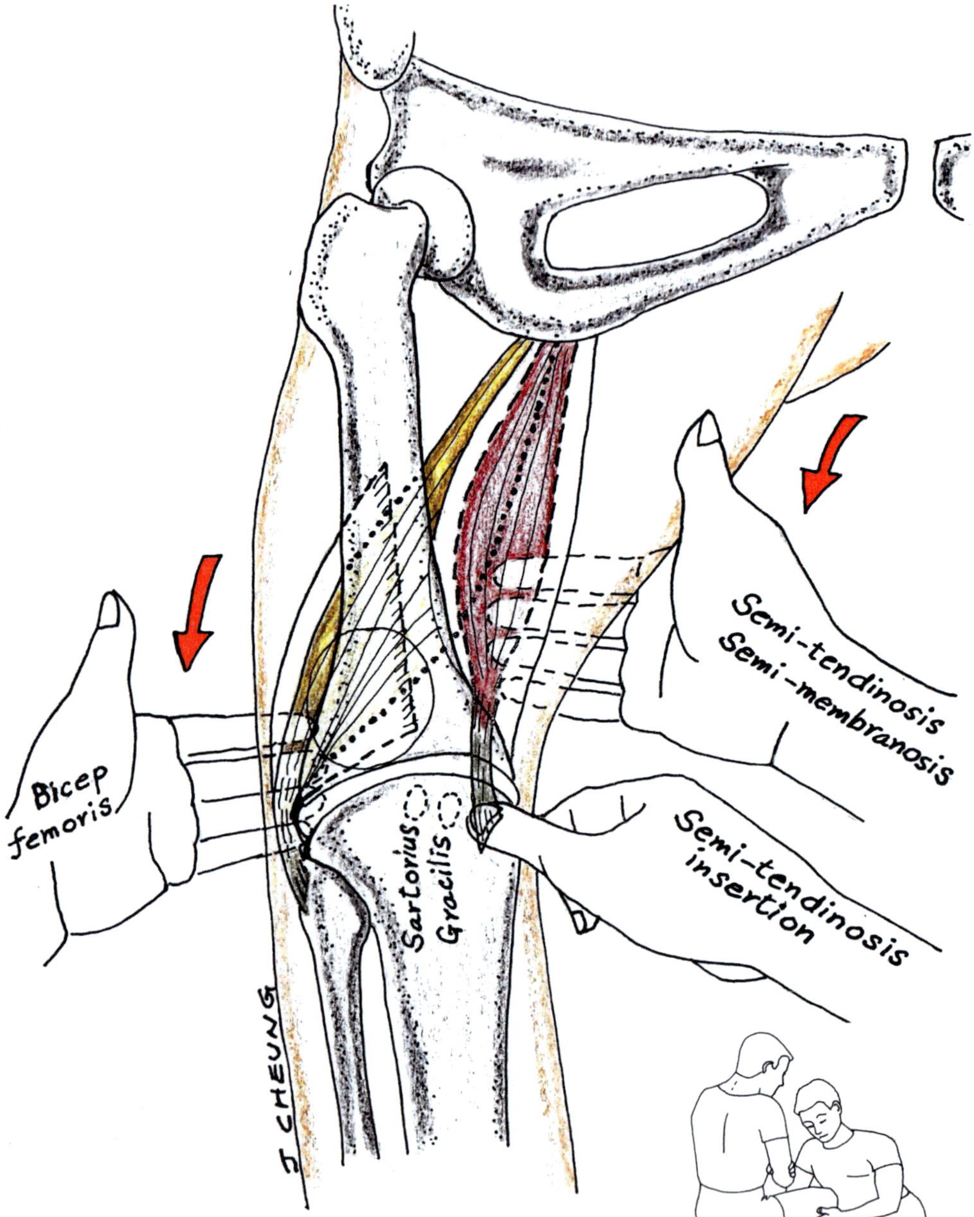

Figure 44: Palpation diagram for the hamstring TrPs

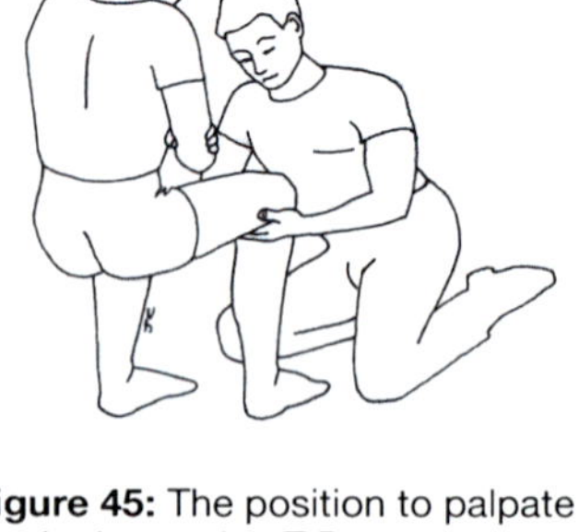

Figure 45: The position to palpate for the hamstring TrPs

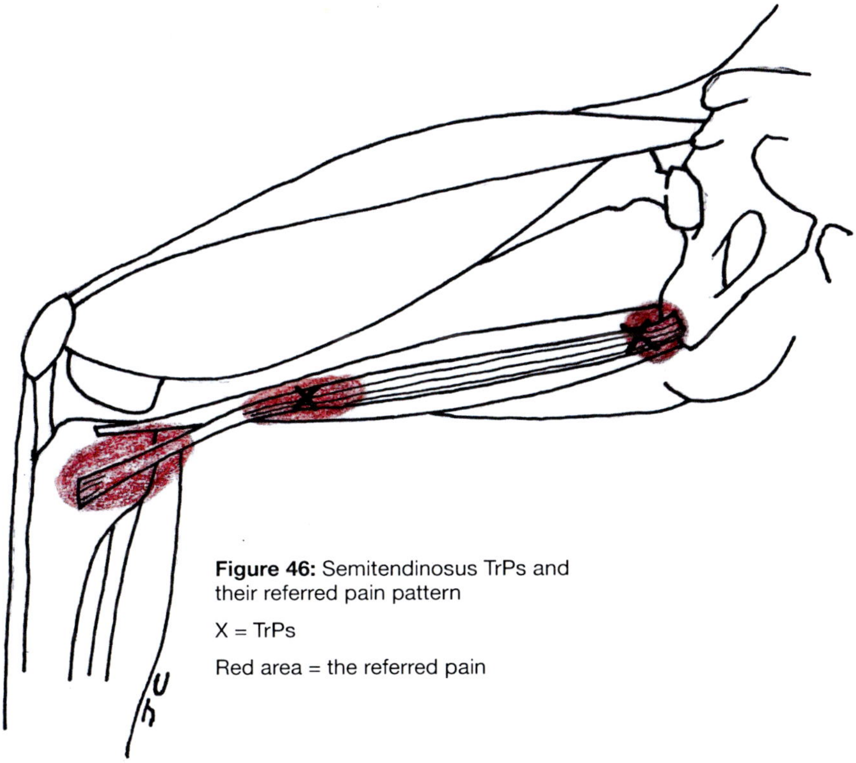

Figure 46: Semitendinosus TrPs and their referred pain pattern

X = TrPs

Red area = the referred pain

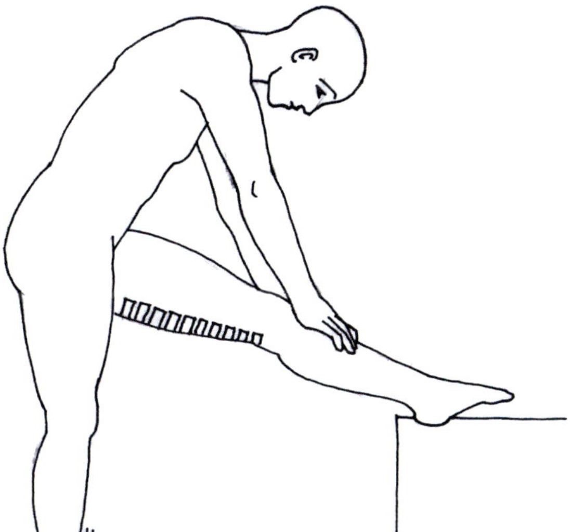

Figure 47: A useful stretch for the hamstrings

CASE STUDY 7: Multiple muscular pains – gracilis, gastrocnemius, hamstring and right subscapularis TrPs, treated with YNSA

HISTORY: A 65-year-old female business owner presented with a three-year history of multiple muscular cramps and severe associated pains. She was diagnosed to have multiple myeloma and was being treated with lenalidomide, a drug related to thalidomide. While her disease was stable and not progressing, she was suffering from multiple side effects. Besides symptoms of extreme tiredness, diarrhoea (three times a day) and nocturia (three times a night), she experienced severe cramping and pain in her calves, hamstring, right subscapularis and diaphragm. These pains were constant, at 4/10 to 5/10 during the day and 10/10 at night. The sleepless nights added to her low energy level.

REASONING: A common side effect of lenalidomide is deep vein thrombosis (DVT). The patient's calf pain could have been a result of DVT, however, it was already being constantly monitored by her oncology team. Rather, the pain appeared to be a neurotoxicity caused by the lenalidomide.

EXAMINATION: The patient had a high pain threshold, but on palpation, extremely tender TrPs were found in the gracilis, gastrocnemius, hamstring and right subscapularis.

INVESTIGATION: None necessary.

TREATMENT: The patient was treated with YNSA, active points of the diaphragm area, gracilis in the J somatotope were needled in addition to the gastrocnemius, hamstring and right subscapularis. An active point in the vicinity of the bladder in the J somatotope was also needled.

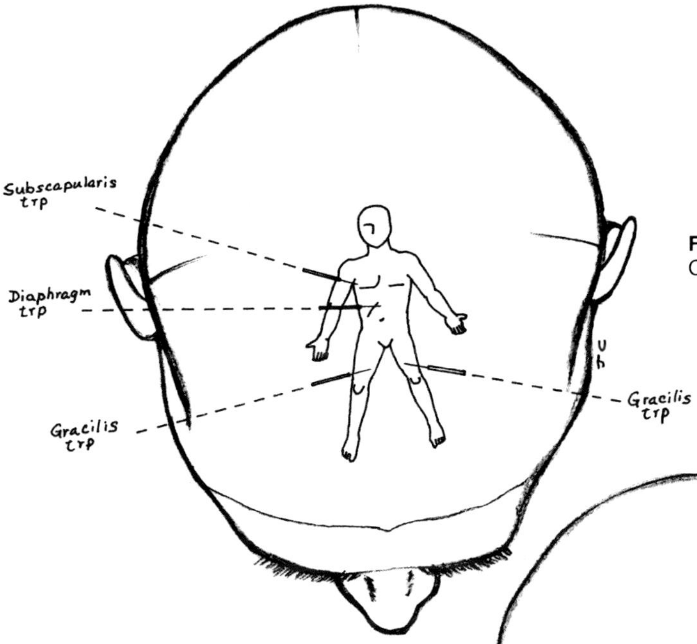

Figure 48: TrP treatment for Case Study 7 (J somatotope)

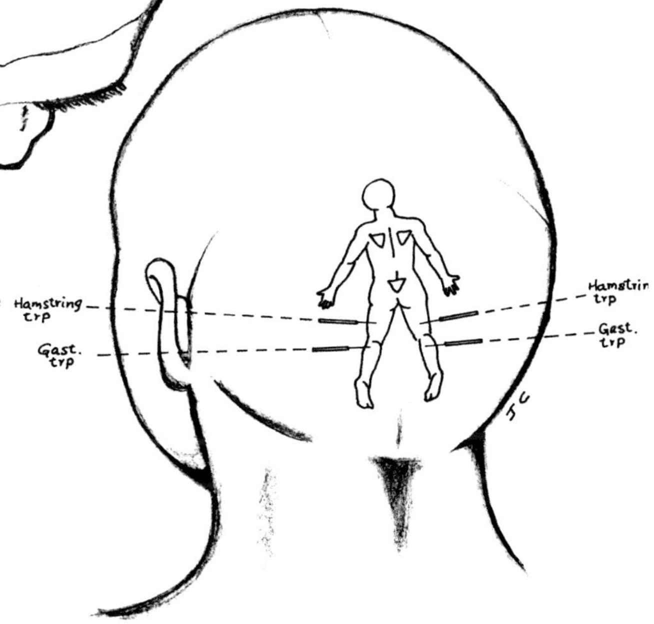

Figure 49: TrP treatment for Case Study 7 (K somatotope)

OUTCOME: Surprisingly, the pain in the right subscapularis and diaphragm cleared with several treatments, after persisting for three years. The other pains gradually improved over ten weekly treatments. After the ten sessions, she described the pain in her legs as minor, she was sleeping through the night and the nocturia had subsided. Her TrPs were still evident but much milder in the gracilis, gastrocnemius and hamstring, and were not troubling her like before. We decided on continuing the treatment every two weeks while she stayed on the lenalidomide.

NB. The patient's diarrhoea and extreme tiredness also cleared with traditional Chinese acupuncture (not YNSA). There are some GPs, anaesthetists/pain specialists and oncologists who use acupuncture regularly to help cancer-related pain and symptoms as a supportive therapy to mainstream cancer treatment.

THE POPLITEUS AND ITS TrPs

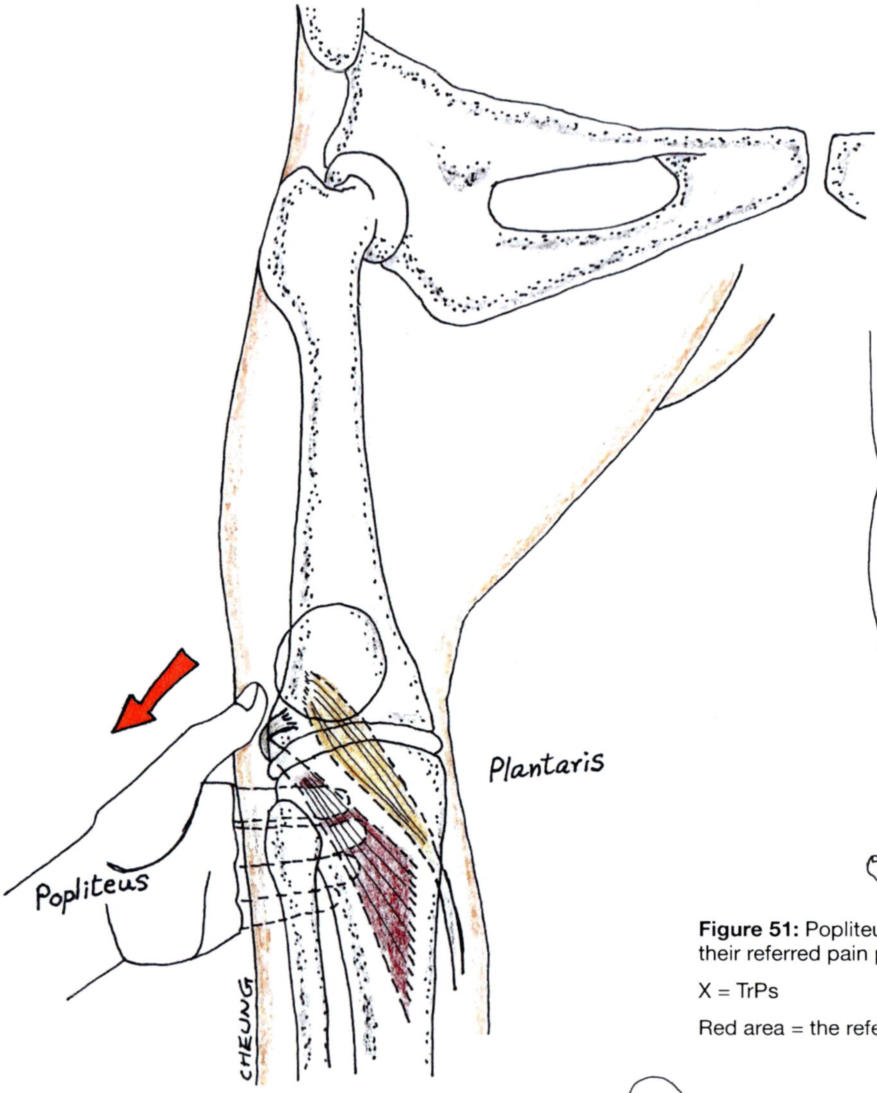

Figure 50: Palpation diagram for the popliteus TrPs

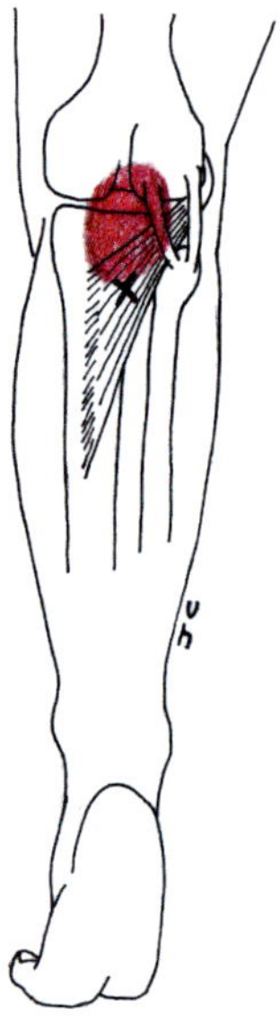

Figure 51: Popliteus TrPs and their referred pain pattern

X = TrPs

Red area = the referred pain

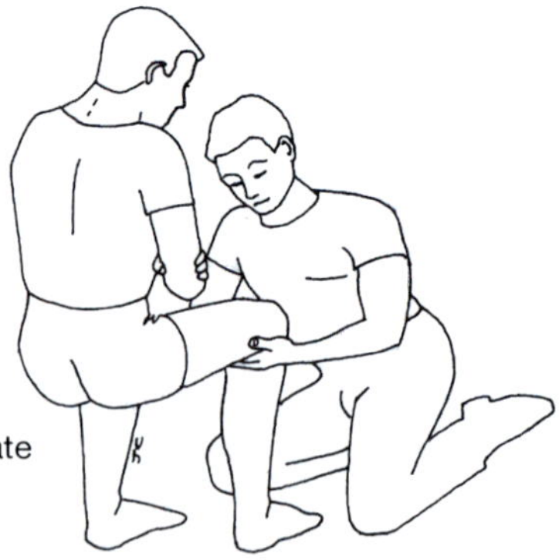

Figure 52: The position to palpate for the popliteus TrPs

CASE STUDY 8: Right knee pain – popliteus TrP, treated with YNSA

HISTORY: A 76-year-old female presented with a two-week history of right knee pain. She went to the gym twice a week and it occurred after riding on a stationary bike and pedalling backwards. The pain was sharp, in the posterior aspect of her right knee. She rated the pain as 5/10 and it was affecting her walking. The patient had no pain when she sat or lay down and no prior knee pain. Her GP examined her briefly and ordered an X-ray and ultrasound, which respectively showed moderate OA and a Baker's cyst. The GP thought the bike riding might have aggravated the OA or the Baker's cyst and gave her some NSAID to try. As the medications didn't help, she sought a second opinion.

REASONING: A Baker's cyst is usually asymptomatic unless it ruptures, which is uncommon. With the sudden onset of symptoms and no previous history of arthritic pain, her pain was unlikely due to the X-ray finding of OA. It pointed instead to a muscular strain in the popliteus, plantaris or gastrocnemius.

EXAMINATION: Swelling was present in both knees but no effusion. She was afebrile. Tests for meniscal injuries were normal. Careful palpation revealed very localised and tender TrPs on the popliteal muscle, which was most likely the cause of her pain.

DIAGNOSIS: TrP of the popliteus.

INVESTIGATIONS: None necessary.

TREATMENT: The patient was treated with YNSA (the active points for the popliteal muscle on the K somatotope).

OUTCOME: The patient made progressive improvement and was pain-free after four treatments. Falls in the older age group are very common, especially with existing pain; she was warned about the danger of falls and to limit her walking until the condition improved.

CASE STUDY 9: Left knee pain – semitendinosus, gracilis and vastus medialis TrPs, treated with YNSA

HISTORY: A 57-year-old female office worker presented with a ten-year history of left knee pain and intermittent knee swelling. The pain had increased in the last month from a VAS of 2/10 to 6/10 and appeared to be more consistent and localised to the anterior aspect of the knee. She could no longer take her regular short walks and negotiating stairs was painful, both going up and down. The patient's previous MRI had shown moderately severe left knee tibiofemoral and patellofemoral OA. There were no recent injuries or falls, no prolonged morning stiffness and no history of locking. Other aspects of the patient's history that are useful in assessing older patients with pain syndromes – such as breast cancer and bowel cancer screening, cervical screening, bone density, vitamin D and calcium levels – were normal.

She was seen by her GP and a rheumatologist and underwent different tests and treatments. Blood tests for inflammatory joint disease were negative, NSAID did not help, and thigh muscle strengthening exercises from a physiotherapist proved too painful. Ultimately, the patient was diagnosed with severe OA and told there was no cure. The patient thought she was destined to have increasing disability and pain from her knee in the years to come.

REASONING: With a relatively sudden increase in pain, OA as the main cause was possible but unlikely. There was no history of trauma and the history didn't support meniscal or ligamentous injuries. Inflammatory joint disease had been ruled out. With the long history of knee pain and OA, patellofemoral pain syndrome (PFPS) was likely. Again, TrPs as a possible contributing factor had to be considered.

EXAMINATION: Some wasting of the vastus medialis on the left side was noted. There was no joint effusion, meniscal tear tests were negative. The patella ligament was not tender. Tests for PFPS (the Tilt test and Clarke's test) were negative. Upon palpation, there were very tender areas over the distal end of the vastus medialis, gracilis and the semitendinosus. It was particularly tender at the distal insertion sites of the left semitendinosus and gracilis, and the patient felt that those tender spots were the cause of her knee pain.

DIAGNOSIS: TrPs of the above muscles were the main cause of the pain, but she did have mild PFPS.

INVESTIGATIONS: None necessary.

TREATMENT: Interestingly, while the trigger points along the length of the muscles were very tender, patients usually don't report the pain being there; they mainly only locate it at the attachments at the knee area. She was treated with YNSA – the semitendinosus, gracilis and vastus medialis insertion sites near the knee of the J somatotope as well as the active point of the semitendinosus muscle on the K somatotope was needled. The G1 point near the mastoid process was active and a press needle was placed there with significant additional improvement. The G point in the YNSA system is excellent in treating knee problems as well (Fig. 53).

THE YNSA G POINT, USED FOR TREATING KNEE PROBLEMS

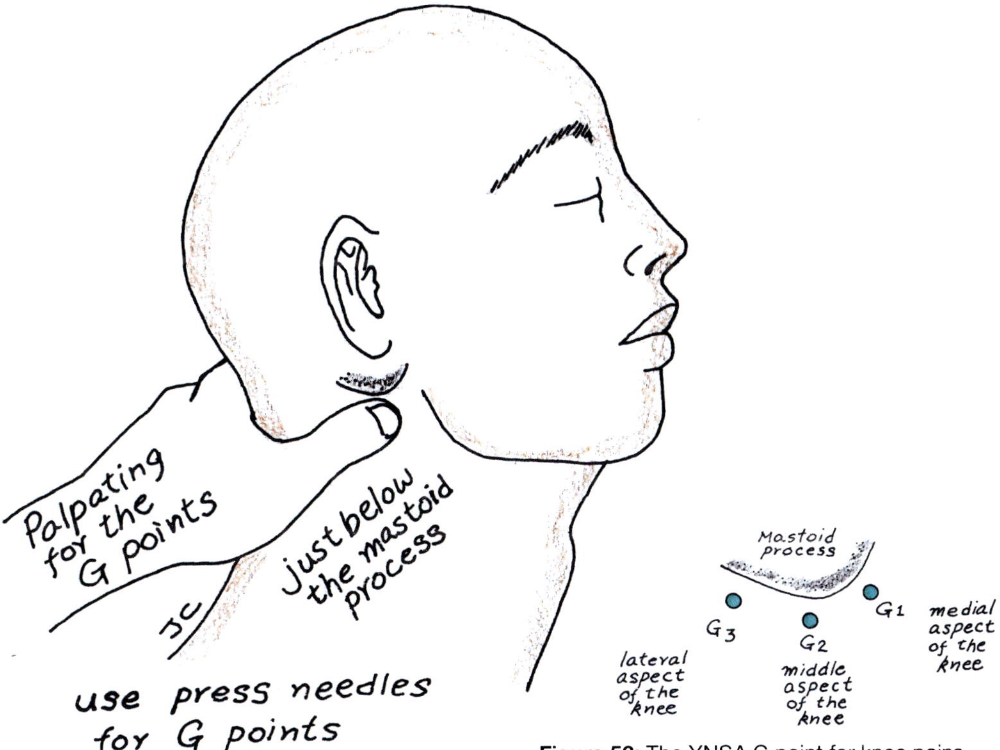

Figure 53: The YNSA G point for knee pains

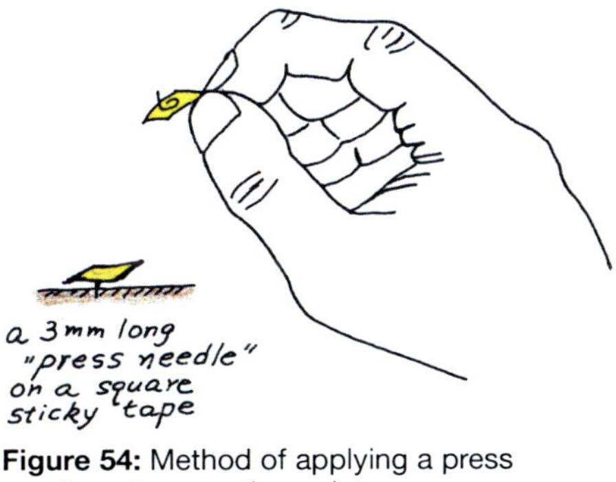

Figure 54: Method of applying a press needle onto an active point

NB. Only press needles can be used in the G points. Acupuncture needles must not be used due to the proximity of important structures here.

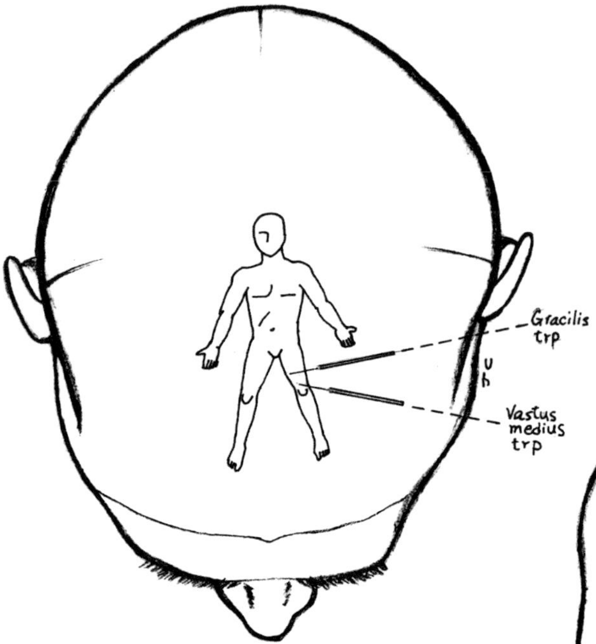

Figure 55: TrP treatment for Case Study 9 (J stomatotope)

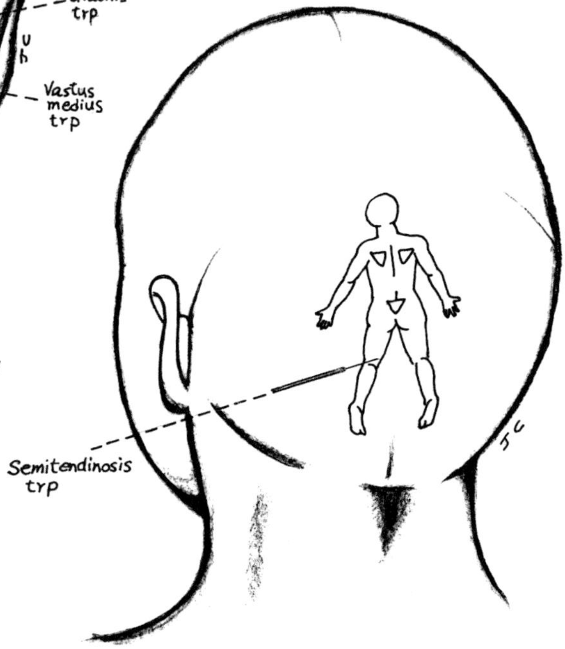

Figure 56: TrP treatment for Case study 9 (K stomatotope)

OUTCOME: After three weeks of twice-weekly treatments, her knee pain vastly improved. VAS was now 2/10 and she was able to return to some gentle walking. As the knee pain was much improved, she could then do her stretching and strengthening exercises better and, hopefully, slow down the progression of her patellofemoral OA. OA and TrPs can coexist, the latter were probably caused by the OA. In this case study, the TrPs became the main cause of her pain. By addressing the TrPs, the main pain was relieved. It was also important to address the weak vastus medialis with some supervised strengthening exercises so that progression to more severe patellofemoral OA may be arrested.

NB. This case study illustrates that significant pain has to be alleviated first, otherwise the planned exercises – even though appropriate – would be too painful to do or maintain.

THE SOLEUS AND ITS TrPs

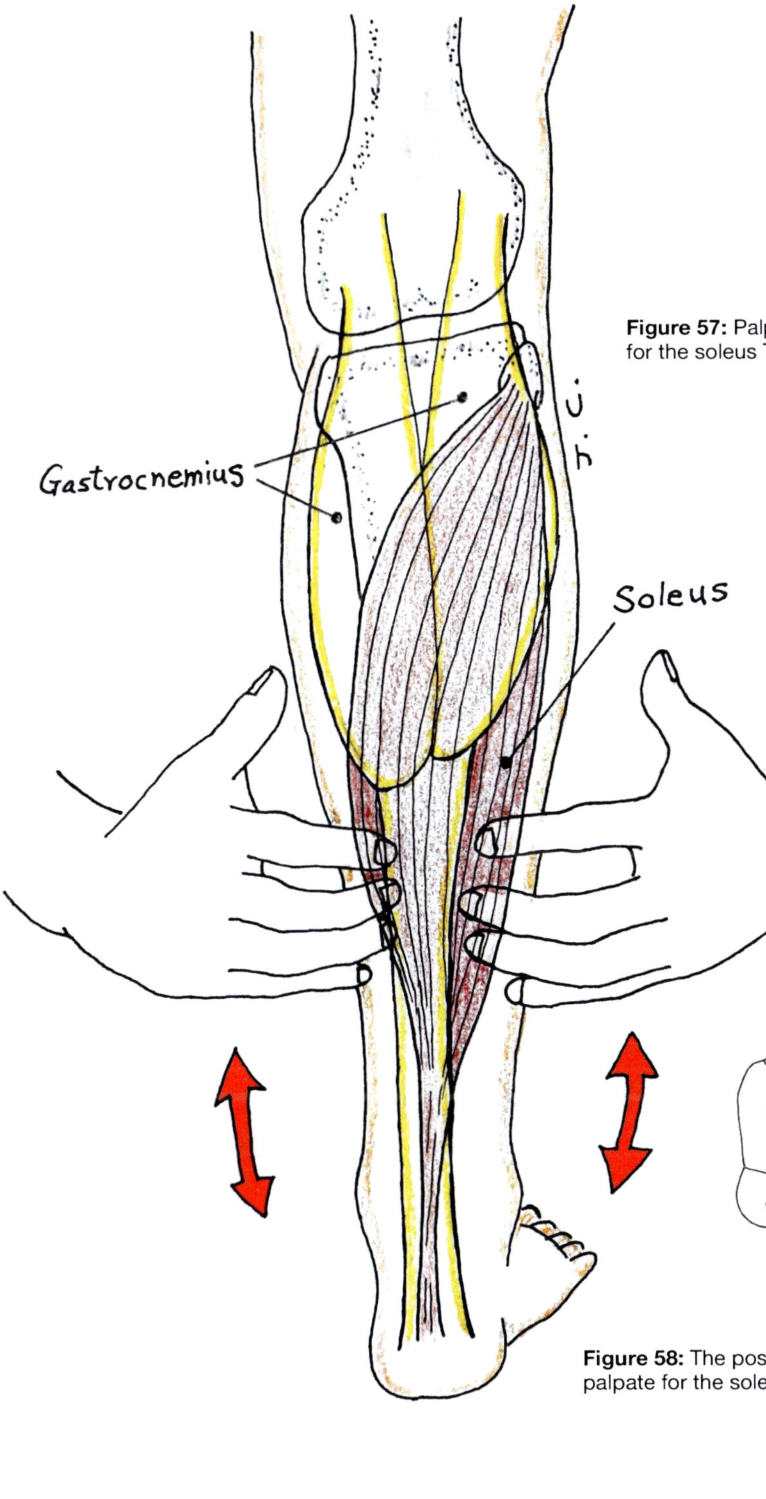

Figure 57: Palpation diagram for the soleus TrPs

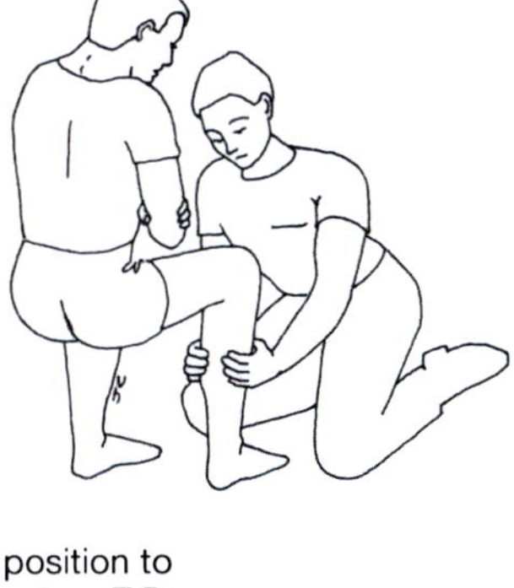

Figure 58: The position to palpate for the soleus TrPs

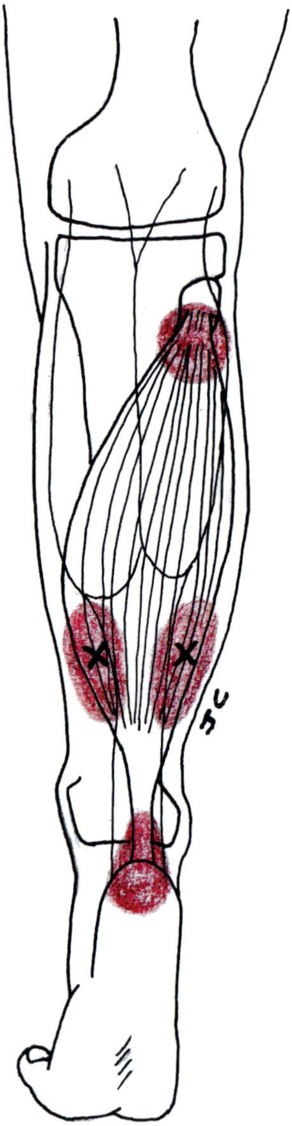

Figure 59: Soleus TrPs and their referred pain pattern

X = TrPs

Red area = the referred pain

NB. There are many causes for plantar heel pain syndromes. It is always worthwhile to palpate for TrPs in the gastrocnemius and the soleus, which can cause heel pain.

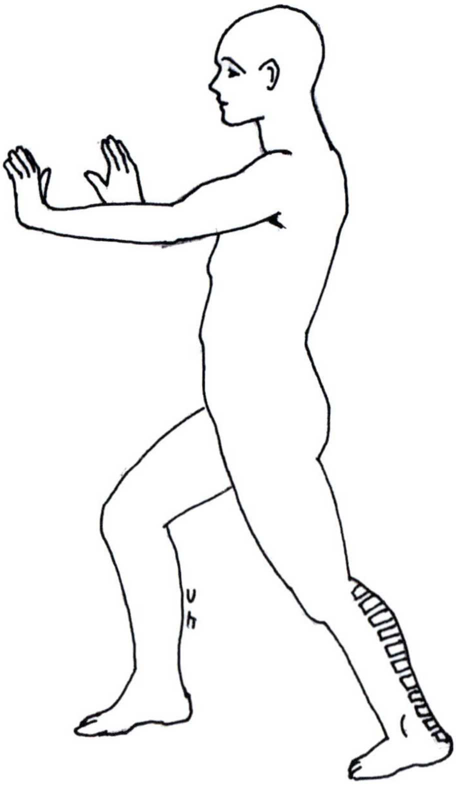

Figure 60: A useful stretch for the soleus and gastrocnemius

CASE STUDY 10: Left heel pain – peroneus TrPs, treated with YNSA

HISTORY: A 52-year-old female office worker presented with a six-month history of severe left heel pain. The pain was in the centre of the heel and also over the lateral aspect of the heel. The patient rated it as 6/10 and reported it was worse in the morning and had stopped her from her usual daily walks. She had a BMI of 28 and the pain started when she had increased her walking to lose some weight. She had numerous medical conditions but none related to the heel pain. A plain X-ray and MRI showed a thickened plantar fascia and a moderate calcaneal spur. The patient had tried a course of NSAID, physiotherapy treatments, an exercise program, orthotic insert and podiatry treatments.

REASONING: She had numerous imaging and different treatments which hadn't helped. TrPs that can cause heel pains need to be examined.

EXAMINATION: A slightly thickened but non-tender Achilles tendon. There was no localised tenderness over the plantar fascia or the heel area. However, very tender TrPs were found at the lateral, lower aspect of the soleus and along the length of the peroneus longus.

DIAGNOSIS: TrPs of the soleus and peroneus longus.

INVESTIGATIONS: None necessary.

TREATMENT: She was treated with YNSA, active points were located for the soleus, peroneus longus and heel in the K somatotope. Immediately after the needle insertions, the soleus and peroneus TrPs were noticeably improved.

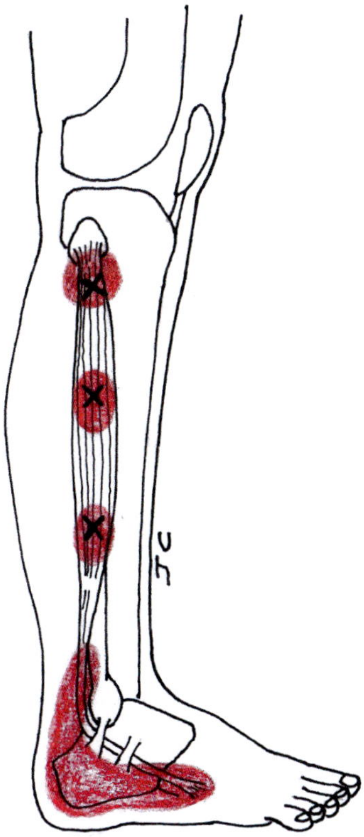

Figure 61: Peroneus longus TrPs and their referred pain pattern

X = TrPs

Red area = the referred pain

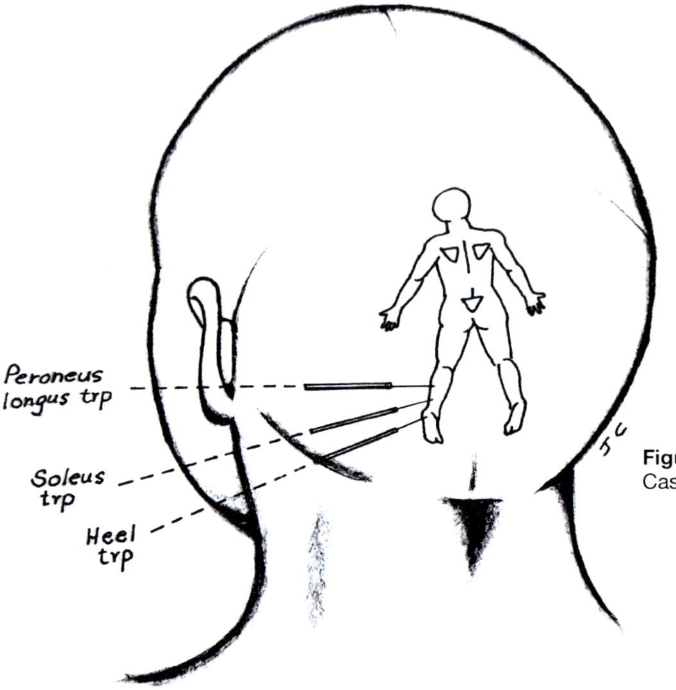

Figure 62: TrP treatment for Case Study 10

OUTCOME: Her pain improved with each treatment and she was pain-free after six weeks. The patient was encouraged to return to the regular stretching program prescribed by her physiotherapist.

Tips: TrPs in the lateral or medial aspect of the body can be located in the K or J somatotopes. If one is not effective, try the other somatotope.

Plantar heel pain affects 10% of the population in their lifetime;[72] it is a complex, multifactorial condition involving multiple tissues. Specific entities such as Achilles tendinopathies, bursitis, plantar fascia tears and calcaneal stress fractures should be excluded first. Investigations of plantar heel pain often involves X-ray, ultrasound and MRI. The presence of calcaneal spurs is not a clear indication for it to be the cause of pain. Studies have shown 10–63% of calcaneal spurs are asymptomatic.[73] Thickening of the plantar fascia correlates well with plantar heel pain, as studies have found that fascia thickening of >4 mm is 100 times more likely to have plantar heel pain,[74] but it is still not indicative of it being the cause or indeed the sole cause of pain. After taking all that into consideration, we were left with plantar fasciitis and muscular TrP referring pain to the heel area. From my experience, it is always worthwhile to look for TrPs in the gastrocnemius and the soleus muscles, and eradicate them (especially if there is no localised tenderness in the plantar fascia and the heel area).

Exercises and manual therapies should be the first-line treatment for problems in the gastrocnemius-soleus-Achilles tendon-plantar fascia complex. However, studies on their efficacies are rare compared to more invasive methods.[75]

A SUMMARY OF A PROPOSED APPROACH TO A PATIENT PRESENTING WITH KNEE PAIN

1. Attempt to reach a diagnosis through a thorough history. Remember that the causes of knee pains are highly positional and, by noting the site of the pain, one can narrow down the possibilities.
2. Rule out any red-flag diagnosis.
3. Carry out a targeted examination to confirm diagnosis and exclude other possibilities.
4. If appropriate, include palpation for trigger points around the knee region. They may be the main or partial cause of the pain. With practice, it will take a few minutes (Fig. 63).
5. Order appropriate imaging or other investigations. Tests should not take precedence over – or replace – the above steps. Try not to order unnecessary tests that would not change the management plan. Tests often show multiple pathologies that are not the cause of the problem and can confuse the diagnostic process.
6. Plan treatment with the aim to cure or improve the condition, rather than just treating the pain.

Finding trigger points (TrPs) and treating them successfully can

- **eradicate the pain completely (when the TrPs are the cause);**
- **improve some of the pain (as the TrPs cause some of the pain);**
- **exclude TrPs as the cause of the pain, then moving on to consider other possible diagnoses; and**
- **often avoid expensive imaging or invasive treatments.**

NB. There are often many instances when a pain syndrome is wrongly diagnosed to be from knee osteoarthritis (OA) or meniscal tear when the cause of pain is primarily from TrPs. However, just because significant TrPs are found in a patient, it doesn't always mean that it is the diagnosis. The TrPs may be secondary to another condition. Often multiple conditions can coexist.

It is worth remembering that diagnoses are static entities whereas a patient's condition changes and evolves with time. A patient with osteoarthritic knee pain may evolve to develop significant muscular TrP pain, overshadowing the original OA pain. Someone with mainly TrP pain may evolve to develop a bursitis; or, after eradicating the TrP pain in a patient, an underlying OA pain or bursitis pain may become more evident. As TrPs are very common and readily treatable, it is still worthwhile eradicating them first.

PALPATION FOR TRIGGER POINTS IN THE KNEE REGION

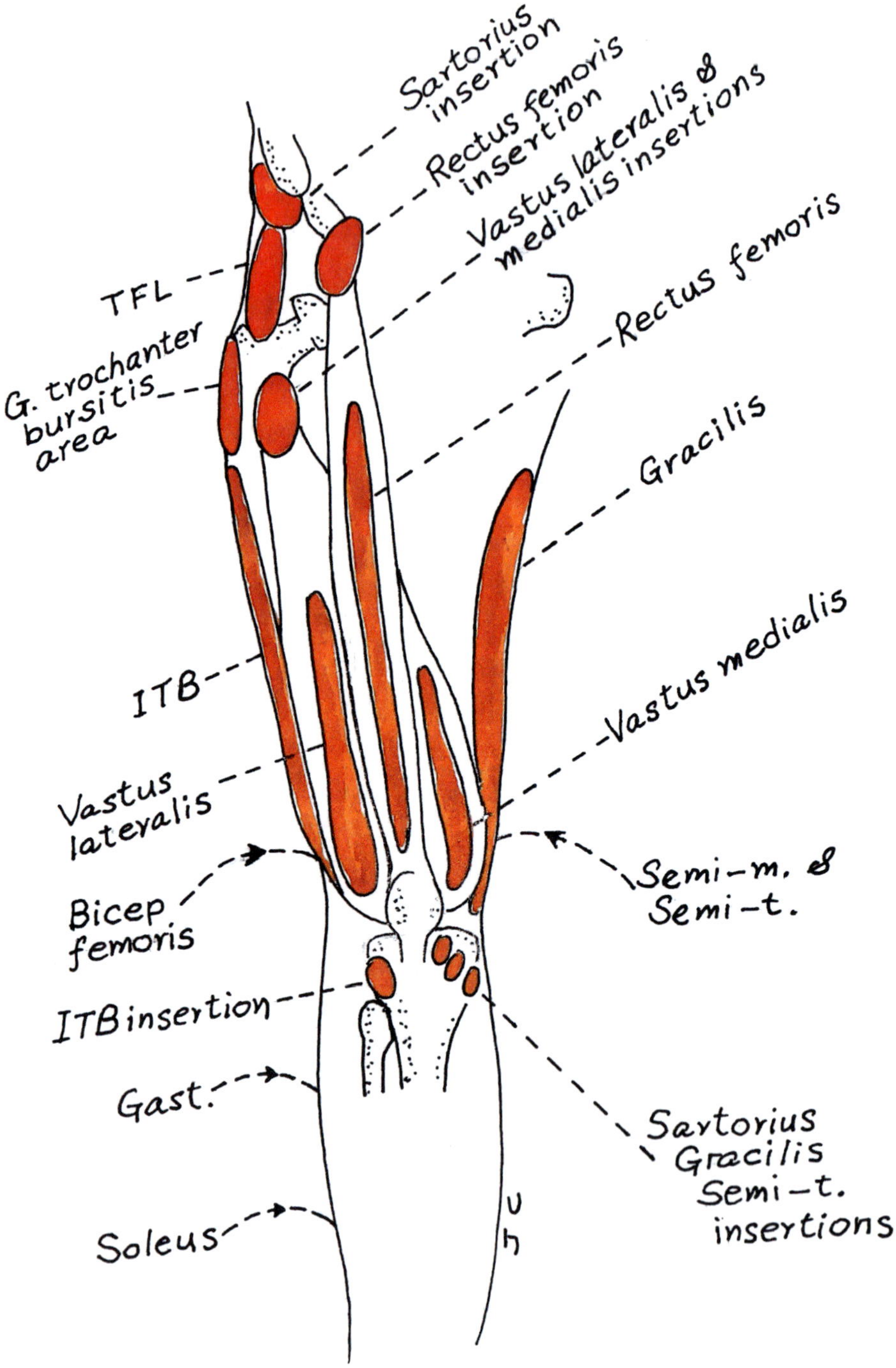

Figure 63: Palpation for TrPs in the knee region

SOME STRETCHES FOR THE KNEE REGION

Stretches need to be felt in the designated muscles, and all adjacent muscles should be relaxed to target it. Stretches should be maintained for eight breaths or 30 seconds and repeated if necessary. Encourage patience – stretches should be done daily.

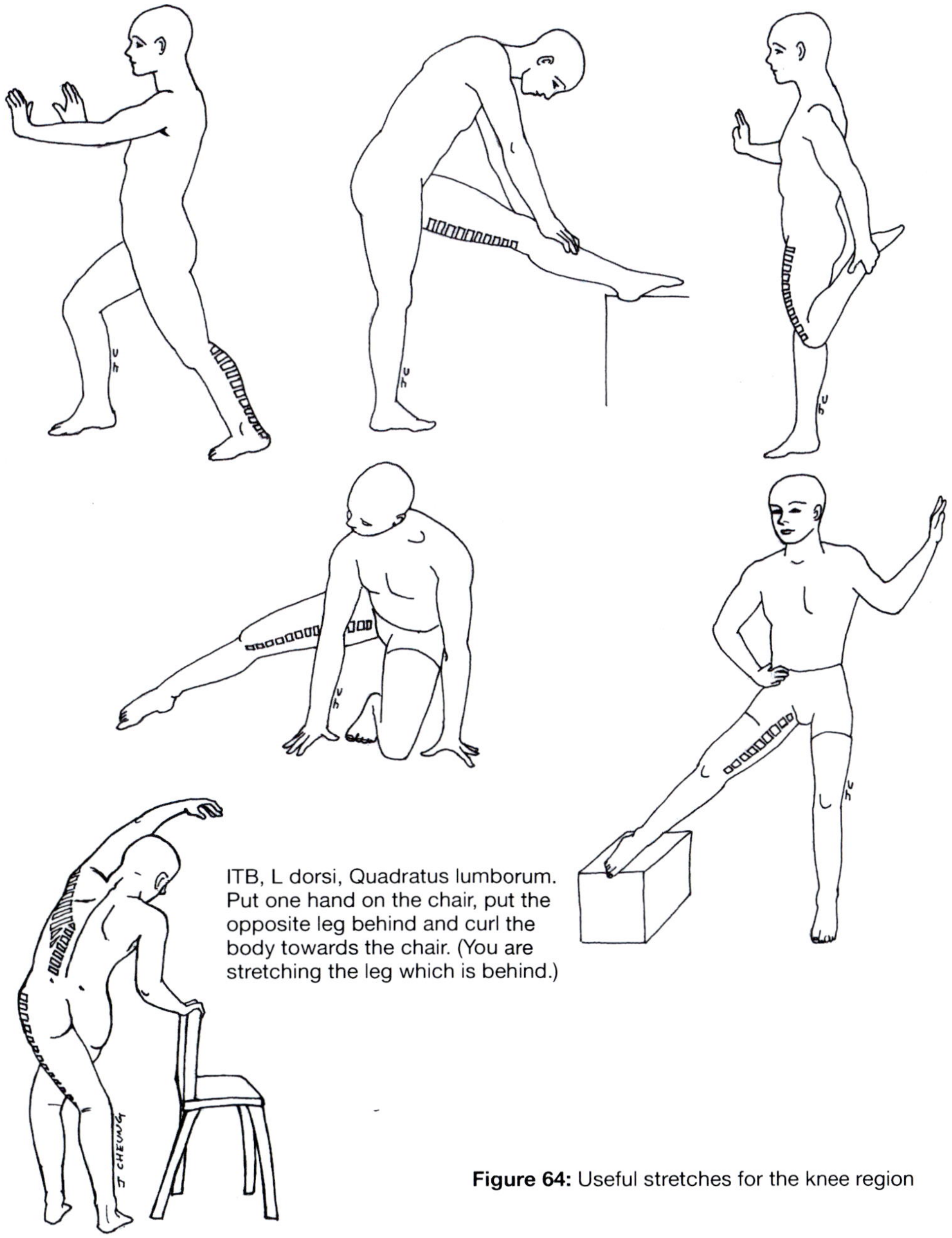

ITB, L dorsi, Quadratus lumborum. Put one hand on the chair, put the opposite leg behind and curl the body towards the chair. (You are stretching the leg which is behind.)

Figure 64: Useful stretches for the knee region

SOME STRENGTHENING AND BALANCING EXERCISES FOR THE KNEE

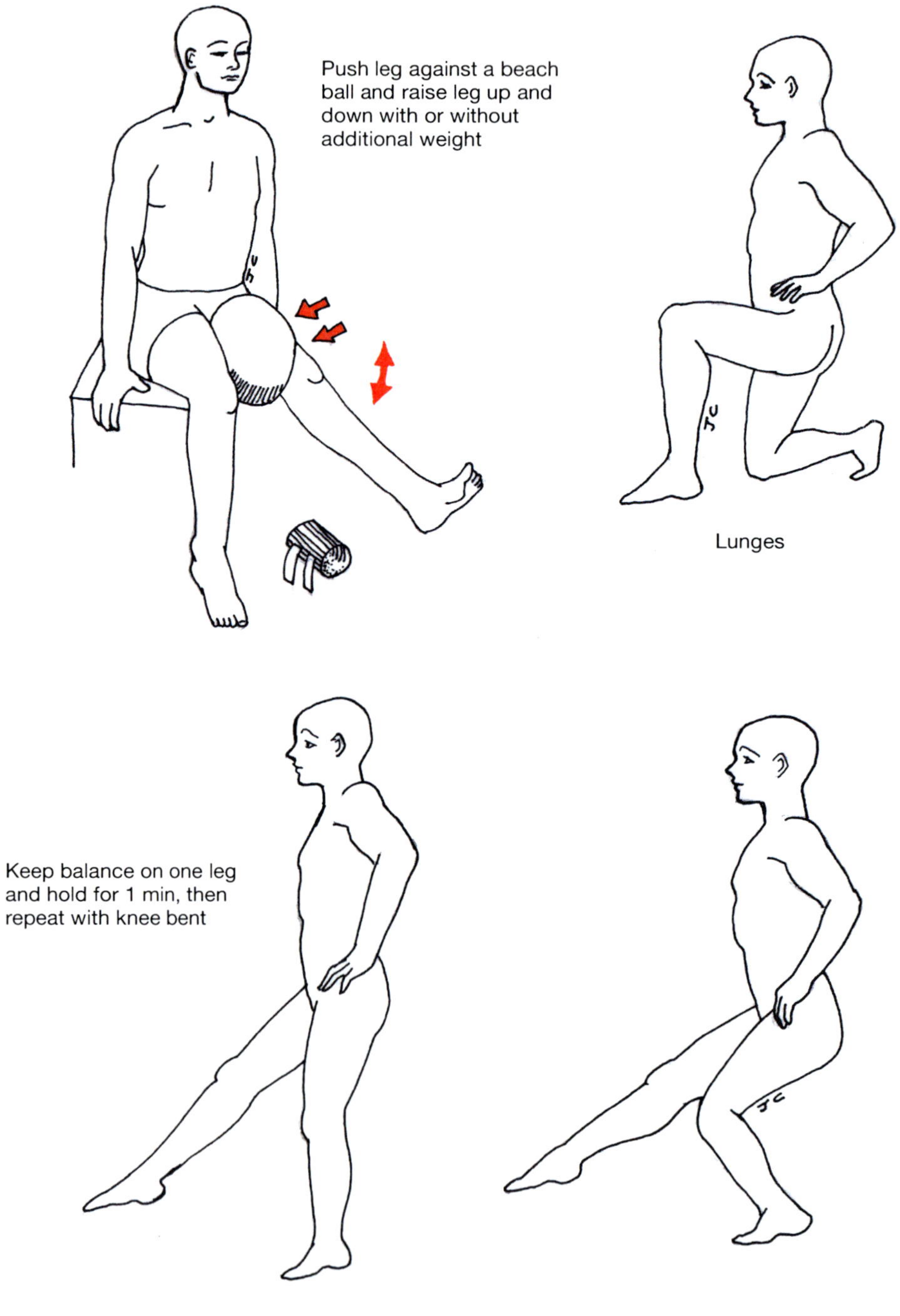

Figure 65: Useful strengthening and balancing exercises for the knee region

3. THE LOWER BACK AND THE UPPER THIGH REGION

Briefly, this chapter will cover the following aspects:

Musculoskeletal (MSK) problems account for about 20% of GP presentations and, of these, lower back pain (LBP) is the most common.[76] LBP has a lifetime prevalence of 39.9% +/- 24.3%.[77] **The most common causes of LBP are muscular strain/ mechanical;** they are usually self-limiting and resolve without intervention. Approximately 50% will resolve within 1–2 weeks and 90% within 6–12 weeks.[78] The LBP which presents to GPs are likely to be more severe or chronic cases.

FRAMEWORK OF QUESTIONING IN LOWER BACK PAIN SYNDROMES

A framework of questions is useful when approaching pain syndromes. With practice, a mental framework of questioning will become automatic.

1. Are there any **red flags?** e.g. unstable fractures, urgent neurological presentations (cauda equina), urgent vascular presentations (aortic aneurysm), acute/serious infections and undiagnosed malignancies.
2. Is it a **fracture?** Any history of trauma or sporting injuries causing possible fractures. Bear in mind that injuries can occur without any trauma in the older age group e.g. spondylosis, vertebral compression fractures, spondylolysis, spondylolisthesis.
3. Could the patient's **employment, sports and activities** have contributed to the presenting problem? e.g. a handyman building a stone retaining wall.
4. Is it an **inflammatory joint disease?** e.g. Psoriatic arthritis, reactive arthritis/Reiter's syndrome.
5. Is it **gout?**
6. Is it **infective?**
7. Is it a **tumour (benign or malignant), or a cyst**?
8. Is the pain originating from the **sacroiliac joint?**
9. Is the pain coming from **neighbouring structures?** e.g. hip joint pathologies, greater trochanteric bursitis.
10. Is the pain coming from **distal pathologies?** e.g. renal colic causing back pain.
11. Is it a **neuralgia?** e.g. from the sciatic nerve, pudendal nerve, post herpetic neuralgia.
12. Is it a **radiculopathy?** Is it **spinal canal stenosis?**
13. Is it **osteoarthritis?**
14. Is it a **muscular strain?**

CAUSES OF LOWER BACK PAIN

SPONDYLOSIS

An entity with numerous definitions, it is generally defined as a degenerative condition of the vertebral disc, vertebral body and/or associated joints of the spine.[79]

VERTEBRAL COMPRESSION FRACTURE

Vertebral compression fracture accounts for 4% of all LBP causes, consisting of traumatic and osteoporotic.[80] Osteoporotic vertebral compression fractures (OVCF) are common in the older age group. Osteoporosis is common, affecting up to 6.2 million Australians over the age of 50 years. One in three women and one in five men in Australia will experience an osteoporotic fracture.[81] It can be asymptomatic or symptomatic with severe back pain, often lasting four weeks. It may not be preceded by any trauma. Imaging will show wedging and/or vertebral body height reduction of >20%. Pain control includes NSAIDs and short-term opioids, and anti-osteoporotic drugs may be used for pain control as well.[82] The emphasis of OVCF should be preventive rather than treatment.[83] When we assess a patient at any age, we should look at their diet, calcium intake, vitamin D level and how much weight-bearing exercises they do. In the older age group, consider a screening DEXA bone density scan or a base-line thoracic and lumbar spine X-ray. Have they had a minimal trauma fracture already? Are they a falls risk?

SPONDYLOLYSIS

It is defined as anatomical defect of the pars interarticularis. While genetic disposition plays a part, it is mainly caused by mechanical factors, therefore more common in young athletes. In the setting of bilateral pars defects, forward movement of the caudal vertebra may occur, a condition known as isthmic spondylolisthesis. The prevalence of spondylolysis is estimated to be 5–11.5% and isthmus spondylolisthesis to be 4–8% in adulthood.[84] As not all spondylolysis is symptomatic, it is often an incidental finding. In more advanced diseases, lower back pain is common, often worse with lumbar extension, which loads the pars. Radiculopathies can occur. Investigations include X-ray, CT scan, MRI and radionuclide imaging (planar bone imaging and SPECT).[85] It is advisable to refer patients with spondylolysis to a spinal specialist for initial assessment. In mild cases, conservative treatment of activity modification and physical therapies are used, while surgical treatment is reserved for more advanced cases.

SPONDYLOLISTHESIS

It refers to the relative displacement of the upper and lower vertebrae, usually at L4/5 or L5/S1. The aetiology is multifactorial, including congenital, mechanical (sport related), trauma and degeneration. Degenerative spondylolisthesis being the most common as discs, facet joints, ligaments and muscles degenerate. The incidence is 4–6% in children and 5–10% in adults.[86] It is more common in females. In children, the symptoms can be LBP and buttock pain. These pains are worse with activities and lumbar extension. In adults, the symptoms can be LBP, radiculopathies and possible cauda equina syndrome. Treatment includes conservative management of physical therapies and, in severe cases, surgical intervention. Not all degenerative spondylolisthesis progresses; in one study, the progression rate ranged 12–34% in up to 25 years of follow-up, which is important in counselling patients suffering from degenerative spondylolisthesis.[87]

Axial spondyloarthritis (axSpA) is defined as an inflammatory arthritis of the spine and sacroiliac joints (SIJs). It is divided into non-radiographic axial spondyloarthritis (nr-axSpA) and ankylosing spondylitis (AS). Since X-ray takes 5–10 years to show the SIJ erosive changes in AS, patients presenting with axial and SIJ inflammatory arthritis but no X-ray evidence of erosion are classified as having nr-axSpA, which is considered to be a precursor of AS. AxSpA has a prevalence of 0.3–1.4%.[88] The presenting features are insidious in onset, often affecting people <40 years of age, with lumbar and alternating buttock pain. It is worse with rest and relieves with activity. There is a prolonged morning stiffness >30 minutes.

The X-ray request should be a plain anteroposterior pelvis views, as dedicated SIJ views have high inter-reader variations. MRI may show presence of bone marrow oedema in the SIJ, however, that can be present in high-level athletes and postpartum women. HLA-B27 (human leukocyte antigen B27) is positive in 50–80% of patients with axSpA, but it is also present in 7–9% of healthy Caucasian populations.[89] ESR (erythrocyte sedimentation rate) and CRP (C-reactive protein) can be raised or normal and is often the latter in earlier phases of the disease. Treatments include NSAIDs and physical treatments, and tumour necrosis factor inhibitors (TNFi) are often required.[90]

PSORIATIC ARTHRITIS

The prevalence of psoriatic arthritis (PsA) in the general population is low, at 0.1–0.25%, but in patients with psoriasis the prevalence is 23.8%.[91] PsA has an oligoarticular and a polyarticular pattern, with distal interphalangeal joint involvement being more common than other forms of inflammatory arthritis. Inflammation of other musculoskeletal tissues can occur, with enthesitis (67%) and dactylitis (12–39%). Axial PsA is observed in 5–28% of patients at diagnosis, increasing to 70% with late-stage disease. The prevalence of axial disease in isolation with psoriatic arthritis has been reported to be 7–17%.[92] The sacroiliac joints can be involved as well. Clinical presentation follows other inflammatory arthritis, with morning stiffness >30 minutes, joint pain aggravated by rest and relieved by exercises. PsA patients are usually seronegative, CRP can be normal or abnormal. Treatments include the usage of conventional synthetic disease-modifying antirheumatic drugs (csDMARDs) and TNFi.

REACTIVE ARTHRITIS/REITER'S SYNDROME

Reactive arthritis (ReA) is an inflammatory joint disease secondary to a localised infection at a distance from the affected joint(s). The incidence is estimated at 1–1.5% after a digestive infection, and 4–8% after a genital chlamydia infection. The duration of the arthritis is usually limited to 6–12 months. However, in 30% of cases, duration can last for more than 6 months, and 15–30% evolve to chronic arthritis or spondyloarthritis.[93] Typically, it involves an acute asymmetrical oligoarthritis of the large joints of the lower limb. Axial arthritis can occur at the cervical, thoracic and lumbosacral spine, as well as sacroiliitis. Lower back pain and buttock pain are typically worse at night. There is prolonged morning pain and stiffness, worse with rest and improves with activities. There can be enthesitis in the Achilles tendon and plantar fascia. Dactylitis can occur up to 40% of ReA.[94] ESR and CRP are usually elevated in the acute phase but normalise during the chronic phase. HLA-B27 has been reported to be positive in 90% of patients with ReA.[95] Investigations include X-ray and MRI. Treatment includes antibiotics when the infection is still present as well as NSAIDs, csDMARDs and TNFi.

GOUT

Axial gout has been estimated to be present in 14–35% of patients with gouty arthritis.[96,97] It commonly affects the lumbar spine and can affect the SIJ as well. Symptoms include back pain and radiculopathy. Imaging includes CT scan evidence of erosions in the facet joints and/or tophi. It is thought to be under-diagnosed.

INFECTIVE (OSTEOMYELITIS, SEPTIC ARTHRITIS, DISCITIS, ABSCESS)

Be aware of infective causes when there is fever, raised ESR and/or CRP.

MALIGNANCY (PRIMARY, METASTATIC)

Primary bone tumours of the spinal column are rare, comprising 5% of all primary skeletal tumours.[98] The majority of these tumours are benign, with malignant tumours accounting for 20% of cases. Overall, spinal metastases are the most common malignant spinal tumours (MST). The most common sites of these are from lung, breast, prostate and renal cell carcinoma. Symptomatic MST are found in 10% of cancer patients, while MST is present in 70–90% of patients with breast or prostate cancer. Common symptoms are pain, which occurs in 95% of cases, and neurological deficits in 75–85%. MST are found mostly in the thoracic spine (60–80%), followed by lumbosacral spine (15–30%) and cervical spine (10–15%).[99]

BENIGN TUMORS AND FACET JOINT SYNOVIAL CYSTS

Primary bone tumours of the spinal column are rare, comprising 5% of all primary skeletal tumours. The majority of these tumours are benign, with malignant tumours accounting for 20% of cases.[100] Most facet joint synovial cysts are asymptomatic and are found incidentally. Symptoms can occur when they impinge on adjacent nerve roots, causing radiculopathy. In rare cases, they can rupture, haemorrhage or become infected.

SACROILIAC JOINT (SIJ) PATHOLOGIES

SIJ pathologies cause pain in the SIJ and lumbar region. SIJ pathologies include mechanical strain, arthritis, axial spondyloarthritis, reactive arthritis, psoriatic arthritis, gout and infection. Pathologies in the lumbar spine, SIJ, hip joint and all the related muscular and ligamentous structures can cause overlapping pain patterns in the area. History, examination and multiple SIJ clinical tests play a limited role in determining whether the pain is coming from the SIJ.[101,102] Imaging of the SIJ, whether it is X-ray, CT scan or MRI often show osteoarthritic changes but they may not be the cause of the pain. Bone scan with SPECT can be useful but is still not completely specific. It remains a challenge for the clinician to determine the cause of pain in the SIJ region.

OSTEITIS CONDENSANS ILLI (OCI)

OCI can be defined as sclerotic bone lesion in the iliac side of the sacral iliac joint, it is often bilateral. The aetiology remains unknown. The prevalence in the general population is 0.9–2.5%.[103] OCI is more common in females under 40, during or after pregnancy, but it can also occur in nulliparous women and men. Symptoms include lower back, lateral hip or pelvic pain. Investigations including X-ray, CT, MRI and SPECT can also be used. Inflammatory markers such as ESR and CRP are normal, HLA-B27 antigen is absent in the majority of patients. There is no specific treatment for OCI except for the reassurance that it is a relatively benign condition and that regression of symptoms occurs in most patients given time. Physical therapy and NSAIDs can be used to relieve symptoms.[104]

LBP COMING FROM NEIGHBOURING STRUCTURES

1. Hip and knee joint pathologies – for example, OA and labral tears – can refer pain to the buttocks, groin, anterior thigh and knee. It is always useful to examine the hip joint in patients with LBP. At times, LB and hip joint problems can co-exist. Hip and knee pain can result in an antalgic gait which would aggravate LBP. Therefore, they have to be addressed as well.

2. Greater trochanteric bursitis is estimated to affect between 10% and 25% of the population[105] and is often caused by obesity, poor gait and walking dynamics. It is characterised by pain over the greater trochanter, which can radiate to the groin, down the lateral thigh and gluteal regions. The patient usually cannot sleep on the affected side. The condition shares some features of other causes of sciatica.

3. Abdominal and pelvic pathologies can refer pain to the lower back. For example, renal colic, pyelonephritis, endometriosis, aortic aneurysm, tumours and malignancies.

LUMBAR RADICULOPATHY

The incidence is estimated to be 3-5% of all lower back pains.[106] Age and degeneration are the primary risk factors and there is a male preponderance. Lumbar radiculopathy affects men often in their 40s and women in their 50s and 60s. The pathology involves compression or irritation of the nerve root caused by a disc bulge or herniation, ligamentum flavum hypertrophy, or other factors that narrow the neural foramina or lateral recesses. These factors may include disc height reduction, vertebral osteophytic encroachment, facet joint arthritis, or facet joint synovial cysts.[107] On rare occasions, the nerve root can be compressed extra-foraminally by a lateral disc herniation from a lower level.

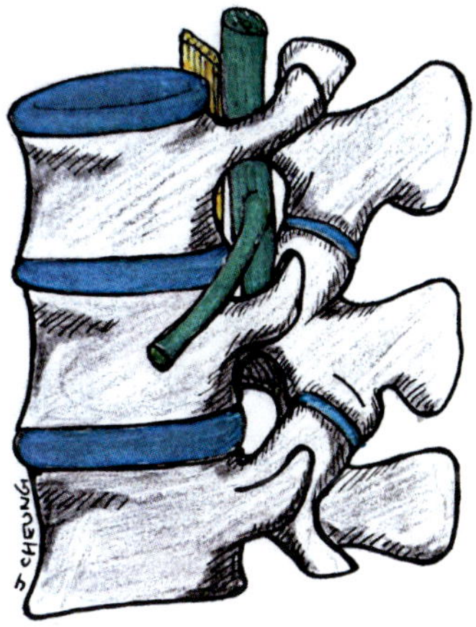

Figure 66: Diagram of lumbar nerve roots

History

The patient presents describing a sharp shooting pain down their leg, which typically increases with coughing or sneezing. There may be parathaesia as well, both corresponding to the dermatome involved. There may be muscle weakness, corresponding to the myotome involved.

In radiculopathy, when the nervous tissue is irritated by firm structures like the disc, osteophyte, cyst or ligamentum flavum, the pain would tend to be more constant and severe than would be from the sciatic nerve being irritated by a softer structure like the piriformis muscle (piriformis syndrome), or from a myofascial pain referred from a nearby muscle e.g. the gluteus medius (see Table 1).

Table 3: The Most Common Vertebral Levels Affected in Lumbar Radiculopathies

Nerve Root	L4	L5	S1
Motor weakness	Extension of quadriceps	Dorsiflexion of great toe and foot	Plantar flexion of great toe and foot
Screening examination	Squat and rise	Heel walking	Walking on toes
Reflexes	Knee jerk diminished	None reliable	Ankle jerk diminished

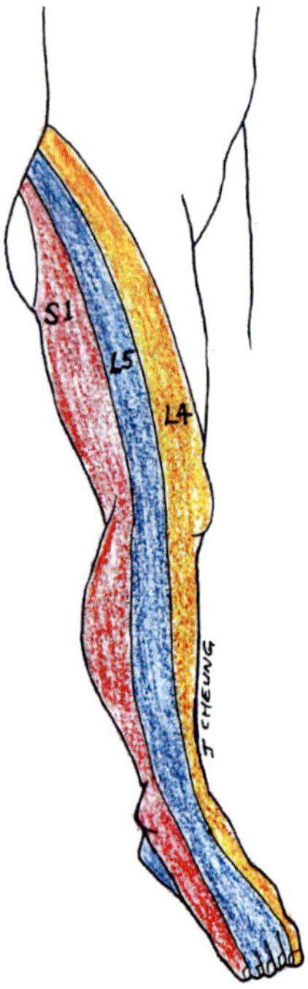

Figure 67: Lumbar L4, L5 and S1 dermatomes

Examination

Test for abnormalities in muscle strength, reflexes and skin sensation.

Straight leg raising and Lasegue's sign may be positive. It is a very sensitive but not very specific nor reliable test for lumbar radiculopathy e.g. it can be positive with tightness in the hamstring.[108]

Investigation

CT and MRI. If signs and symptoms are severe and non-conservative intervention is imminent, MRI should be advised instead of CT to conserve patient radiation exposure.

Diagnosis

Strong indicators include pain and paraesthesia (reported or observed) over the dermatomes as well as reflex changes and muscle weakness corresponding to the affected myotome. As many other conditions can cause pain radiating down the leg (facet joint arthropathy, piriformis syndrome and other myofascial pain from gluteus medius, gluteus minimus, etc.), pain distribution would need to fit the dermatome (see Table 1). Findings in CT and MRIs, unless significant and obvious, may not be conclusive and can often include multiple probable sites of impingements. It is important to always treat the patient, not the radiological findings.

Treatment

If there are red-flag features (cauda equina syndrome, significant and progressive muscle weakness, severe 10/10 pain after a reasonable time), this would necessitate prompt or urgent surgical intervention of spinal decompression. In the absence of these, a conservative approach can be taken first, with the patient reviewed and followed up and a treatment plan tailored to response.

Pharmacology A trial of NSAIDs, anti-convulsant (gabapentin 300–1200 mg three times a day), tricyclic antidepressant (amitriptyline or nortriptyline 25–150 mg daily) can be used.

Manual Therapies and Exercise Programs This can also be trialled. The safest option is physiotherapists with a special interest in radiculopathy work and some have postgraduate training in 'manipulative therapy', using techniques such as the McKenzie Method.[109,110]

Injection The next step would be targeted CT-guided injection, whether it is intra-facet, transforaminal or epidural. This can be both therapeutic and diagnostic, to determine whether the targeted injection at the specific level is successful in relieving the pain. It is usually performed by interventional radiologists who specialise in such procedures. CT-guided injections are a safe procedure, however, the risks are more substantial in patients on anticoagulants.

Surgery As far as the decision of surgical intervention goes, the severity of the pain often determines the choice and timing. It is always reassuring to refer to and work with a neurosurgeon who is interested in trialling other modalities before embarking on surgery. A 2020 systemic review comparing early surgery to conservative treatment found that surgery is probably superior in improving pain and function in the short to medium term but makes no difference in the long term.[111]

Opioids They should not be used routinely in LBPs and are not recommended for chronic pain from any causes. Between 2016–2017, one or more prescriptions of opioids were given to 3.1 million Australians (13% of the population), with 1.5% of the population using opioids on a daily basis.[112] At present, there are about 240 different prescription preparations of opioids in Australia. Everyday three people die of opioid overdose (70% are related to prescribed opioids) and 150 are hospitalised for non-fatal opioid poisoning or overdose.[113] As doctors, it is critical we prescribe opioids with the utmost care and only in necessary circumstances, in order to avoid and limit the ever-increasing opioid use disorder.

SPINAL CANAL STENOSIS OF THE LUMBAR SPINE

It is defined as narrowing of the lumbar spinal canal and/or the neural foramina, resulting in the compression of the spinal nerve roots. The most common cause is degenerative, a combination of disc protrusion, facet joint hypertrophy, osteophyte impingement, hypertrophy of the ligamentum flavum and spondylolisthesis. It affects 11% of US adults. It is of interest that, while 20% of people over 60 have imaging evidence of canal stenosis, 80% of these are asymptomatic.[114] Symptoms include pain in the lumbar spine, buttocks, thigh, lower leg and feet. Presentation tends to be insidious. Paraesthesia and poor balance may occur, along with symptoms of neurogenic claudication. This condition is characterised by pain that worsens with lumbar extension (e.g. walking), as it reduces the space in the spinal canal and neural foraminae. The pain is typically relieved by sitting and adopting a position of lumbar flexion. Examination may reveal a wide-based gait and a positive Romberg sign. Lumbar extension, standing and walking exacerbates the pain; flexion relieves it. There may be sensory deficits and reflex changes. In severe cases, the patient may present with cauda equina syndrome. Imaging includes CT scan and MRI. In non-serious cases, treatment includes conservative manual therapy of mobilisation, stretching and strengthening. NSAIDs, gabapentin and duloxetine can be trialled.

Epidural steroid injection can help in the short term. For patients with cauda equina syndrome, urgent surgical intervention is indicated. In one study of 146 patients with lumbar spinal canal stenosis not treated with surgery, a three-year follow-up showed that one-third reported improvement, 50% experienced no change and 10–20% reported deterioration.[115]

LUMBAR SPINE OSTEOARTHRITIS AND LUMBAR FACET JOINT ARTHROPATHY

Lumbar spine OA involves the zygapophyseal (facet) joints and the intervertebral joints. It is estimated to constitute 6% of all lower back pains.[116] **There are far too many instances when patients are given a diagnosis of OA** for their lower back pain simply due to the imaging findings. Most clinicians would agree that the pain and dysfunction of an arthritic joint deteriorates very gradually. Consequently, if a patient presents with a relatively sudden onset of pain or a sudden increase of pre-existing pain, with or without a history of injury, we cannot just assume it is from OA. I believe that, only after the **soft tissue causes of lower back pain** have been firstly addressed, can we entertain OA being the cause of it. Lumbar facet joint arthropathy is estimated to affect 15% of patients with chronic lower back pain.[117]

History

Onset is usually insidious with predisposing factors including disc degeneration, spondylolisthesis and old age. The facet joint capsules are richly supplied with nociceptors, which when stretched or compressed elicit back and/or leg pain. Patients were given facet joint saline intra-articular injections, and resulted pain patterns recorded. Upper lumbar facet joint arthropathy tends to refer pain to flank, hip, groin and upper lateral thigh. Lower lumbar refers pain to buttock, lateral and posterior thigh, lower lateral leg and groin. The distributions do not fit dermatomes, as in radiculopathies. The pain tends to be more axial and does not usually include the extremities. The pain distribution of intervertebral joints/disc degeneration and injury is thought to be similar to that of facet joint arthropathy.

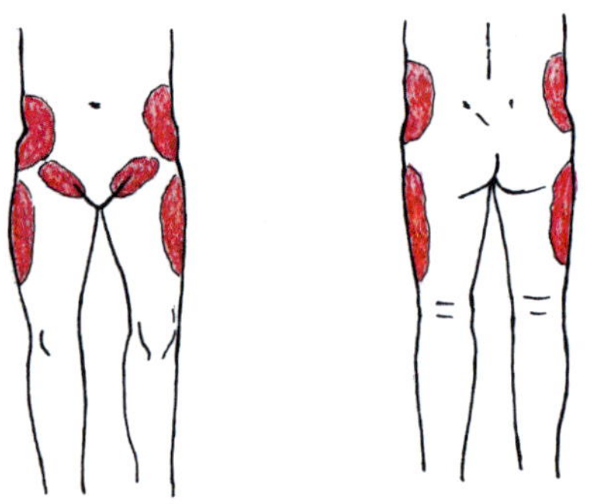

Figure 68: Areas of referred pain from upper lumbar facet joints

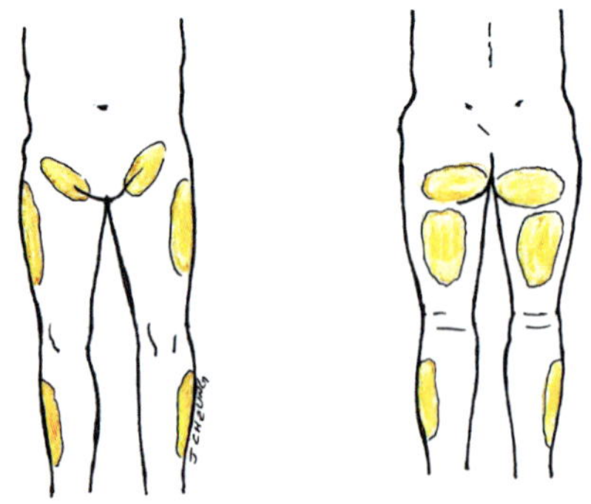

Figure 69: Areas of referred pain from lower lumbar facet joints

Examination

There may be localised tenderness on palpation of the affected facet joints and the overlying intervertebral muscles. Examination should exclude other conditions (see Table 1).

Investigation

Investigation involves plain X-ray, CT, MRI and bone scan. In many instances, X-ray, CT or MRI would show multiple-level facet joint arthropathy, making it difficult to determine which one is causing the pain. If a CT-guided facet joint injection is contemplated, then a bone scan with single-photon emission computed tomography (SPECT) would help to clarify which facet joint(s) are 'hot' (detecting dynamic osteoblastic activities active with inflammation) and which to inject. However, it still may not be 100% reliable.

Diagnosis

Diagnosis of OA as the cause of a pain should not be made purely from imaging findings. All other conditions like muscular strain, inflammatory joint diseases, renal pathologies etc should be considered first. I believe a diagnosis of OA should be made after excluding all other possible conditions.

Treatment

A multimodal approach of conservative therapy of NSAIDs, manual therapy and an exercise program for a reasonable period of time e.g. six weeks. Failing that, CT-guided corticosteroid and LA intra-articular injection can be considered. If the diagnosis is confirmed by medial branch block of the designated facet joint, medial branch radiofrequency ablation or cryoablation can be used.

The most common lower back pain syndromes in general practice are lumbar radiculopathy, lumbar spine osteoarthritis and lumbosacral muscular strain (trigger points). These three conditions share some common features in that the pain can be in the lumbar, gluteal, sacroiliac joint and hip regions; and can radiate down the leg. However, there are clinical features that can help us to differentiate them. Please refer to Table 1.

While OA, radiculopathy, trigger points and neuralgias share some common features, they can be differentiated (see Table 1).

Table 1: Different Neuromuscular Pains

	Nerve root impingement	**Peripheral nerve entrapment**	**Facet joint arthropathy**	**Muscular myofascial trigger points**
Distribution of pain	Fits the dermatomes, tends to include the extremities in distribution	Area innervated by the nerve, can radiate along the course of the nerve	Fits the facet joint pain distributions, tends to be more axial in distribution, rarely passes the elbow or knees	The affected muscles, their attachment sites and adjacent areas (these can overlap with other causes of pain e.g. TrPs in Latissimus dorsi overlapping with C8 radiculopathy)
Nature of pain	Tends to be more constant, tends to be severe	Tends to be more constant, tends to be severe	Worse on movements, especially in extension and rotation (when the facet joints are loaded)	Tends to be intermittent, tends to be less severe, pain can be aggravated by certain movements when the affected muscles are activated
Numbness	Possible	Possible	Usually not	Possible
Muscle weakness and associated clumsy movements	Possible	Possible	Nil	Nil
Reflex changes	Possible	Rarely	Nil	Nil
Tenderness on palpation on the painful area	Nil	Can be tender at the site of impingement	Can be tender on the facet joint and the overlying intervertebral muscles	Tender trigger points of the relevant muscles
Useful clinical examination/tests	Reflexes, power, sensation	Reflexes, power, sensation	Localised tenderness on palpating over the facet joints, extension – rotation test	Palpation of all the muscles in the painful area and adjacent muscles

Dr Joe Cheung

NB. The pain distribution of intervertebral joints/discs degeneration and injury is thought to be similar to that of facet joint arthropathy.

LUMBOSACRAL MUSCULAR STRAIN

LBP caused by muscular strain or dysfunction is, without doubt, the most common musculoskeletal problem presenting to clinicians, estimated to be 70% of all LBP.[118] The diagram below examines the lumbosacral muscles and their TrPs involved in LBPs. **From my experience, the most common muscle strain (TrPs) causing LBP are the quadratus lumborum, the gluteal muscles and the piriformis.**

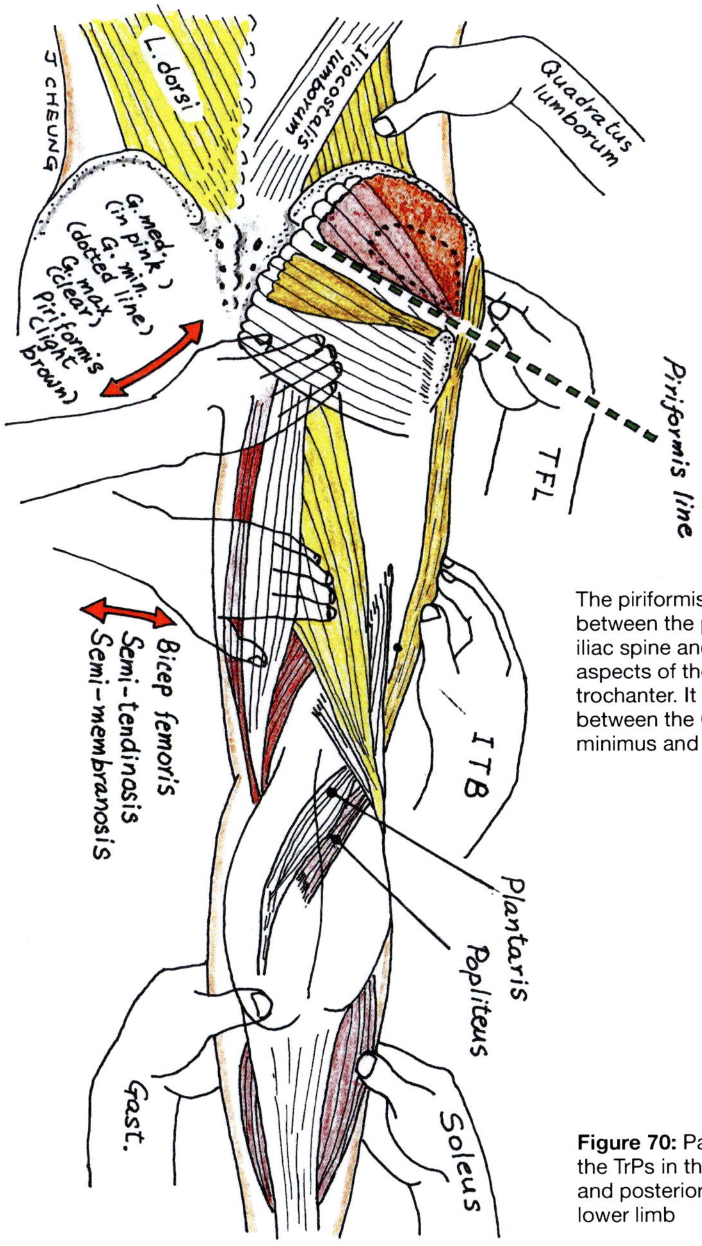

The piriformis line – A line drawn between the posterior inferior iliac spine and the superior aspects of the greater trochanter. It demarcates between the G medius, G minimus and the piriformis.

Figure 70: Palpation diagram for the TrPs in the lower back region and posterior aspect of the lower limb

POSITION OF THE PATIENT AND EXAMINER WHEN PALPATING THE LOWER BACK AND UPPER THIGH REGION

The gluteals, piriformis, and quadratus lumborum are thick and deep muscles. In order to look for their TrPs, you need to put your body weight behind the palpating fingers with overlapping hands (fingertips in line for better coverage), and apply some oil to increase the sensitivity. The examiner should facilitate this by rocking their body forwards and backwards

The hamstrings and the ITB are thick and deep structures as well. In order to palpate for their TrPs, you need to put your body weight behind the palpating hands and use the heel of your palms to detect the TrPs. A small amount of oil would increase the sensitivity.

NB. From my experience, in any lower back pain syndromes, **TrPs in the hamstring and the ITB, when detected, need to be treated** in order to settle mechanical LBP. Improving the TrPs in the hamstring and ITB appears to have a flow-on effect to other lumbar muscles. Perhaps it is because some of these muscles are in the same myotomes.

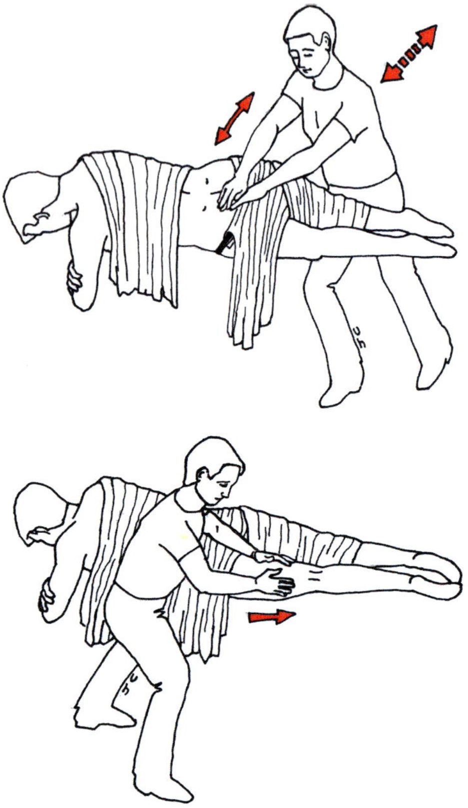

Figure 71: The position to palpate for the lumbar muscles, hamstrings and ITB TrPs

NB. Three short videos on TrP palpation techniques for the knee, lower back, neck/ shoulder regions are available on YouTube under joecheungYNSA, or visit http://www.joecheung.com.au

CASE STUDIES ON LOWER BACK AND UPPER THIGH PAIN

Most of the case studies (with only a few exceptions) utilise the modality of YNSA for treatment, and are only intended for readers who are interested in or practise the modality of acupuncture.

THE SARTORIUS AND ITS TrPs

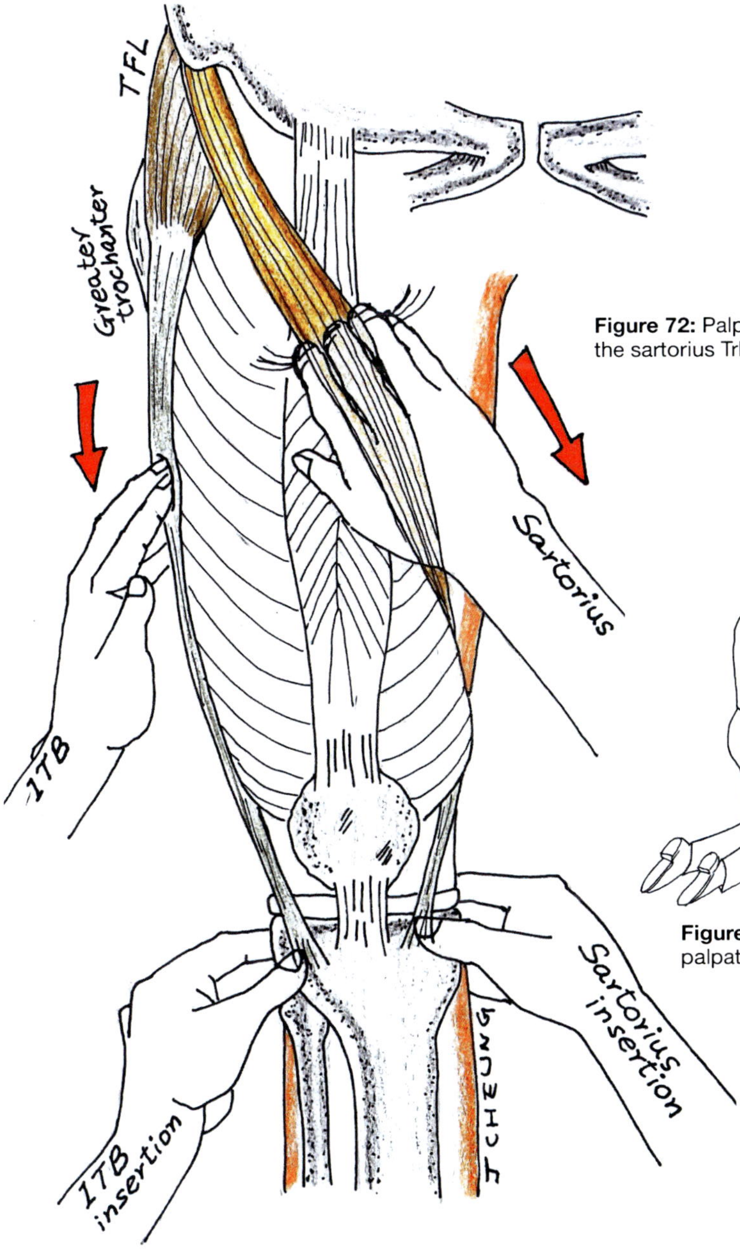

Figure 72: Palpation diagram for the sartorius TrPs

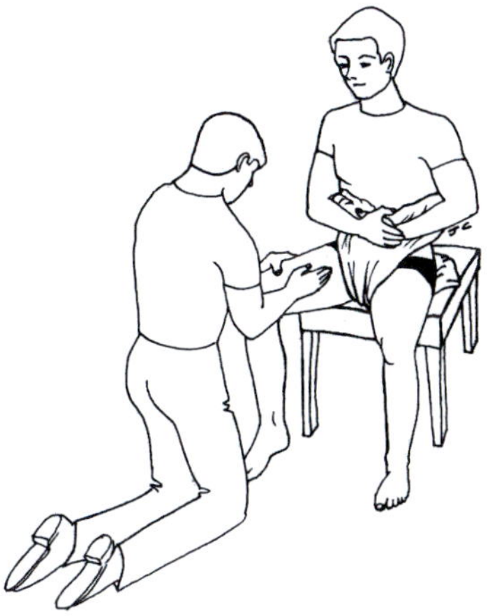

Figure 73: The position to palpate for the sartorius TrPs

CASE STUDY 11 (left hip pain – sartorius and gracilis TrPs, treated with YNSA)

HISTORY: A 53-year-old female presented with a one-year history of intermittent left anterior hip area pain. She pointed at the anterior superior iliac spine area as the site of her pain. The pain was rated at 2/10 and so uncomfortable while walking that the patient avoided it. The patient did not recall any injury, there was no past history of hip joint problems or any other joint pains, and no prolonged morning joint stiffness. X-ray of the hip showed no evidence of OA.

REASONING: The hip joint would have to be looked at carefully for any pathologies. When a pain is aggravated by a specific movement, muscular strain would be a likely cause. It was reassuring that the X-ray did not show any lytic or sclerotic lesions.

EXAMINATION: ROM was normal in the hip joints. Palpation in the destinated area of pain showed very localised tender TrPs in the proximal attachment of the sartorius and also midway along it. Some minor TrPs were found in the left gracilis as well.

INVESTIGATIONS: None necessary.

DIAGNOSIS: TrPs in the sartorius

NB. It is of interest that some TrPs which occur seemingly without any significant injuries can persist for a long time.

TREATMENT: The patient was treated with YNSA and active points of the sartorius muscle on the J somatotope were needled, as was the gracilis. After the needle was inserted, the palpable tenderness of the sartorius improved instantly.

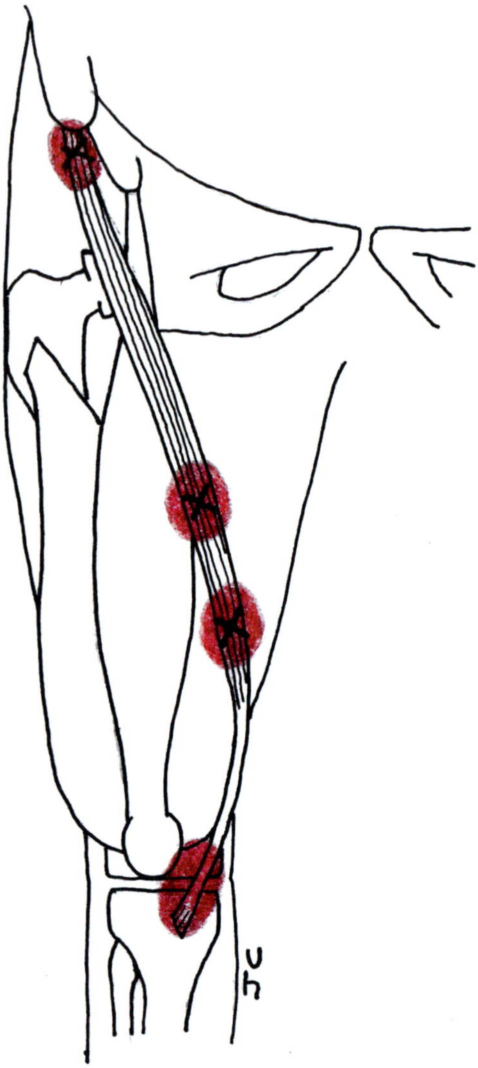

Figure 74: Sartorius TrPs and their referred pain pattern

X = TrPs

Red area = the referred pain

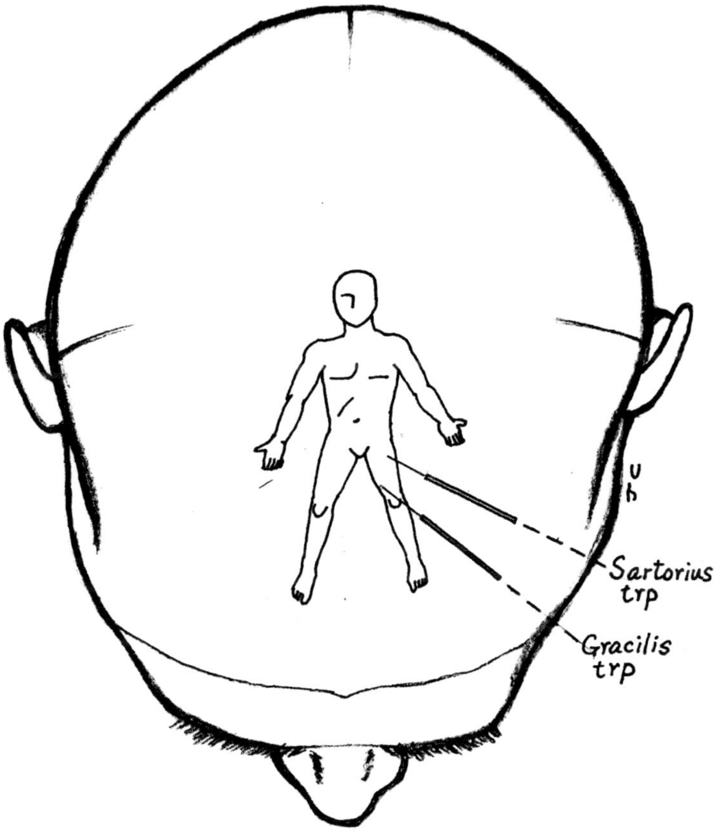

Figure 75: TrPs treatment for Case Study 11

OUTCOME: Her pain improved with each treatment and she was pain-free after four weekly treatments.

NB. I feel very strongly that, in any examination, we should include careful and purposeful palpation at the site of pain.

THE ADDUCTOR MAGNUS AND ITS TrPs

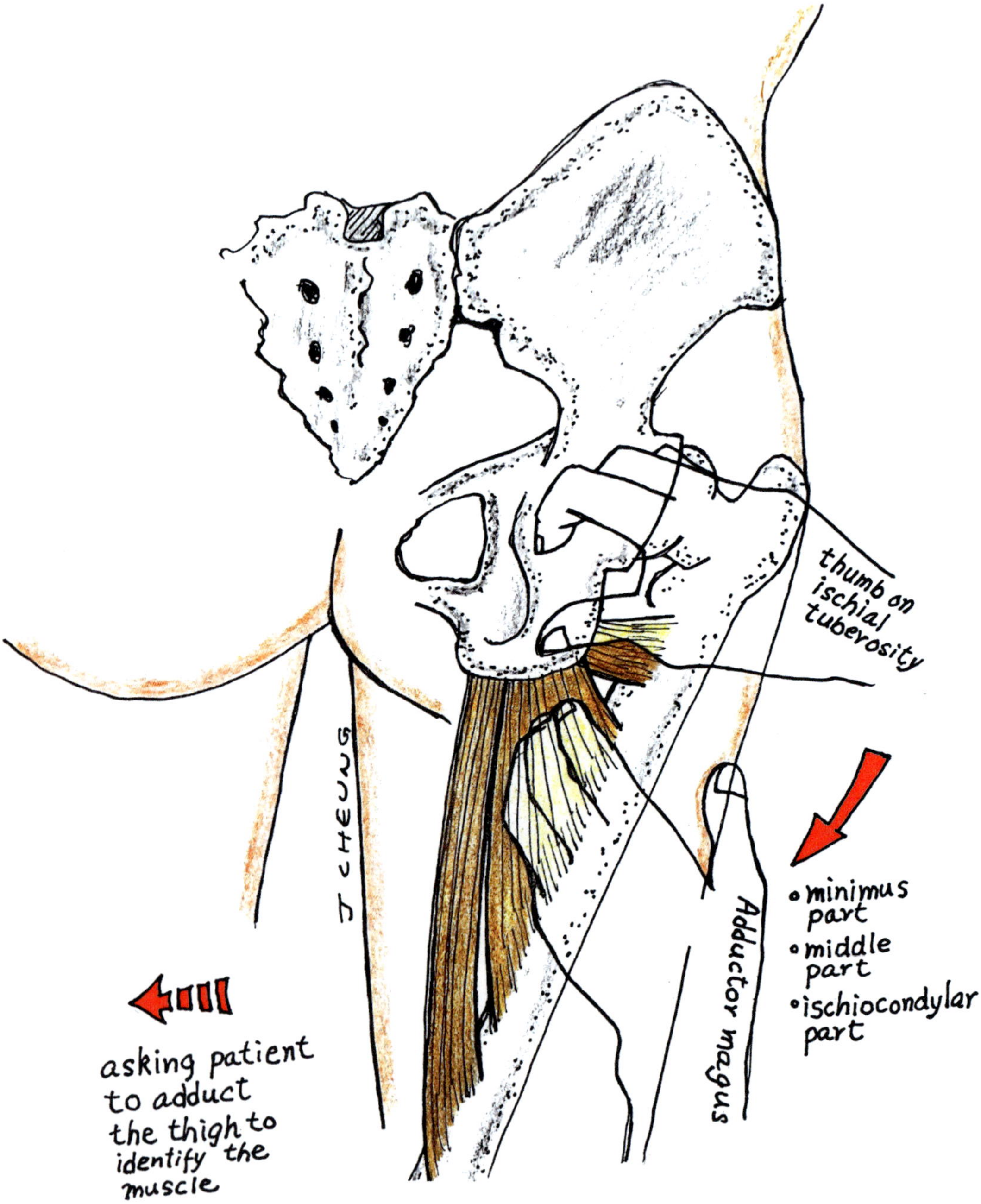

Figure 76: Palpation diagram for the adductor magnus TrPs

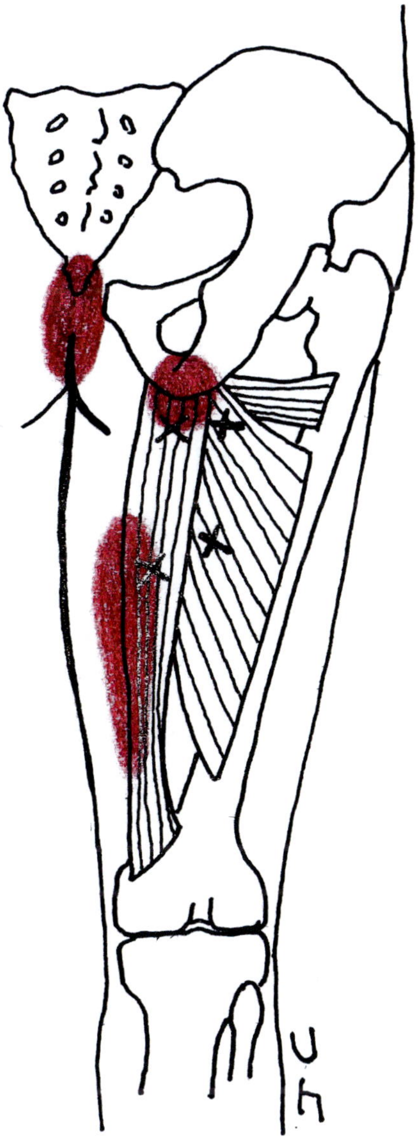

Figure 77: Adductor magnus TrPs and their referred pain pattern

X = TrPs

Red area = the referred pain

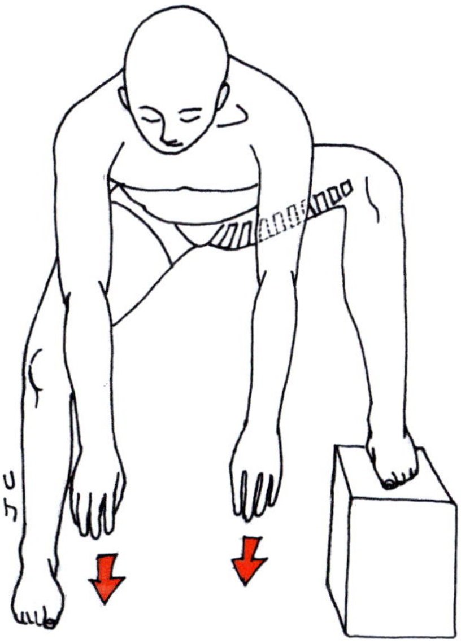

Figure 78: A useful stretch for the adductor magnus

THE HAMSTRING AND ITB AND THEIR TrPs

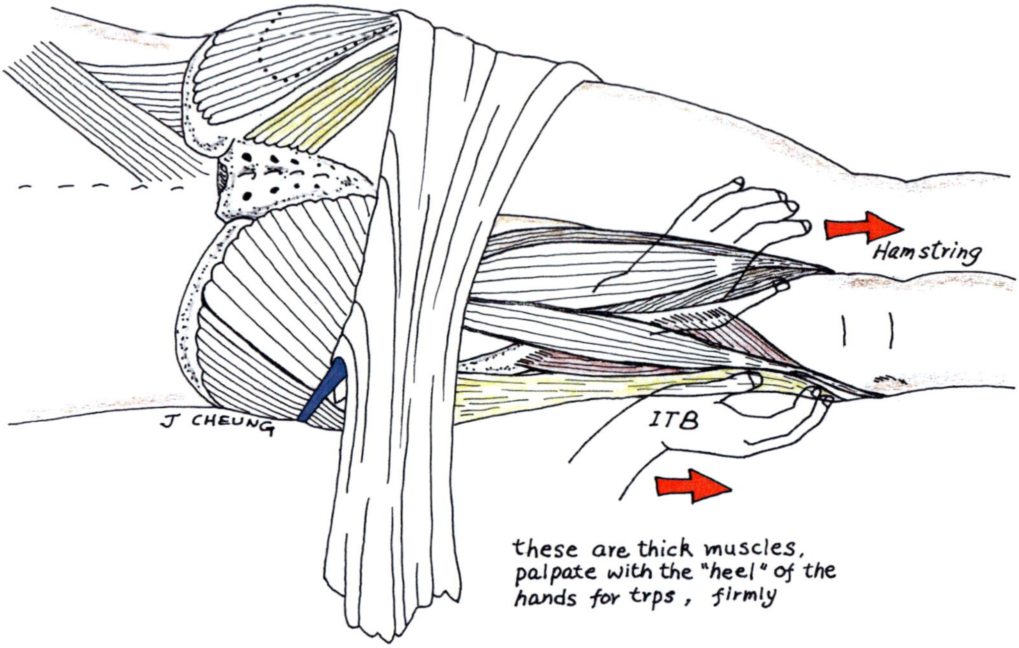

Figure 79: Palpation diagram for the hamstring and ITB TrPs

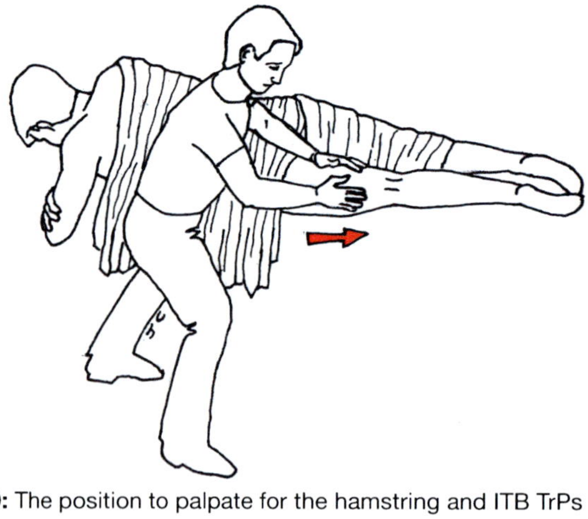

Figure 80: The position to palpate for the hamstring and ITB TrPs

NB. The only way to examine these thick muscles is to have the patient lying prone and direct your body weight onto the palpating hands. Applying a little amount of oil would increase the sensitivity in palpation. For any lower back pain, we should palpate for TrPs in the quadratus lumborum, gluteals, piriformis, hamstring and ITB, which are commonly involved.

Figure 81: Palpation diagram for the hamstring and its proximal attachment of the hamstring TrPs

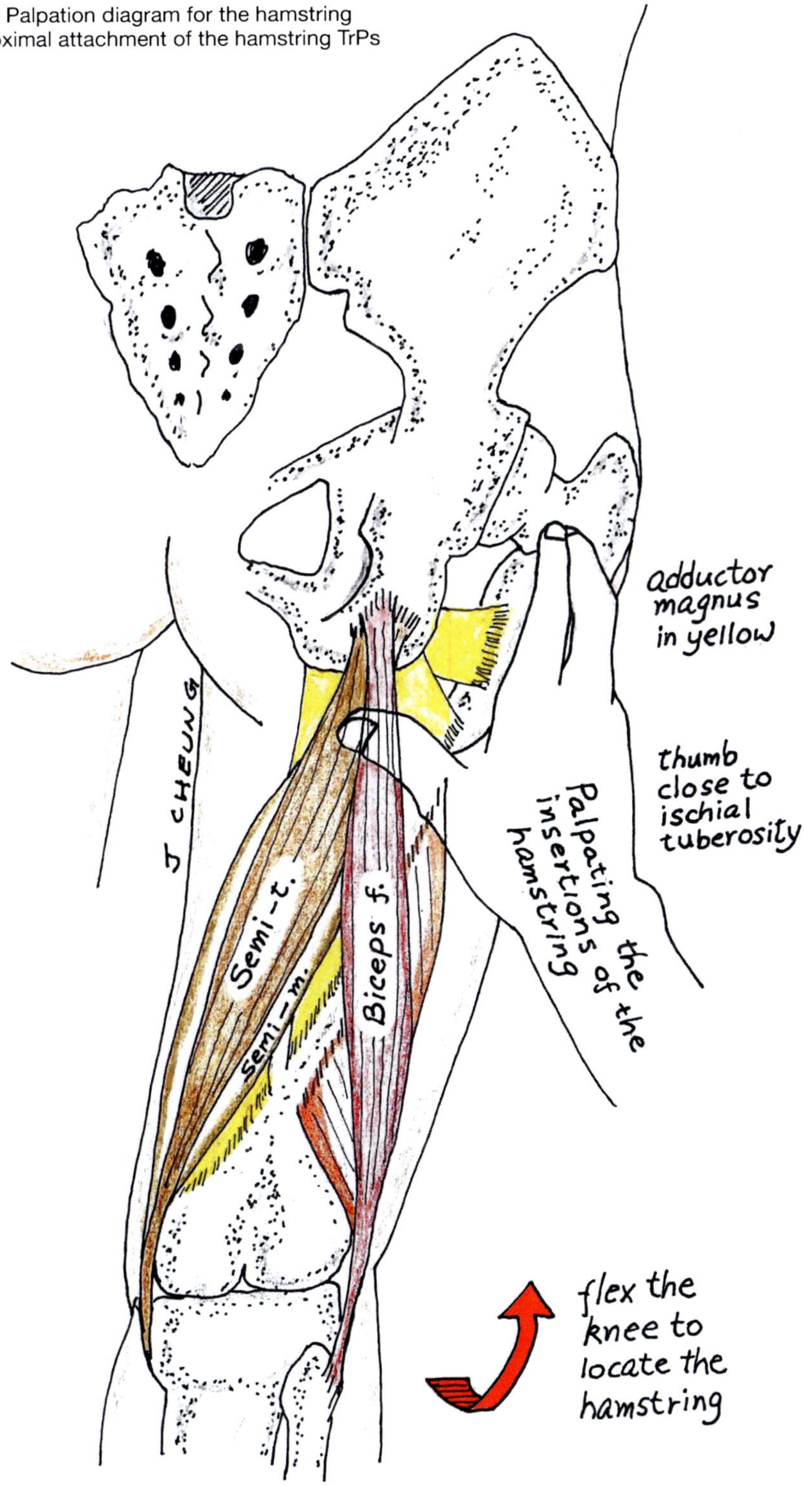

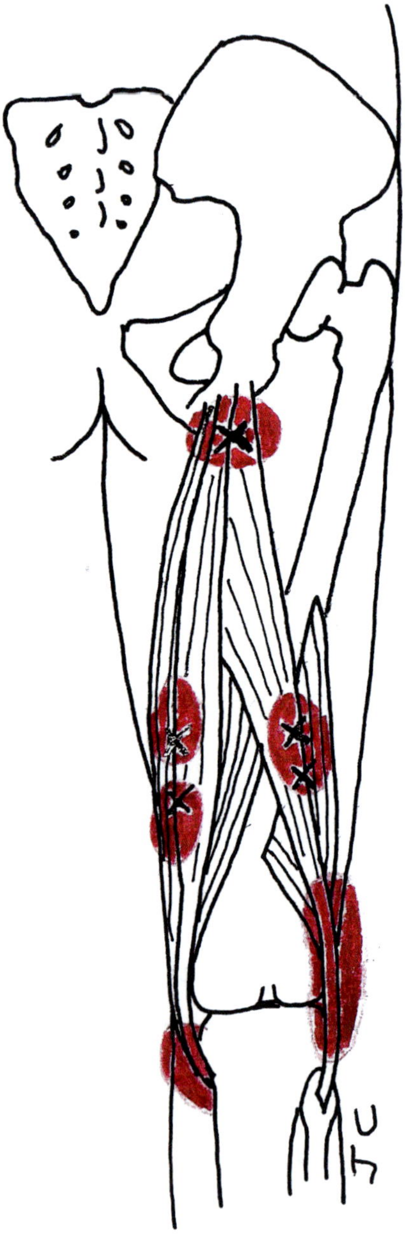

Figure 82: Hamstring TrPs and their referred pain pattern

X = TrPs

Red area = the referred pain

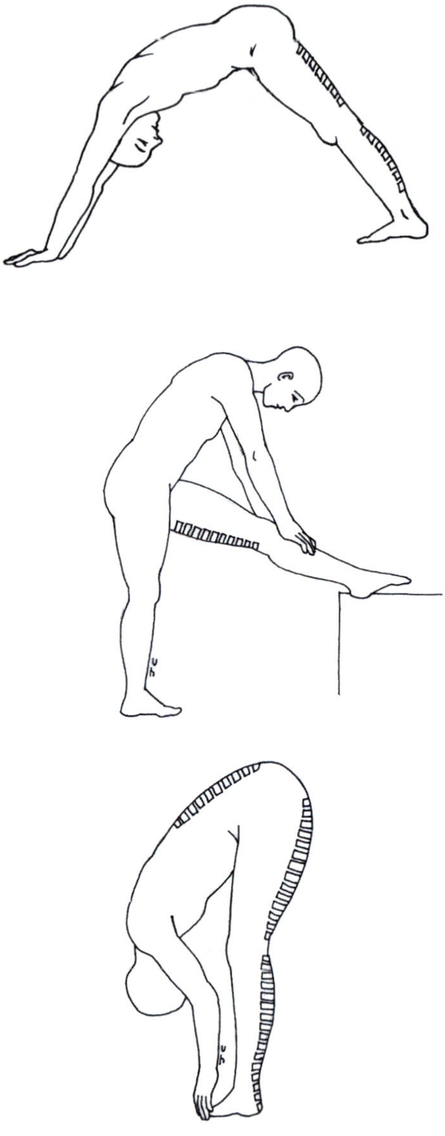

Figure 83: Useful stretches for the hamstring

CASE STUDY 12 (right gluteal and rectal area pain – adductor magnus and hamstring TrPs, treated with YNSA)

HISTORY: A 58-year-old, male office worker presented with a six-week history of intermittent deep right groin pain and in the rectal area. He rated it as 5/10 in severity. He also complained of a five-year history of low-grade pain on his right buttock whenever he sat. He was a keen walker and would frequently walk for 10–15km on the weekend. He had a few accidents when he had jarred himself but had never sought medical attention. There were no urinary symptoms, his GP examined him and checked his urine and prostate. He was told that he had no inguinal hernia. A colonoscopy and a colorectal consultation yielded normal results. X-ray of his hip and lumbar MRI was normal except for some minor OA. He had no significant past medical problems.

REASONING: It was reassuring that red-flag diagnoses had been excluded. As the history pointed to the possibility of an injury and there was pain localised to the gluteal region, TrPs in the area should be palpated for.

EXAMINATION: He was thin and tall in body build and was walking in some discomfort. He had normal movement of his hips and targeted examination showed very localised TrPs in the proximal attachment of his right adductor magnus (the minimus and middle parts) and his right hamstring. The former probably caused his groin, rectal symptoms and the latter had caused his more longstanding pain upon sitting on his ischial tuberosity. A tear in either muscle was possible, but a decision was made to treat the TrPs first before ordering more imaging.

DIAGNOSIS: TrPs in the proximal adductor magnus and hamstring

INVESTIGATIONS: MRI of the ischial tuberosity area would help if the trial of treatment failed.

TREATMENT: He was treated with YNSA, and active points were found and needled on the K somatotope on the adductor magnus (two points) and hamstring (one at the proximal insertion area and one on a TrP further down the hamstring).

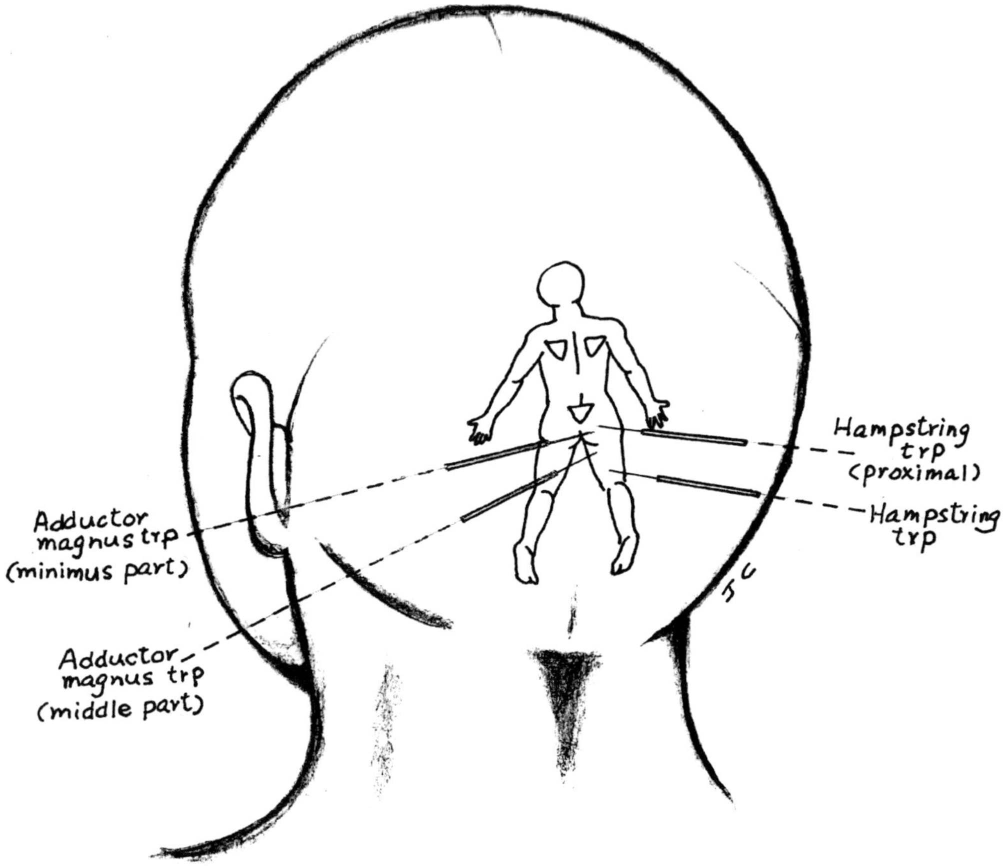

Figure 84: TrPs treatment for Case Study 12

OUTCOME: The patient experienced immediate improvement to his pain by about 20%. The adductor magnus TrP cleared after four weekly treatments, as did his groin and rectal symptoms. The hamstring needed another four weekly treatments as it was more chronic.

DISCUSSION: People with a slight build are more likely to injure or tear muscles.

THE GLUTEALS, PIRIFORMIS, QUADRATUS LUMBORUM AND THEIR TrPs

NB. Tuck the towel inside the underpants, which allows the examiner to move the towel up and down securely in order to palpate the lumbar and gluteal muscles.

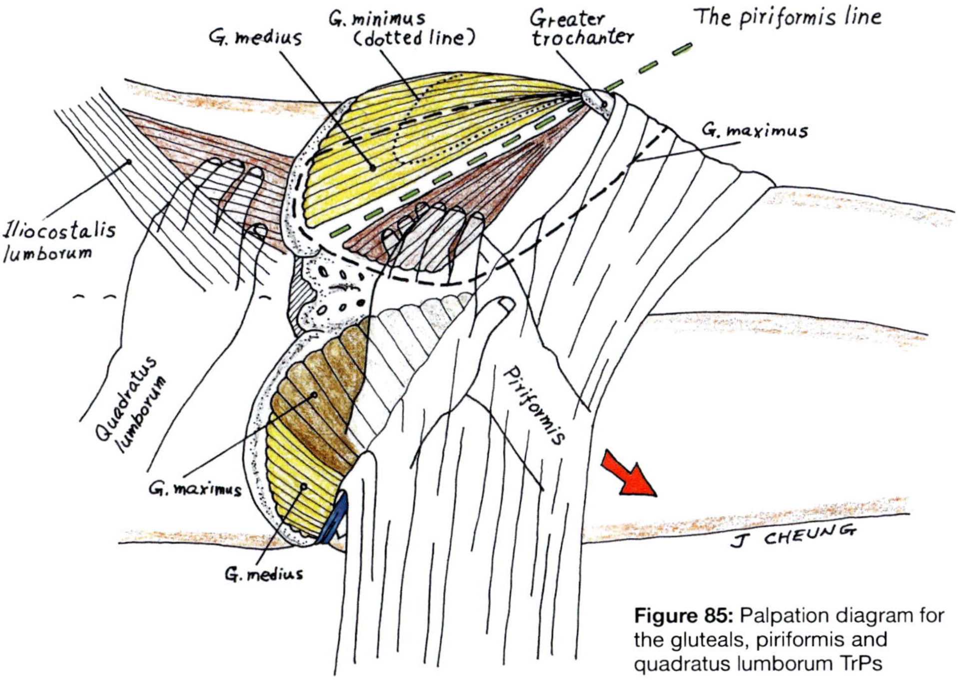

Figure 85: Palpation diagram for the gluteals, piriformis and quadratus lumborum TrPs

NB. The only way to examine these thick muscles is to have the patient lying in the prone position and to direct your body weight onto the palpating hands. Applying a little amount of oil will increase the sensitivity in palpation. For any lower back pain, we should palpate for TrPs in the quadratus lumborum, gluteals, piriformis, hamstring and ITB, which are commonly involved.

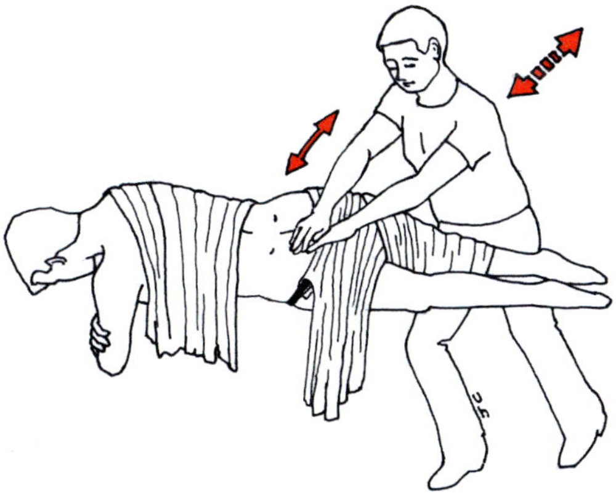

Figure 86: The position to palpate for the gluteals, piriformis and quadratus lumborum TrPs

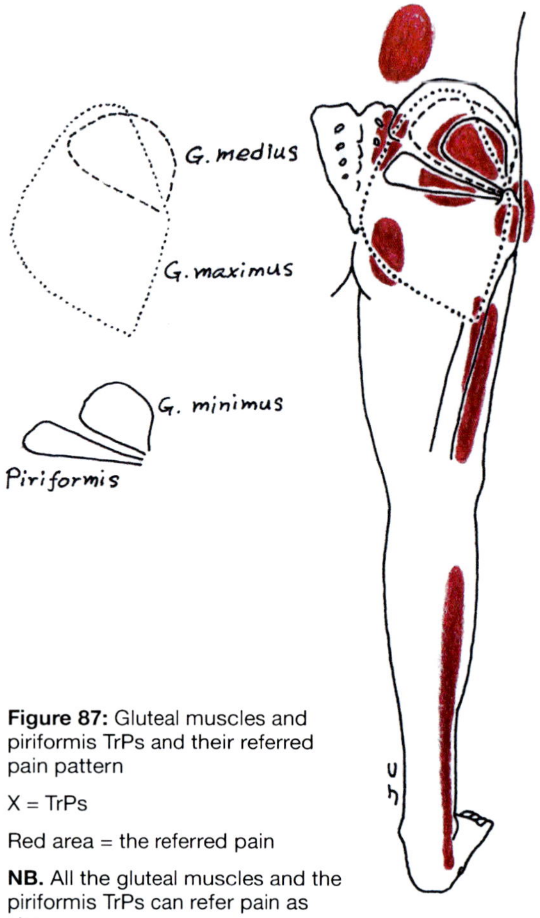

Figure 87: Gluteal muscles and piriformis TrPs and their referred pain pattern

X = TrPs

Red area = the referred pain

NB. All the gluteal muscles and the piriformis TrPs can refer pain as shown.

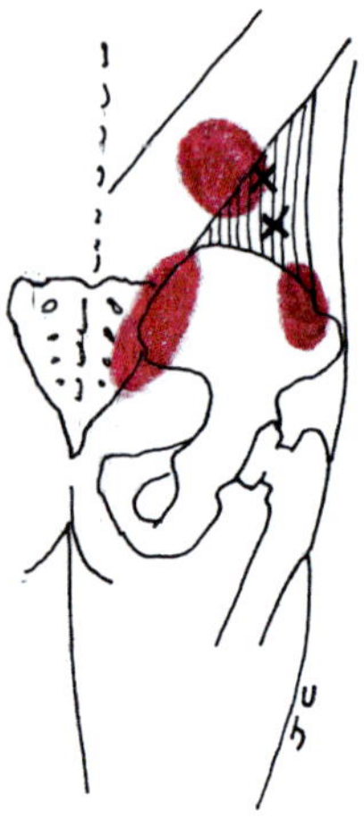

Figure 88: Quadratus lumborum TrPs and their referred pain pattern

X = TrPs

Red area = the referred pain

NB. There are many instances in which pain in the sciatic distribution its treated as a radiculopathy when it is actually referred from muscle TrPs or from neuralgia/nerve entrapment. If the diagnosis is not definitive, it is always worthwhile to palpate for possible TrPs that can cause pain down the leg (see Table 1).

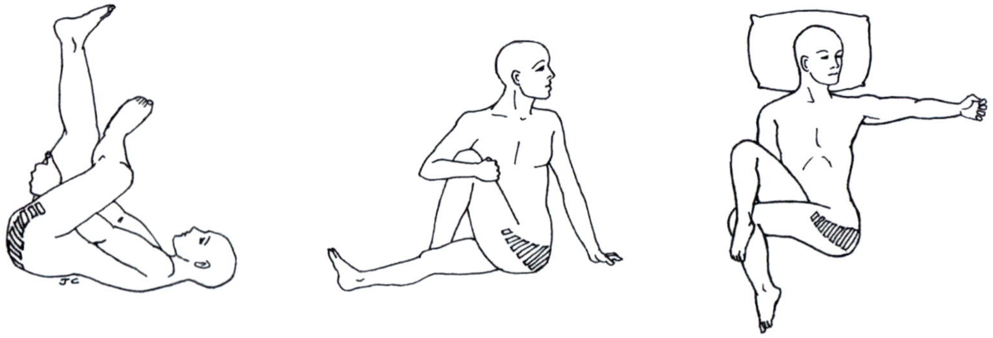

Figure 89: Useful stretches for the gluteal muscles

THE ILIOPSOAS AND ITS TrPs

Iliopsoas dysfunction can refer pain to the lumbar and anterior thigh region; it usually occurs in sporting activities like running and kicking. It can be tested by the 'modified Thomas test', which involves having the patient lying supine with the buttock on the edge of the bed, one hip fully flexed and the testing hip pushed downwards in extension by the examiner. It can also be palpated deep in the abdomen for tenderness.

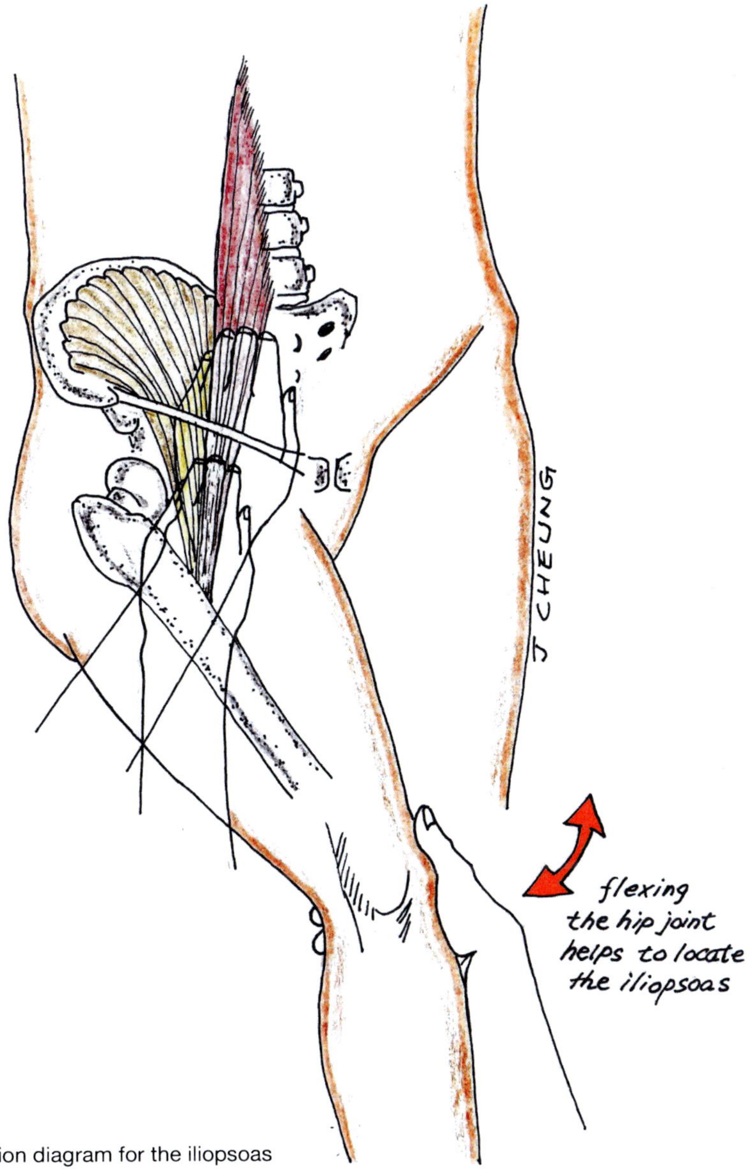

Figure 90: Palpation diagram for the iliopsoas

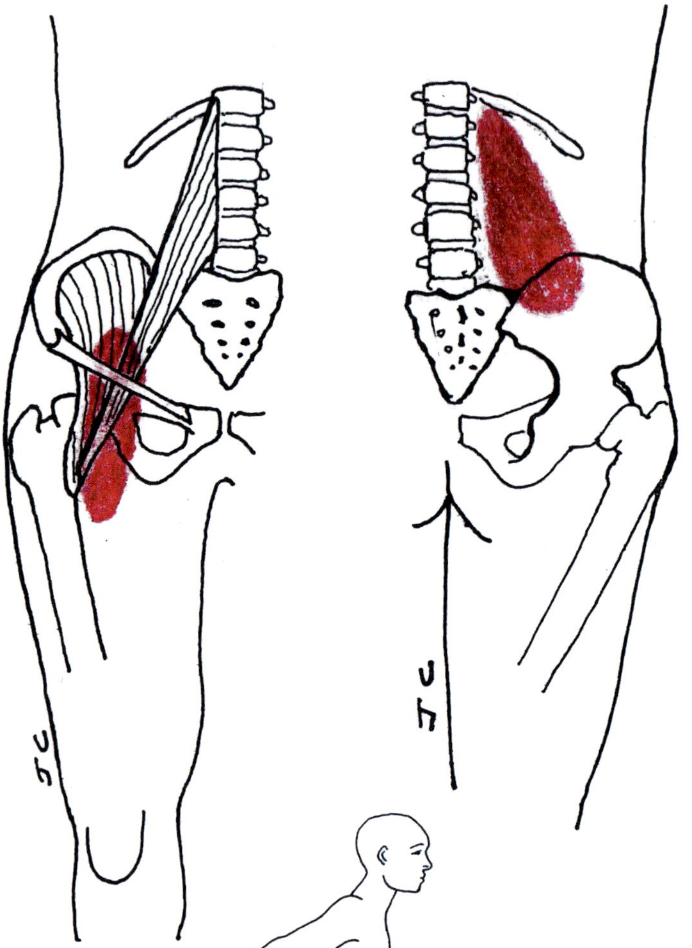

Figure 91: Iliopsoas TrPs and their referred pain pattern

X = TrPs

Red area = the referred pain

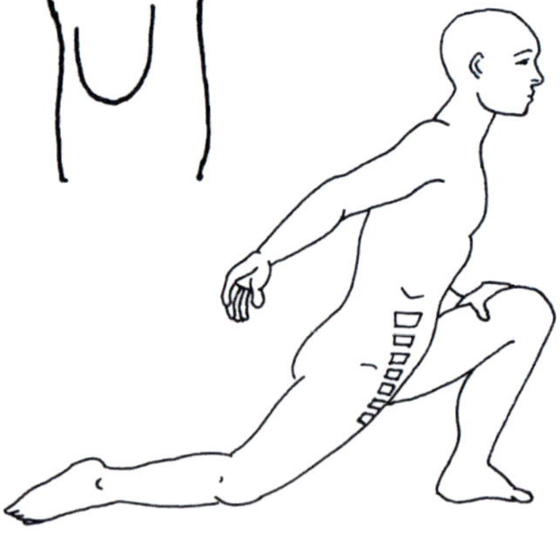

Figure 92: A useful stretch for the iliopsoas

Dysfunction and trigger points in **the thoracolumbar paravertebral muscles** can also cause LBP. These consist of a superficial group/erector spinae of long-fibre longitudinal muscles (longissimus thoracis, iliocostalis thoracis, iliocostalis lumborum) and a deep group of short diagonal muscles (semispinalis, multifidus, rotators, at successive deeper levels). These TrPs are best palpated with the patient seated and head drooping down, which relaxes the usually taut paravertebral muscles. Using some massage oil or soluble bath oil makes the task easier and is important to increase sensitivity of palpation.

CASE STUDY 13 (right sciatic distribution pain – piriformis and hamstring TrPs, treated with YNSA)

HISTORY: A 75-year-old female presented with a four-week history of 6–7/10 pain over the right gluteal, lateral thigh and lower leg area. There were no falls or trauma and she did not suffer from any significant LBP prior to this presentation. The pain was not constant, occurring mainly on walking and she was largely pain-free in bed and when sitting. There was no weakness or parathaesia, pain was not exacerbated by coughing and there was no bowel or bladder incontinence. In the week before presentation, she had also noticed some pain in her left lower leg at the lateral aspect. Her past history included lumpectomy for breast cancer 20 years ago and osteoporosis on treatment with denosumab. The patient recalled her GP examining her briefly and ordered a lumbar spine MRI, which showed generalised facet joint arthropathies and disc bulges, causing possible multiple bilateral foraminal stenosis. It also reported a 6x3 mm right-sided facet joint synovial cyst at L2/3, causing marked subarticular recess effacement, likely to cause irritation or impingement of multiple descending nerve roots. The patient was referred to see a neurosurgeon and, at this point, sought a second opinion.

REASONING: Not all pain radiating down the leg in the sciatic nerve distribution is due to radiculopathies. Unfortunately, it is a common assumption. Given the pain was intermittent and aggravated by very specific movements, it made radiculopathy less likely (see Table 1). There was no parathaesia or muscle weakness either. It pointed more to a muscular cause. Given the past history of osteoporosis and breast cancer, a spontaneous minimal trauma fracture, lytic and sclerotic lesion needed to be excluded (which was achieved by her recent MRI).

EXAMINATION: Her reflexes, muscle power and sensations were normal, as were the patient's hip joints. There were very tender and localised TrPs at the right piriformis and hamstring and also at the left lateral soleus.

DIAGNOSIS: The diagnosis was that of TrPs at the piriformis and hamstring, causing the pain in the right sciatic distribution. The patient had also strained her left soleus from the antalgic gait, thus, causing the left lower-leg pain.

INVESTIGATIONS: MRI performed already

TREATMENT: The patient was treated with YNSA, with points on the right piriformis, right hamstring and left soleus used in the K somatotope.

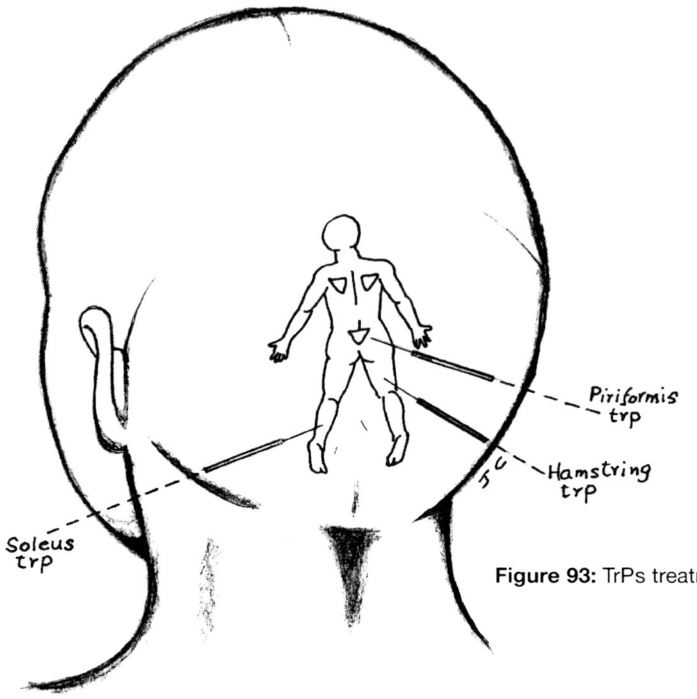

Figure 93: TrPs treatment for Case Study 13

OUTCOME: After six weekly treatments, she was completely pain-free. The patient was given a fact sheet on lower back and leg stretches.

NB. It often surprises me when patients with pain radiating down the leg or arm with some imaging backings are often treated as radiculopathies – even when neither the history nor examination support the diagnosis. TrPs in the piriformis and gluteal muscles often mimic radiculopathies and facet joint arthropathies. The differentiating aspect is that the pain from radiculopathies tends to be more constant and severe in nature, follow the dermatome distributions and can have associated parathaesia, weakness and reflex changes; whereas pain caused by TrPs tends not to be constant nor severe and occurs when the specific muscles are activated. Pain caused by facet joint arthropathies tends to be more axial in distribution and rarely past the knee or elbow (see Table 1). Palpating for possible TrPs in the relevant muscles often helps to seal the diagnosis and avoid expensive investigations and invasive interventions. A practical approach is to clear the TrPs first, before considering other diagnoses.

Finding TrPs and treating them successfully can

- **eradicate the pain completely (when the TrPs are the cause);**
- **improve some of the pain (as the TrPs cause some of the pain);**
- **exclude TrPs as the cause of the pain, allowing the consideration of other possible diagnoses; and**
- **often help to avoid expensive imaging or invasive treatments.**

CASE STUDY 14 (lower back, gluteal pain, urinary symptoms and vaginal/clitoral pain – piriformis, hamstring and quadratus lumborum TrPs, treated with YNSA)

HISTORY: A 52-year-old female presented with a very complicated history of (i) two months of bladder pain/spasm with intermittent frequency and urinary retention, (ii) vaginal pain, (iii) two years of low-grade chronic right lower back and gluteal pain (diagnosed as a L5/S1 radiculopathy two years ago). She also had a past history of renal calculi, three very difficult births, chronic constipation and two anal fissure operations. She was investigated by her GP, her colorectal surgeon, a gynaecologist, then extensively by a urologist, with various diagnoses of renal colic, recurrent renal calculi and interstitial cystitis. On careful questioning, it appeared that the urinary and vaginal symptoms were preceded by three months of intensive bike riding at the gym to lose weight. The exact location of the vaginal pain was at the clitoris and vaginal canal.

REASONING: As the only nerve supply to the clitoris and vaginal canal is the pudendal nerve, a provisional diagnosis was made of pudendal neuralgia rather than a myofascial pain caused by the right piriformis. A search in literature showed that as the pudendal nerve courses through the sacral-pelvic region, entrapment can occur. A common site is when it passes next to the piriformis (the most common being between the sacrospinous and the sacrotuberous ligament).[119,120] It was likely that the intensive bike riding on ill-fitting bike seats had aggravated the piriformis, which apparently can happen to keen bike riders.

EXAMINATION: She had normal reflexes, muscle power and sensation. There were very tender TrPs of the piriformis, right more than left, right quadratus lumborum and hamstring.

DIAGNOSIS: Pudendal neuralgia possibly caused by TrPs in the piriformis.

TREATMENT: The patient was treated with YNSA, points in the right piriformis, quadratus lumborum, and hamstring in the K somatotope were needled once weekly.

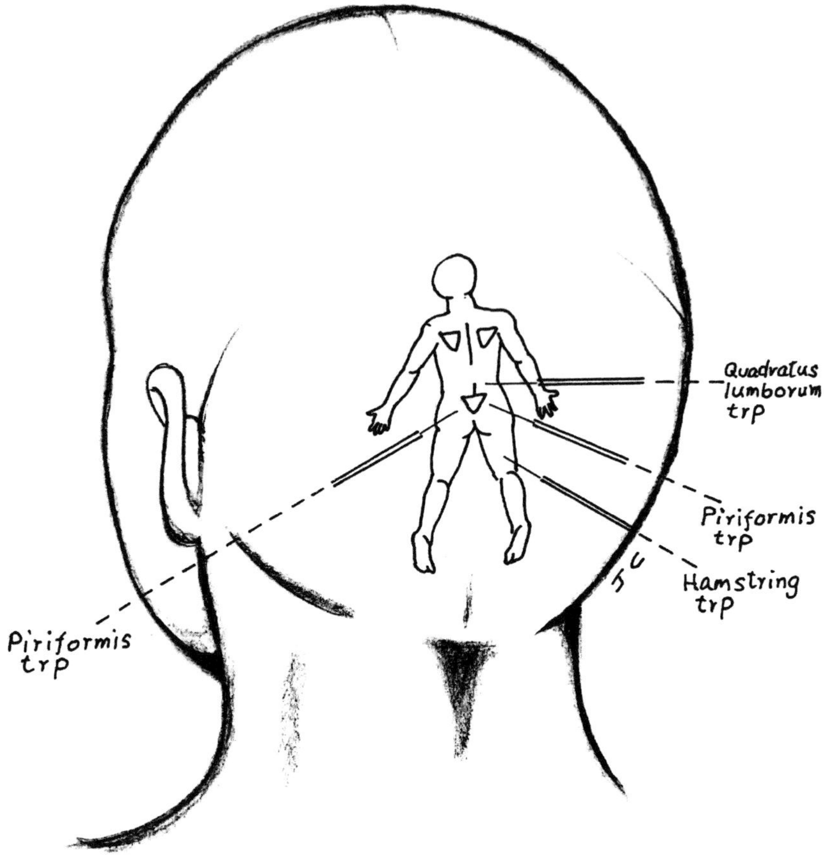

Figure 94: TrPs treatment for Case Study 14

OUTCOME: She gradually improved, with some weeks better than others. As her symptoms were very distressing, and we were hoping to avoid a pudendal nerve block, we persisted for three months. At the end of that time, she was 95% better. Interestingly, on the days when her constipation problem deteriorated, or when there was prolonged sitting, the clitoral pain recurred albeit mildly.

CASE STUDY 15 (right sciatic distribution pain piriformis and hamstring TrPs, treated with YNSA)

HISTORY: A 75-year-old female presented with a three-year history of severe 8/10 pain over the right gluteal region. She described some radiation of pain descending to the posterior thigh region. There was no parathaesia or lower leg weakness. Coughing or sneezing did not aggravate the pain. There was no change in her bowel or bladder control. She did not recall any falls. The pain was not constant and was worse sitting in the driving position or sitting upright with the legs straight down. Interestingly, sitting in bed with the legs straight was painless. There was little pain lying down. Walking on level ground was all right but not on uneven ground. She could not remember clearly, but the pain seemed to start after her right hip replacement (posterior approach) three years prior.

She saw the hip surgeon about it in the follow-up appointments and was told to persist with physiotherapy and rehabilitation exercises. She had a DEXA bone density test, which was normal. Lumbar spine MRI showed probable multiple-level nerve root impingement. She had been prescribed tapentadol SR 50mg bd (and tapentadol 50mg bd PRN) for her pain, which she had been taking for the last two years. She had two ultrasound-guided corticosteroid injections to the greater trochanter, which did not help. She was seen by two neurosurgeons, both felt that it was a nerve root impingement. One had offered a discectomy with a 75% success rate predicted. Not wanting surgery, she saw a pain specialist who decided that the pain was caused by a facet joint arthritis. It appeared that, without a trial of CT-guided medial branch block, he did a medial branch radiofrequency ablation. This did not help the pain. In the follow-up appointment, and seeing that the previous procedure had not worked, he offered to do a sacroiliac joint injection himself and booked her in to do that. At that point, the patient sought another opinion.

REASONING: What did not support the diagnosis of radiculopathy was that the pain was intermittent and there was no parathaesia nor weakness. The fact that it was so specifically aggravated by certain movements and leg positions pointed more to a possible muscular problem. Referred pain from lumbar facet joint arthritis could radiate to the posterior thigh but is usually not aggravated by leg positions. The MRI excluded osteoporotic fracture, lytic and sclerotic lesions, which was reassuring in her age group. It was of interest that the pain appeared to have started after the hip replacement, which called for further investigation.

EXAMINATION: The patient was in obvious discomfort sitting upright, muscle power, reflexes, sensations were all normal. There was muscle wasting in her right gluteals. The Spring test for the SIJ was negative. Her hip internal rotation was very painful. On careful targeted palpation over the gluteal region, her pain was precisely localised to the piriformis muscle, most intense being at the distal insertion site. 'That's it! That's my pain!' she exclaimed, excited that someone had 'found' her pain.

DIAGNOSIS: Not having witnessed any hip replacement performed before, I rang an orthopaedic surgeon, who explained, 'The piriformis is divided in a posterior approach hip replacement, then reattached. At times, inflammation can occur at that site, resulting in a piriformis syndrome. Corticosteroid injection often works, and in rare occasions the intensely inflamed piriformis has to be surgically divided to stop the pain.' As a result, the patient's pain was diagnosed to be an intense inflammation at the distal end of the piriformis.

TREATMENT: She was treated with YNSA; points for the piriformis and hamstring in the K somatotope were used. Unfortunately, no lasting improvements occurred after four treatments. She was then referred to a hip orthopaedic surgeon for further management and treatment. The site of inflammation at the piriformis was injected with corticosteroid twice, without lasting results.

INVESTIGATIONS: None necessary.

OUTCOME: At the time of writing, the patient was still in pain and undecided about a possible open exploration of the piriformis.

NB. While all the doctors involved had examined the patient, it appeared that none had palpated her designated painful area. It is not good practice deciding on invasive interventions purely relying on imaging. The process should be a thorough history to diagnose – or at least narrow the differential diagnoses – followed by **targeted** physical examination with **palpation,** to confirm a diagnosis. Imaging should mainly play a supportive role.

CASE STUDY 16 (right hip pain – treated with corticosteroid injection)

HISTORY: A 56-year-old, female office worker presented with a two-month history of right outer hip pain, radiating to the gluteal and lateral thigh area. The pain could be felt in the groin at times but no further than mid-thigh. There was no history of falls or trauma but the pain did come soon after a bushwalk. It became more severe, changing from a 4/10 intermittently to a 6/10 fairly constant pain. The pain was particularly severe when getting up from a seated position and when sleeping on the right side. She denied any numbness or weakness of the leg. The pain did not increase when coughing. She denied parathaesia in the leg or foot weakness. There was no past history of any hip or other joint pains. She was overweight at 76kg, BMI 29 and hypertensive. She admitted to not doing any regular exercise. She had regular breast screening and cardiologist check-ups but did not know her calcium or vitamin D levels, and she had not had a DEXA bone density test before. She has had numerous back massages, which did not really help.

REASONING: The diagnosis of greater trochanteric pain syndrome came to mind straight away due to the location of pain, inability to sleep on that side and pain worsening when rising from a seated position. Hip OA and lumbar facet joint arthropathy had to be considered as well. The history did not point to a lumbar radiculopathy.

EXAMINATION: She had definite pain when rising from a seated position, and obviously favoured the good leg when walking. Power, reflexes were normal. Straight leg raising was normal. Internal rotation of the hip joint was painful. The left hip, knees and feet examination were normal. Sharp and severe pain was localised to the right great trochanter, with the patient yelling out upon firm pressure.

DIAGNOSIS: With the findings, greater trochanteric pain syndrome was highly likely, and the history and physical findings were very typical of the condition.

INVESTIGATION: A plain X-ray of the hip and lumbosacral spine would be appropriate to look for evidence of OA, osteoporosis and to rule out lytic and sclerotic lesions.

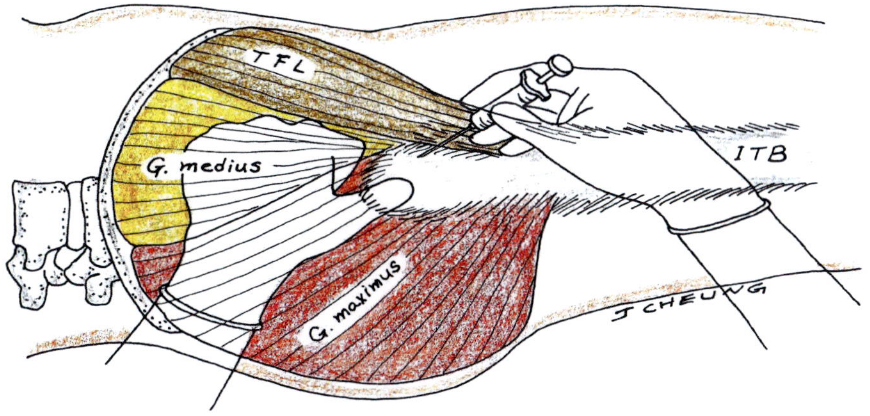

Figure 95: Injection for the greater trochanteric bursitis

TREATMENT: As the patient had very severe pain, and the confidence level of the diagnosis was high, a decision was made to inject the site with LA and corticosteroid (1ml of 2% xylocaine and 2ml of betamethasone 5.7mg/ml). The greater trochanter was palpated all over, carefully and firmly, and two spots of maximal tenderness were selected and injected. This can be performed aseptically in the rooms by palpation or at a radiology centre as an ultrasound guided injection.

OUTCOME: After five minutes, the LA took effect and the patient was almost pain free, which confirmed the diagnosis. The patient reported later that, while the pain returned after the LA had worn off, it was much improved. The patient was instructed to limit her walking for the next three weeks to allow the condition to recover fully. Some stretching exercises for the gluteals, quads and ITB were given. The patient was also encouraged to lose some weight and to start doing regular weight-bearing exercises. DEXA BMD (Bone mineral density) scan, vitamin D and calcium levels should be tested and monitored for women over 50-years-old to prevent against osteoporosis.

GREATER TROCHANTERIC PAIN SYNDROME (GTPS)

The condition is often collectively called greater trochanteric bursitis, which is a misnomer, as pain at the site can include tendinopathy (typically the gluteus medius, gluteus minimus or piriformis), tears and bursitis (which consists of sub-gluteus medius, sub-gluteus minimus, sub-gluteus maximus or trochanteric bursae, and one between the ITB and greater trochanter as well). It is often difficult to determine which is the actual pathology, even by imaging, and multiple pathologies can co-exist. It is thought to be arising from frictional forces between the tensor fasciae latae (TFL), gluteus medius, gluteus minimus, piriformis and the trochanteric bursa. It is not unlike the condition of subacromial bursitis.[121,122]

GTPS has an annual incidence as high as 1.8 per 1000 adults in the primary care setting. While it is seen in all age groups, it most commonly affects patients during their fourth to sixth decades of life, with a female predominance of 2–3 to 1.[123] Trauma, obesity and gait are probable factors. Injection of LA and corticosteroid – either by palpation or guided by ultrasound – works well but predisposing factors need to be addressed, otherwise recurrence is common. It is not a difficult procedure to do and, in some ways, it may be more effective to inject by palpating for the most tender spot(s); as in ultrasound-guided injection, the radiologist may have to choose from numerous active bursae detected by ultrasound. Caution must be exercised with corticosteroid injections, as repeated injections would weaken the muscles and ligamentous structures injected.

CASE STUDY 17 (sacroiliac joint pain)

HISTORY: A 23-year-old male, fit and healthy student presented with a sudden onset of severe 9/10 right sacroiliac joint (SIJ) pain for 24 hours. He played rugby two days before but did not remember sustaining any injury during the game. He also had a fever, rigors and generalised flu-like muscle aches but no respiratory symptoms of any kind. He had no SIJ or lower-back problems previously and no significant past history; system review was normal otherwise.

REASONING: As the site of the pain was localised to the SIJ, possible diagnoses would include SIJ strain and fracture.

EXAMINATION: The patient had difficulty walking due to the SIJ pain. He had a fever of 39 deg Celsius, chest was clear, abdomen was soft, urine analysis was normal and there were no skin lacerations anywhere. Marked localised tenderness was found in the right SIJ. Pain was almost unbearable on doing the 'Springing test'. (This test involves the patient lying prone, the examiner's right hand applying a springing pressure over the apex of the sacrum with the palpating left thumb over the SIJ. The test is positive when the patient reports pain in the SIJ being palpated. The test is objectively unsatisfactory but subjectively useful in testing for SIJ pathologies.)

DIAGNOSIS: The cause of this pain was uncertain, but as the patient was septic and very unwell, he needed to be admitted for assessment.

OUTCOME: Upon admission, his WCC (white cell count) was raised and the CRP was in the 300s. An MRI the following day showed a small fluid collection in the right SIJ, and a subsequent CT-guided aspiration and culture confirmed the diagnosis of septic arthritis in the right SIJ. He was treated with IV antibiotics and a drainage tube inserted into the SIJ. He had a complicated stay in hospital for three weeks, and finally recovered completely.

NB. In acute clinical presentations, certain conditions have to be considered first until proven otherwise. For example, a right iliac fossa pain is appendicitis until proven otherwise, or a lower abdominal pain in early pregnancy is a tubal pregnancy until proven otherwise; so, too, a painful joint or bone with fever is septic arthritis or osteomyelitis until proven otherwise.

CASE STUDY 18 (LBP – treated with CT-guided corticosteroid injection)

HISTORY: A 76-year-old male with mild intermittent LBP became much worse in the last three months. Pain was fairly constant over the right buttock and posterior right thigh. He rated it between 4/10 to 6/10. He had not suffered any trauma or falls. The pain was worse when doing activities to the point that he had to stop gardening and his daily walks. There was no prolonged morning stiffness. He reported no numbness or weakness, and it was not aggravated by coughing. Two weeks of paracetamol did not help.

Past history included X-ray evidence of mild osteoarthritis in his knees and stable ischaemic heart disease. The patient's BMD, vitamin D and calcium levels were normal as was his recent PSA.

REASONING: Differential diagnosis would include OA, TrPs and radiculopathy. The pain distribution and constancy of pain pointed more to OA (see Table 1) .

EXAMINATION: Power, reflexes and sensations were normal, and straight leg raising was normal. ROM on both hips and knees were normal. Some tender muscle knots over the right gluteal muscles and hamstrings. There was no tenderness in the piriformis nor the greater trochanter. Iliopsoas tested normal.

INVESTIGATION: A CT scan of the lumbosacral spine was ordered to exclude osteoporotic fractures, lytic and sclerotic lesions, and to look for facet joint OA. It showed moderate facet joint OA on multiple levels and possible nerve root impingement at L4/5 on the right side and L4/5 on the left side.

DIAGNOSIS: The diagnosis was more likely to be due to facet joint arthritis of the lumbar facet joints than a radiculopathy (due to the pain distribution not really fitting with L4 or L5 dermatomes), with differential diagnoses being muscular strain of the right gluteal muscles.

TREATMENT: He was given a two-week course of NSAIDs, as there were no contra-indication. It might have helped somewhat but not significantly. He preferred not to have acupuncture and was referred to a physiotherapist with interests in manual therapy, to work on his gluteals. When he was reviewed three weeks later, the gluteal tightness had resolved but the pain persisted.

OUTCOME: A bone scan with SPECT (single-photon emission computed tomography) was ordered, showing that the facet joints at L4/5 and less so at L5/S1 on the right side were active. After conferring with the radiologist, CT-guided facet joint injections with LA and corticosteroid were then given, which significantly improved his presenting pains over the next two weeks.

CASE STUDY 19 (L4 nerve root impingement – treated with CT-guided corticosteroid injection)

HISTORY: A home visit was requested by an 84-year-old female who lived with her son. She was fiercely independent and enjoyed a lot of different sports in her younger years. While very determined mentally, she was becoming frail. She reported two days of fairly constant 5/10 sharp pain in the left hip area that was radiating down the anterior thigh and lower leg. There was no history of trauma. She could walk but the pain was affecting her balance. There was no numbness or weakness and she denied any falls. Relevant past medical history included very well-controlled moderate osteoporosis treated with six monthly subcutaneous denosumab; hypertension and breast cancer was successfully treated 15 years ago. The son left the front door unlocked for me to enter when he left for work, as the patient couldn't come to the door easily.

REASONING: The pain was constant and the pain distribution was consistent with an L4 radiculopathy. As OA pain tends not to develop so suddenly, muscular strain was still a possibility. Osteoporotic vertebral fracture, lytic and sclerotic lesions had to be excluded.

EXAMINATION: The patient could get up from sitting and walk but with some difficulty. There were no reflex changes, muscle weakness nor sensation loss.

DIAGNOSIS: The differential diagnoses included minor nerve root impingement, lumbosacral muscular strain, facet joint OA. Osteoporotic fracture and metastasis needed to be excluded as well.

OUTCOME: As there were no imminent red-flag diagnosis present, a lumbar CT scan could be arranged and conservative management planned. However, in her present condition and being alone most of the time, the possibility of a fall was almost a certainty, and the possibility for the fall to result in a fracture (hip, spine or others) was about 10%.[124]

The patient was convinced with great difficulty that she needed to be diagnosed and managed in a hospital setting. She was very concerned with the possibility of being sent from hospital to a nursing home permanently, which was not an unrealistic worry. After organising an ambulance, a phone discussion with the casualty specialist was made, outlining the patient's condition, her living situation and the likelihood of an impending fall. The call was important, as a less experienced casualty doctor assessing her – and given the usual limited available hospital beds – could result in her being sent home and her trip a 'dry run'.

The patient was admitted under a geriatrician who was very proactive. Her pain settled with a combination of a low dose buprenorphine patch and amitriptyline 50mg bd. After investigations with an MRI, the diagnosis was made of a left L4/5 neuroforaminal stenosis and possible L4 nerve root impingement. A CT-guided corticosteroid and LA peri-foraminal injection were given with good results, and she was able to be weaned off her medications. While in hospital, she was given a dedicated backpain exercise and rehabilitation program as she had become deconditioned. The patient was quite mobile when she was transferred to a rehabilitation hospital for a further two weeks, before being discharged home. She was also recommended to attend an outpatient exercise program for the older population, which is dedicated to promote health, activities and falls prevention.

She had successfully avoided a fall and possible fracture and was able to return to an independent life at home.

CASE STUDY 20 (chronic LBP and opioids)

HISTORY: A 43-year-old male with a young family presented for the first time to the practice, requesting a script for oxycodone 40 mg twice a day for his chronic lower back pain (LBP). He said that he had misplaced his tablets and scripts and that his usual GP was away. He stated that the LBP had started two years ago. He had a motorbike accident, in which he was thrown airborne and sustained fractures in the lumbar spine. He had seen multiple specialists and a pain clinic. He had multiple CT-guided nerve root and facet joint injections which did not help. The medications could only bring the usual intermittent 8/10 pain to 3–4/10. He declined further discussions on the LBP or the offer of an examination.

DIAGNOSIS: His pain was aggravated by prolonged sitting and certain movements; it was highly likely that at least some of his pain could be of a muscular/ligamentous origin.

TREATMENT AND OUTCOME: He was displaying obvious drug-related aberrant behaviour. I decided against giving the prescription, knowing that if I did, it would perpetuate his problem and I would have an exponentially increasing number of such patients in the following weeks.

Before I told him my decision, I gave him a script for a nasal Naloxone and instructions, citing some statistics of the incidence of opioid overdose. I told him my decision and that my door would always be open for treatment to assess his pain or help him to reduce and wean off his opioid usage. Before he left, I very briefly mentioned the negative aspects of opioid use disorder. The poor pain control, poor quality of life, hyperalgesia, opioid-induced androgen deficiency, immunity suppression, tolerance, dependency and opioid-induced ventilatory impairment. I also mentioned how he was putting himself, his family and his business at risk. To his credit, he listened to it all, and I sensed that he did not know some of those information. I encouraged him to read the literature on opioid use disorder. As he left, in a bit of a hurry and with some annoyance, I was left sitting in my chair, with a great deal of sadness and a small amount of hope. I told the receptionist not to charge him.

NB. The usage of opioid preparations for cancer pain and palliative care was welcomed in the 1990s, championed by the hospice movement. It is also invaluable in cases of severe acute pain and short-term post-operative pain. However, it is not recommended for chronic pain. At present, there is an over-prescription of opioids and an epidemic of opioid use disorder, and I wonder how history will judge us, the prescribing doctors.

There were 1123 opioid overdose deaths in Australia in 2018[125] (and 47,000 in the USA in 2017[126]). Most are from prescription opioids, 49% of those prescriptions are for chronic pain, and >50% are prescribed by GPs.[127] Pharmaceutical opioids are present in over 70% of opioid-induced deaths.[128] Evidence shows that, for any patients taking >50 mg of opioids a day, a PBS-subsidised nasal Naloxone script should be given. However, only about 9% of the Naloxone nasal spray given out were from a doctor's prescription.[129]

CASE STUDY 21 (lower back pain – quadratus lumborum, gluteus medius and hamstring TrPs treated with manual therapy and stretches)

HISTORY: A 40-year-old male, presented with a one-day history of severe crippling LBP. Pain was sharp, over the right SIJ area, spreading to the right gluteal region and at times felt over the posterior thigh. Any sudden movement would aggravate it, and it was difficult to find a comfortable sleeping position. He denied any weakness in right leg, nor were there any numbness down that leg. The patient denied any trauma or falls. He said that he has had similar episodes before but not as severe. He had taken some ibuprofen, which did not help. He admitted to sitting in front of a laptop for hours on end and had not been doing any exercise for weeks. There was no other significant medical history and he was not overweight.

REASONING: As the pain was aggravated by movement, it was likely to be a muscular strain. SIJ strain was also a possibility. Facet joint arthropathy was unlikely due to his relatively young age. The pain distribution did not point to a radiculopathy.

EXAMINATION: The patient preferred to be standing during the consultation. His reflexes were normal, hip extension, foot dorsiflexion and plantar flexion were normal. After some effort, the patient was able to undress and laid down in a prone position. The Springing test on his SIJ was negative for SIJ dysfunction. However, there were marked tender muscle spasms over his right quadratus lumborum, gluteus medius and hamstrings; his ITB was also very tight and tender as compared to the left side.

INVESTIGATIONS: None planned at presentation.

DIAGNOSIS: The findings did not point to radiculopathy nor SIJ dysfunction. The diagnosis was that of muscular strain and spasm of the gluteus medius, hamstring and ITB.

TREATMENT: The patient was somewhat phobic towards acupuncture needling and requested manual therapies instead. There are many different forms of manual therapies using firm soft-tissue massage techniques on the gluteal, hamstring and ITB for LBP arising from muscular strain. The patient was treated while still lying prone, several minutes of firm massage on the above muscles in turn, and repeated about three times.

OUTCOME: After about 20 minutes, the acute pain settled and the patient was 60% better. After another similar treatment the next day, the patient was 90% better (see the following page for the massage method). He was advised against prolonged periods of sitting from now on. After this episode of crippling pain, he was more motivated to return to his usual weekly tennis. He was also advised to do some daily stretching exercises. It is very satisfying for a clinician to be able to manually and successfully treat a patient presenting with acute pain. It also negates the need to prescribe strong analgesics.

NB. It is not uncommon for the condition of this presentation to become chronic and, if undiagnosed, be labelled chronic LBP generically. Many of these patients are told that they have arthritis because of the radiological findings and be subjected to long-term pain and medications.

A LOWER BACK MUSCLE STRAIN MASSAGE METHOD

This is a back pain massage from traditional Chinese medicine, not so different to massage methods from other cultures. Basically, working on the gluteals, then the hamstrings and the ITB on the same side in succession would loosen all these muscles; interestingly, the lumbar paravertebral muscles are released indirectly as well. It may be that perhaps some of these muscles are all in the same myotome.

Drape the patient as shown. Apply some massage oil or soluble bath oil. Massage the gluteals **on one side** (as shown) with overlapping hands. Keep the pulp of the fingertips in line for more even contact and better results. Do it firmly and with hooked fingertips, up and down, across the 'grain' of the muscles, for 1–2 minutes.

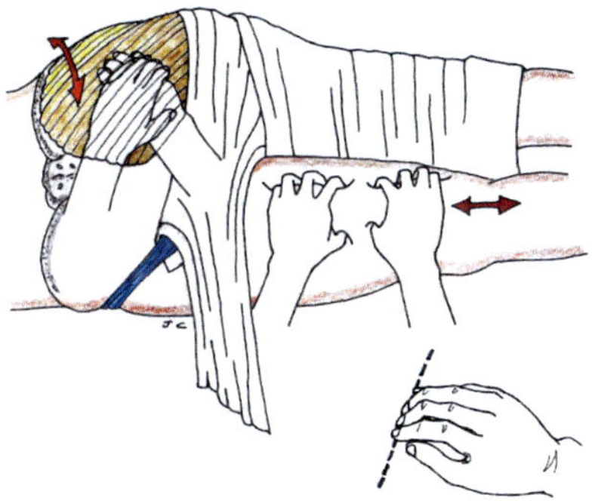

Then work on the hamstrings and the ITB **on the ipsilateral side,** moving up and down as shown with (i) strong fingertip pressure; (ii) squeezing the whole thigh with both hands; and (iii) throwing and shaking the muscles at the same time for 1–2 minutes.

Applying firm pressure with the 'heel' of your palms, push down along the hamstrings and ITB for 1–2 minutes. Then do the same **on the ipsilateral side.**

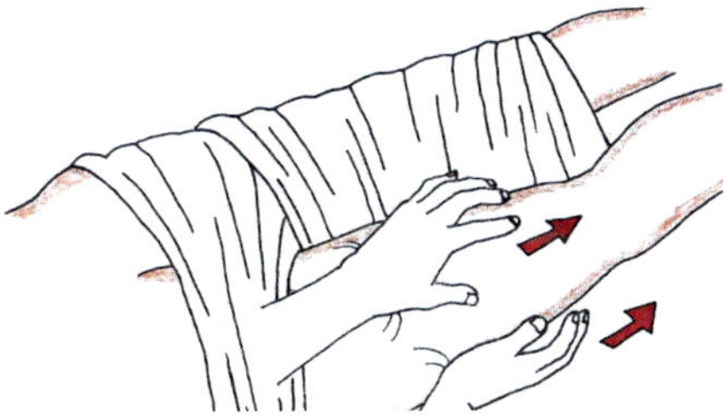

Apply strong pressure by rolling the 'heel' of your hand in a circular motion, downwards for 1 – 2 minutes along the hamstrings. Then do the same on the ipsilateral side.

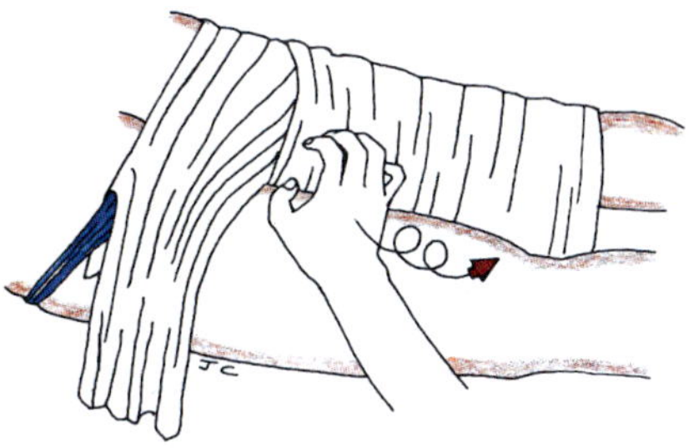

Strike the hamstrings and ITB along their lengths with the edge of your palms, rhythmically (as if beating a drum). Do it for 1–2 minutes.

Grip the hamstrings with one hand, then flop, shake and throw it for 30 seconds.

After working on the hamstrings and ITB, you will find that the gluteals will gradually loosen up a fair bit compared to initially; and working on the gluteals will loosen up the hamstrings and ITB in turn, in a progressive fashion. Repeat the whole process three times on one side, **then do the same thing on the contralateral side.** From my experience, if it is a pure lower back muscular strain, this almost always works.

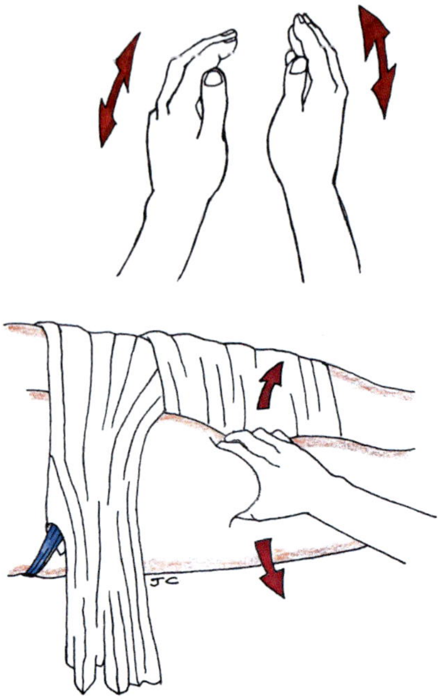

Figure 96: A massage method for mechanical lower back pain

CASE STUDY 22 (right LBP – quadratus lumborum, piriformis and hamstring TrPs, treated with YNSA)

HISTORY: A 45-year-old, female refugee recently arrived in Australia from the Middle East presented with a 10-year history of chronic lower back pain. She described it as an intermittent 7/10 pain in the right lumbar area. The pain would radiate down the back of her thigh and calf but only very rarely. It was present when she was sitting or walking and disturbed her sleep every night. There was no paresthesia or weakness. The pain did not increase with coughing or sneezing. There was no prolonged morning stiffness. She did not remember any falls or accidents prior to the onset of the pain. Her work back in her home country involved sitting for 10 hours, sewing every day without any scheduled breaks. She had no history of any other pains. She had a past history of mild stress incontinence, psychological trauma, anxiety and depression. Life back home, unfortunately, did not include a balanced diet nor any exercise. Recent blood tests showed borderline low vitamin B12 and low vitamin D of 50.

REASONING: As the pain only radiated to the leg rarely and there was no paresthesia or weakness, radiculopathy was less likely. The symptoms would fit OA and also muscular/mechanical causes.

EXAMINATION: The patient was overweight with a BMI of 29. Muscle power, reflexes and sensation were normal. Hip joints were normal. Tender TrPs were found in the right quadratus lumborum, piriformis and hamstrings. On the left side, minor TrPs were found in the piriformis and hamstring. Her core strength was poor.

INVESTIGATIONS: An X-ray of the lumbar spine showed mild anterior wedge of T11, T12 and L1 with approximately 10% height loss but no obvious OA.

BMD showed lumbar spine T score of -0.9, and Femur T scores of 0.4 and 0.

DIAGNOSIS: The patient had BMD evidence of borderline osteopenia and X-ray evidence of multiple osteoporotic vertebral fractures which would need further assessment with an endocrinologist. The LBP was likely due to mechanical/ muscular causes and/or osteoarthritis.

TREATMENT: The patient was treated with YNSA targeting the TrPs listed, once a week.

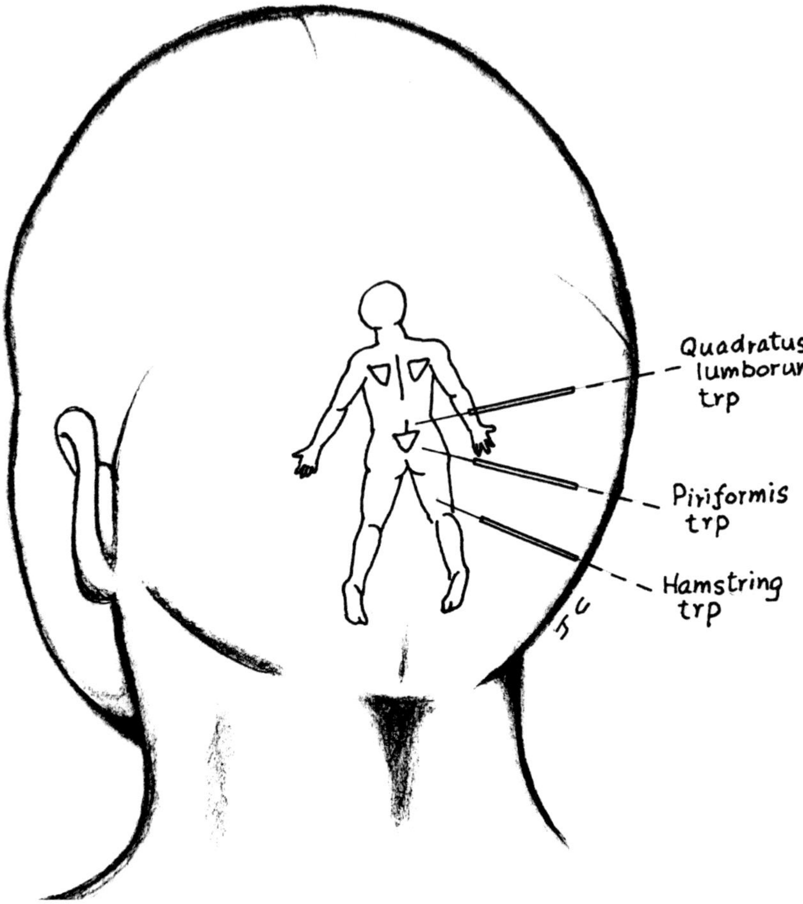

Figure 97: TrPs treatment for Case Study 22

OUTCOME: She improved with each treatment dramatically. After seven treatments, she was pain-free and sleeping through the night. She was also given postural advice, stretching exercises and core strengthening exercises. At the time of writing, two months after the last treatment, she was still pain-free.

I am constantly surprised to find that patients labelled as having chronic lower back pain actually have pain caused by trigger points alone, and YNSA can often resolve these TrPs that have been present for many, many years.

Tips: To treat the lower back and the thick thigh muscles on the posterior aspect with YNSA, the patient needs to be palpated and acupunctured in a prone position. In order to orientate the K and J somatotopes, I would insert an acupuncture needle in the GV 20 point first while the patient is seated because it is much harder to find the GV 20 when the patient is lying down. I would then insert the needles and re-examine the TrPs after the needle insertion, with the patient in the prone position throughout the treatment process.

A SUMMARY OF A PROPOSED APPROACH TO A PATIENT PRESENTING WITH LOWER BACK OR UPPER THIGH REGION PAIN

1. Attempt to reach a diagnosis through a thorough history.
2. Rule out any red-flag diagnosis.
3. Perform an examination targeted to confirm diagnosis and to exclude other possibilities.
4. If appropriate, include palpation for trigger points around the lower back and upper thigh region. They may be part of – if not the main cause of – the pain. With practice, it will take only a few minutes (Fig. 98 and 99). Please keep in mind that the most common causes of LBP are muscular in origin.
5. Order appropriate imaging or other investigations. Tests should not take precedence over or replace the above steps. Try not to order unnecessary tests that will not change the management plan. Tests often show multiple pathologies that are not the cause of the problem, thus, confusing the diagnostic process.
6. Plan treatment with the aim to cure or improve the condition, and not just treat the pain.

Finding trigger points (TrPs) and treating them successfully can

- **eradicate the pain completely (when the TrPs are the cause);**
- **improve some of the pain (as the TrPs cause some of the pain);**
- **exclude TrPs as the cause of the pain, then move on to consider other possible diagnoses; and**
- **often avoid expensive imaging or invasive treatments.**

NB. There are often many instances when a lower back pain syndrome is wrongly diagnosed to be from lumbosacral osteoarthritis or lumbar radiculopathy when the cause of pain is primarily from TrPs. However, just because significant TrPs are found in a patient, it does not always mean that is the diagnosis. The TrPs may be secondary to another condition. Often multiple conditions can coexist.

It is worth remembering that diagnoses are static entities, whereas a patient's condition changes and evolves with time. A patient with lumbosacral osteoarthritic pain may evolve to develop significant muscular TrP pain, overshadowing the original OA pain. Someone with mainly TrP pain may evolve to develop a radiculopathy; or after eradicating the TrP pain in a patient, an underlying OA pain or a minor radiculopathy pain may become more evident. As TrPs are very common and readily treatable, it is still worthwhile eradicating them first.

PALPATION FOR COMMON TRIGGER POINTS IN THE LOWER BACK AND THIGH REGION

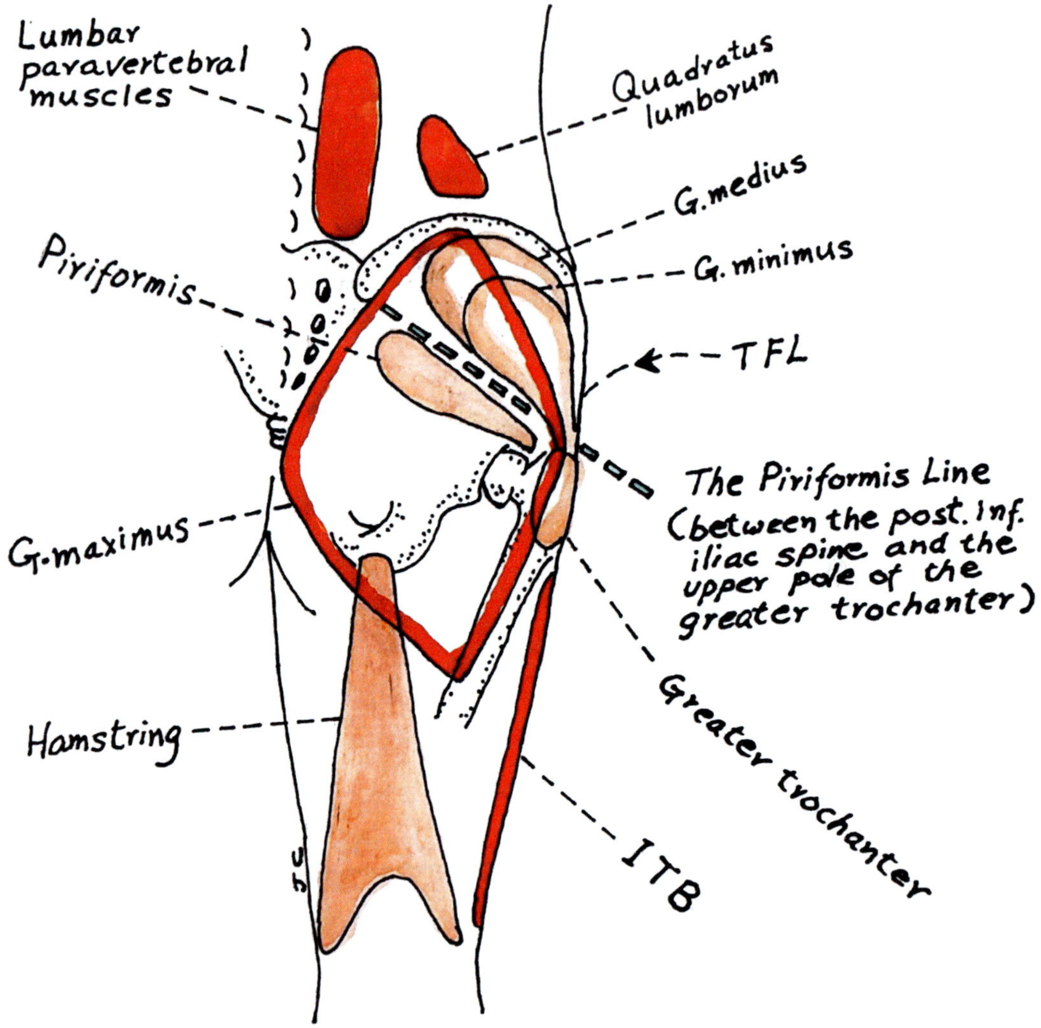

Figure 98: Palpation for TrPs in the lower back and posterior thigh region

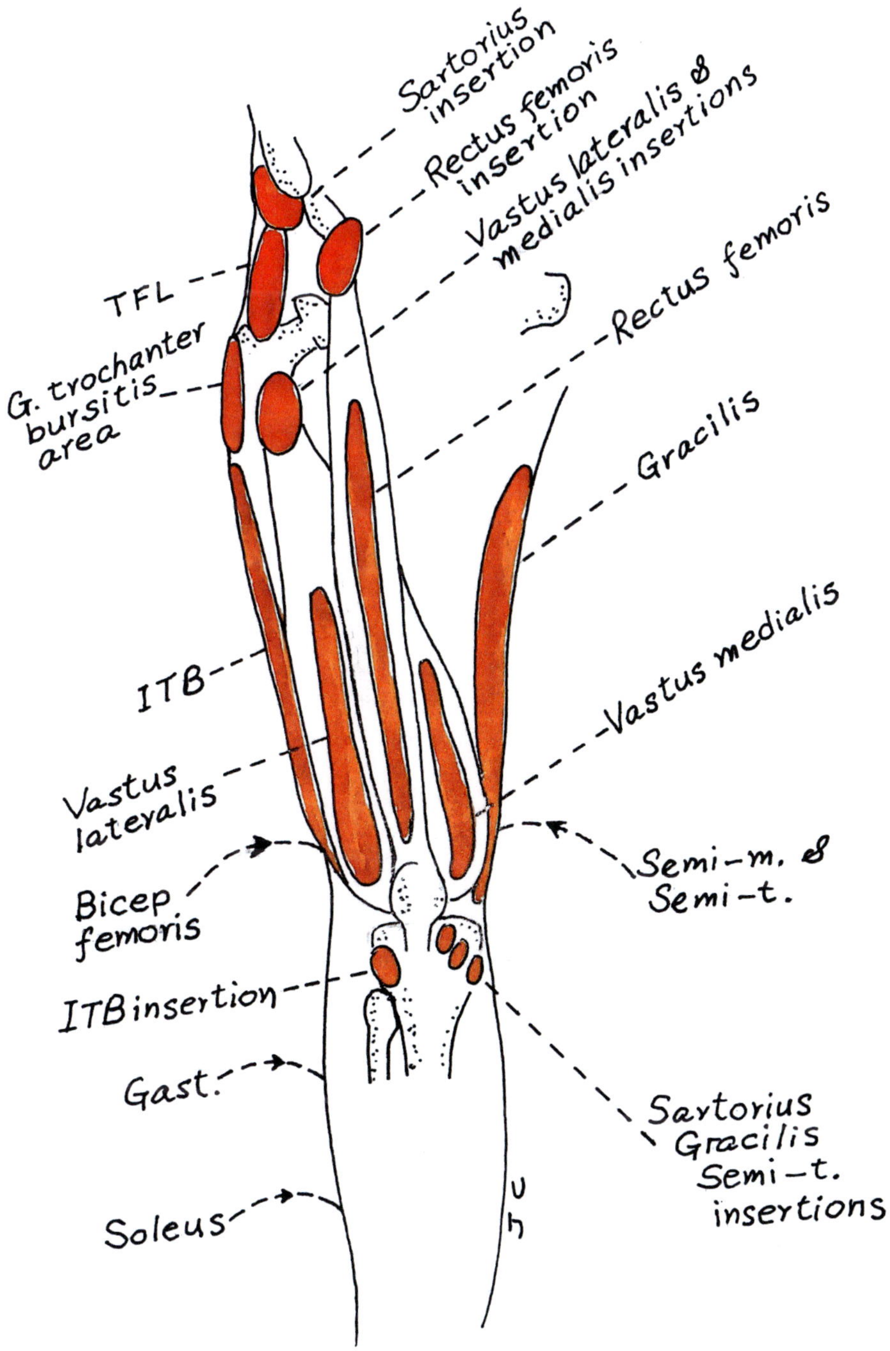

Figure 99: Palpation for TrPs in the anterior thigh region

SOME LOWER BACK STRETCHES

You need to feel the stretch in the designated muscles, relax all the adjacent muscles in order to target it. Maintain the stretch for eight breaths or 30 seconds, repeat if necessary. Be patient, do it every day.

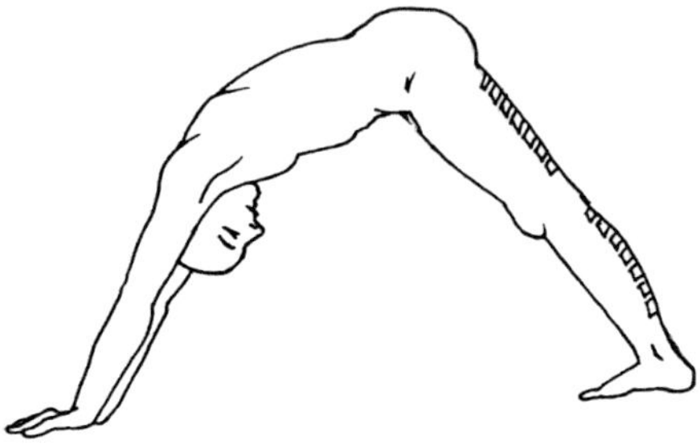

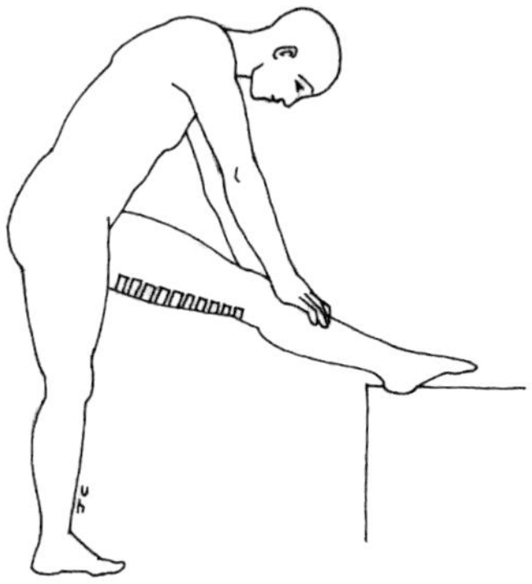

Hamstring, Gastrocnemius

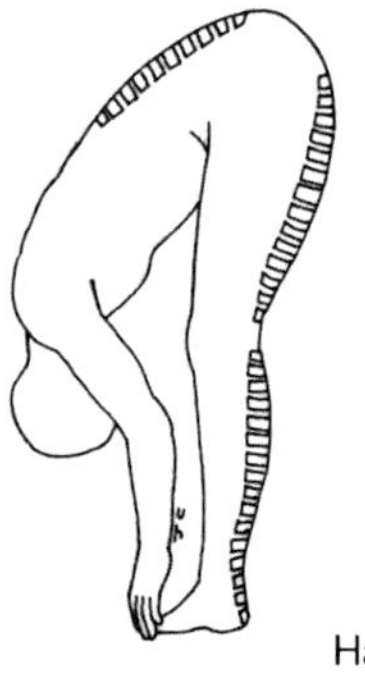

Hamstring,
Gastrocnemius,
Paravertebral, muscles

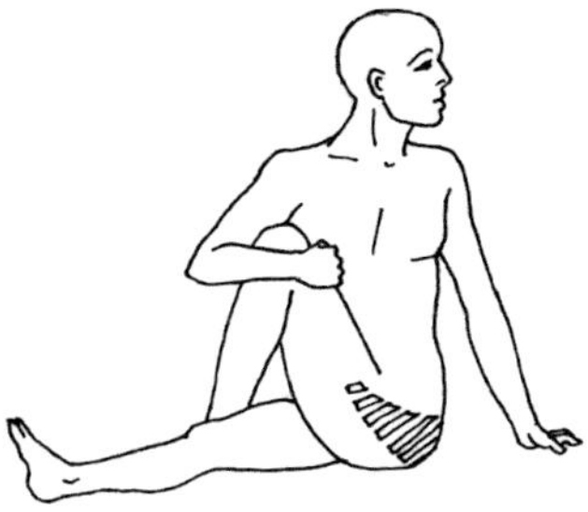

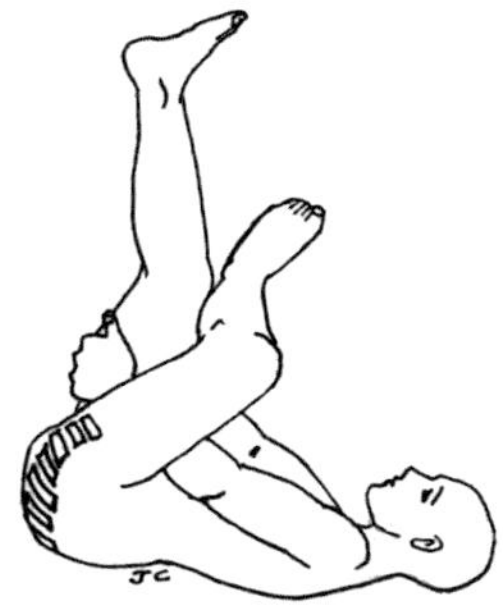

Gluteals, Piriformis

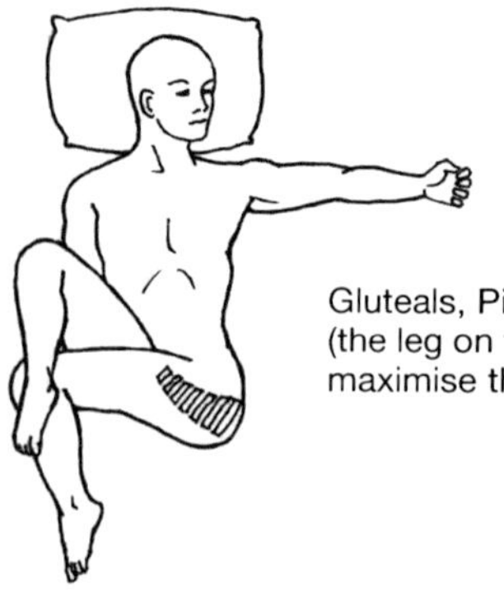

Gluteals, Piriformis, Quadratus lumborum (the leg on top pressing downwards to maximise the stretch)

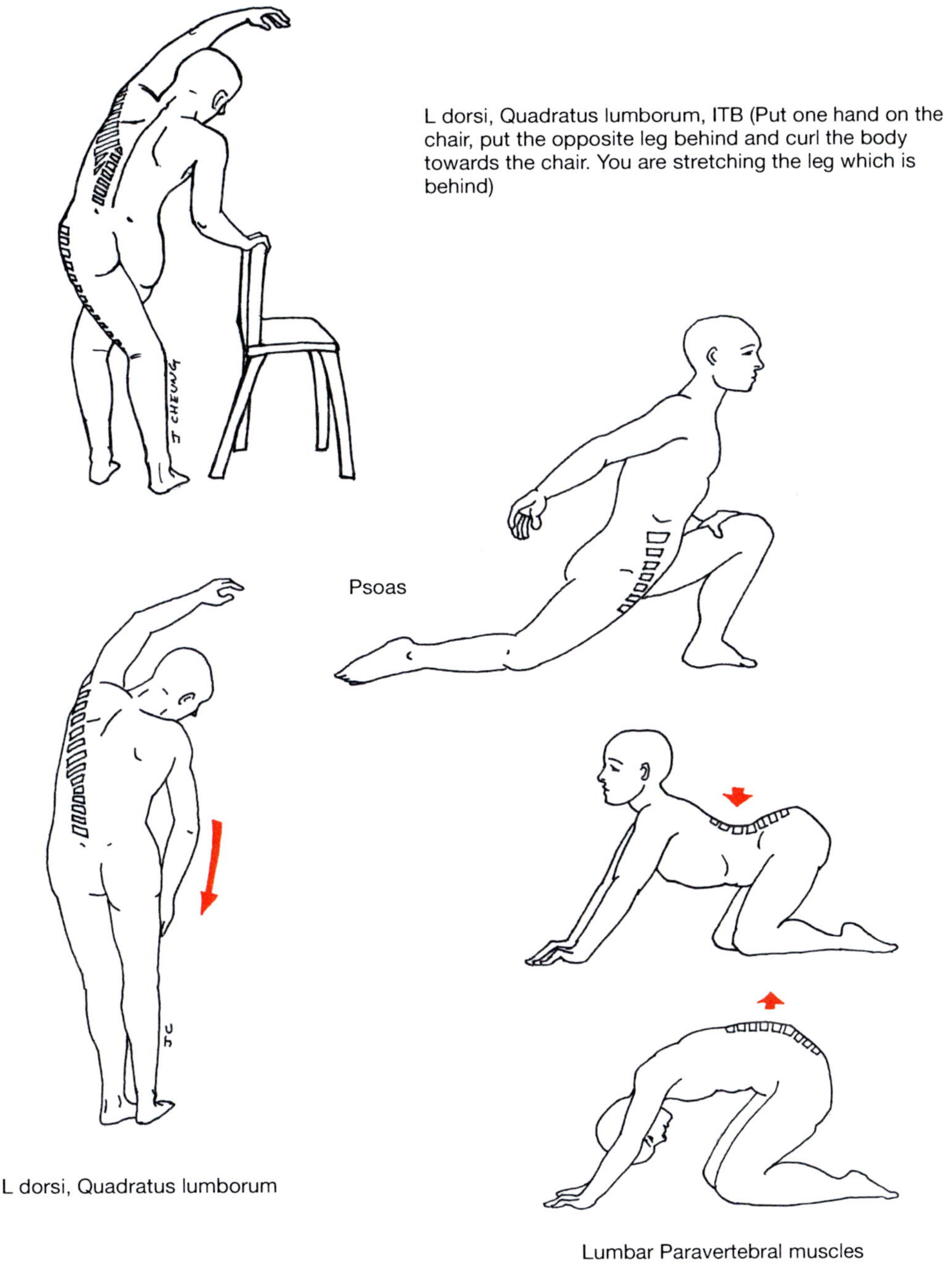

Figure 100: Useful stretches for the lower back region

SOME LOOSENING EXERCISES FOR THE LOWER BACK

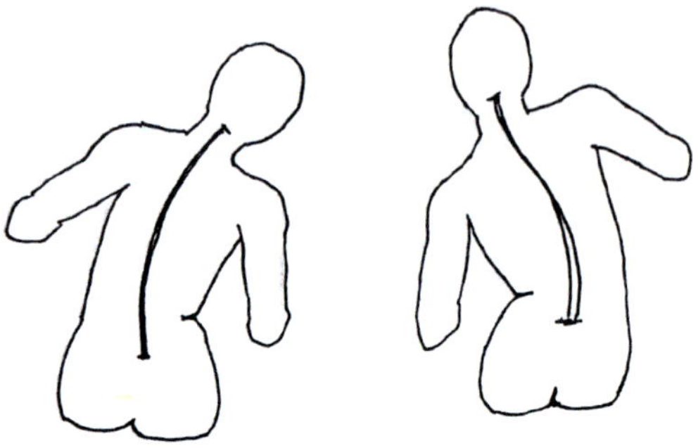

Chalk in the navel, do circles

Imagine you have a piece of chalk stuck in your navel and a blackboard right in front of your tummy, you have to draw a big circle clockwise 10 times and anticlockwise 10 times. While you do the circles, let your head and neck relax and flop with the rhythmic movement – you are actually moving your neck sideways and loosening it indirectly as well.

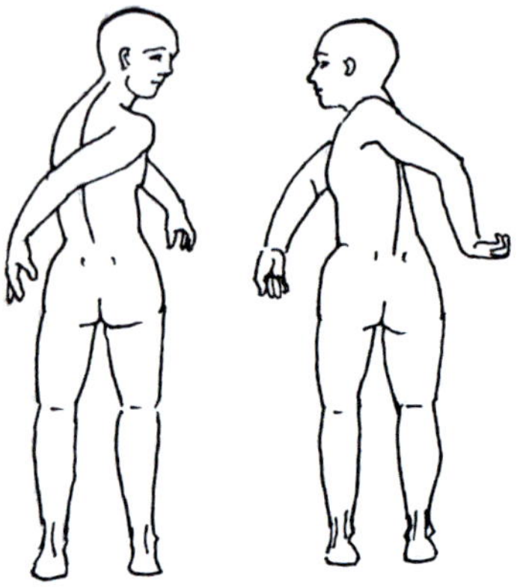

Spinning

With your feet slightly apart, toes gripping the floor, spin your whole trunk one way then the other, using your arms to create the rotational momentum, thereby rotating your whole spine.

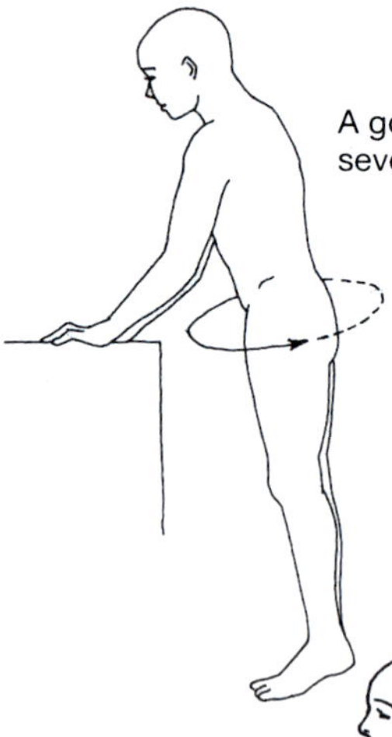

A good exercise for severe lower back pain.

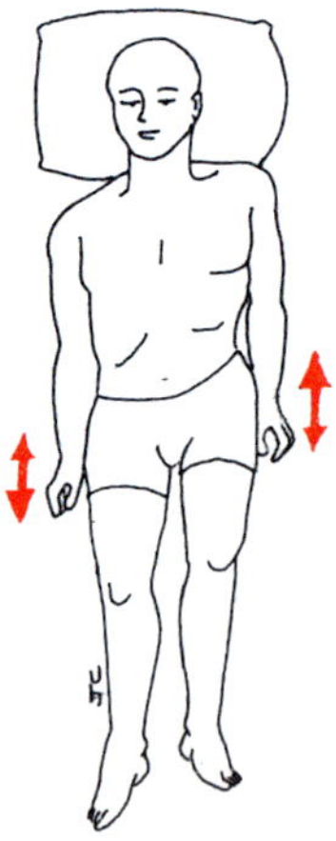

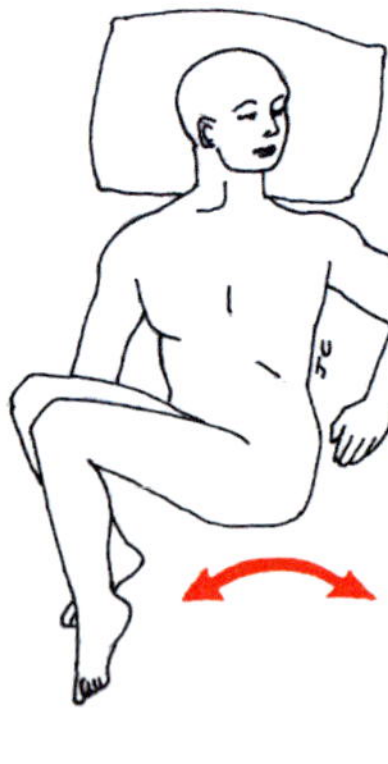

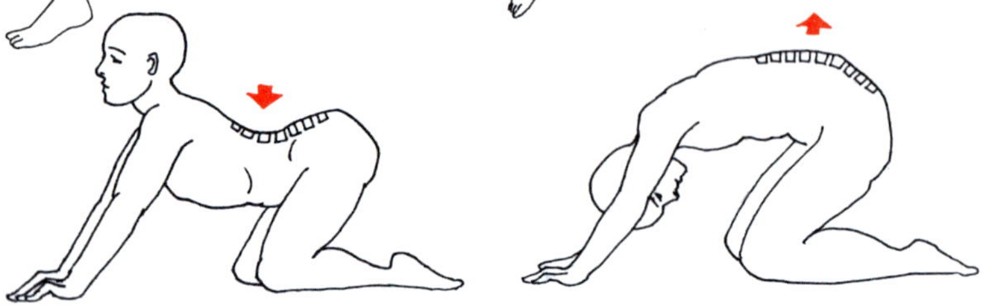

Lumbar Paravertebral muscles

Figure 101: Useful loosening exercises for the lower back

SOME EXERCISES FOR CORE STRENGTH

30 seconds each, repeat four times

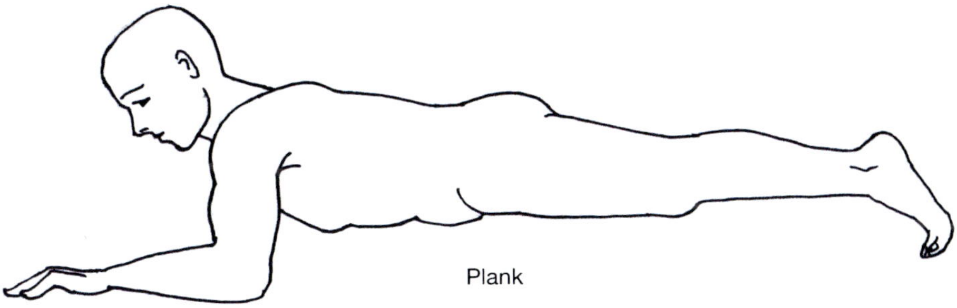

Plank

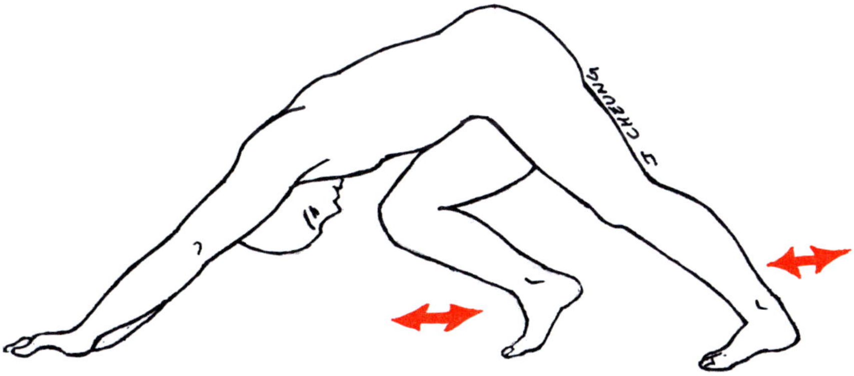

Mountain run

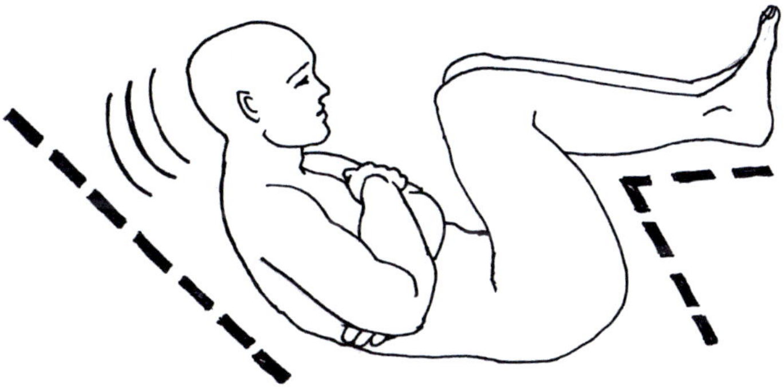

Crunches – keep your upper back elevated, lift your knees up at a 90- degree angle to the floor and try to touch your chin to your knees

Figure 102: Useful exercises for core strength

4. THE SHOULDER AND NECK REGION

Briefly, this chapter will cover the following aspects:

FRAMEWORK OF QUESTIONING IN SHOULDER PAIN SYNDROMES

A **framework of questions** is useful when approaching pain syndromes. With practice, a mental framework of questioning will become automatic.

1. Are there any **red flags?** e.g. unstable fractures, urgent neurological presentations, urgent vascular presentations, acute/serious infection and undiagnosed malignancies.
2. Any history of **trauma or sporting injuries?** Causing possible fractures, joint injuries, muscle and ligament injuries. Bear in mind that injuries can occur without any trauma in the older age group e.g. falling on outstretched hands causing rotator cuff tears.
3. Could the patient's **employment, sports and activities** have contributed to the presenting problem?
4. Is it **infective?** Unexplained pain with fever, abscess, septic arthritis, osteomyelitis.
5. Is it **osteoarthritis?** e.g. insidious in onset, 'I have had this shoulder pain for years', morning stiffness less than 30 minutes, pain worse with activities, improves with rest.
6. Is it an **inflammatory joint disease?** Typically, prolonged morning stiffness of greater than 30 minutes, pain worse with rest, improves with activities, other joint involvement.
7. Is it **gout?** Can affect joints and ligaments, thought to be underdiagnosed.[130,131]
8. Is it a **radiculopathy?** Pain fits the corresponding dermatomes, possible sensory and motor changes.
9. Is the pain from **muscle strain/myofascial trigger points?** This can give rise to referred pain.
10. Is it a **neuralgia?** e.g. neuralgia in the brachial plexus and post herpetic neuralgia.
11. Is it a **tumour (benign or malignant) or a cyst?** e.g. primary or metastatic cancer, synovial cysts.
12. Is the pain coming from **neighbouring structures?** e.g. C5 facet joint arthritis can cause shoulder pain.
13. Is the pain coming from **distal pathologies?** e.g. liver pathologies giving right shoulder pain.

PAIN SYNDROMES OF THE SHOUDLER REGION

OSTEOARTHRITIS OF THE SHOULDER

Shoulder OA can be classified as primary or secondary. Primary shoulder osteoarthritis is the third most common osteoarthritic joint, after knee and hip. Secondary OA occurs after trauma, surgery, inflammatory conditions and osteonecrosis. Shoulder OA affects the glenohumeral joint and the acromioclavicular (AC) joint mostly. Arthritis in the AC joint is the more common of the two but is usually asymptomatic. Symptoms include stiffness and pain, which are worse on activity and improve with rest. Examination shows r**eduction in both active and passive ROM,** whereas rotator cuff disease (RCD) only has restricted active ROM. There may be crepitus on shoulder movement.

It is important to emphasise that, like any other joints, the diagnosis of OA being the cause of pain can only be made after excluding other conditions. If pain comes on relatively suddenly, or if there is a sudden increase in background pain, the pain is unlikely to be due to OA. Pain arising from TrPs can often override the original OA pain and become the dominant pain.

Treatments include conservative treatment of activity modification, strengthening exercises and heat; pharmacological trials of paracetamol, topical and oral NSAIDs; and intra-articular corticosteroid injections. As the shoulder is a non-weight-bearing joint, pain in arthritic shoulder joints is usually not severe. Many patients can live with shoulder arthritis for many years. In severe cases, arthroplasty can be successful. It includes total shoulder arthroplasty, reverse shoulder arthroplasty and shoulder hemiarthroplasty. According to the Australian Orthopaedic Association National Joint Replacement Registry, there were 62,624 knee replacements, 49,169 hip replacements and 7,827 shoulder replacements in 2020.[132]

SHOULDER JOINTS DYSFUNCTIONS

The shoulder joints include the acromioclavicular joint, the coracoclavicular joint, the glenohumeral joint, scapulothoracic joint and the sternoclavicular joints. They can all be subjected to sprains, subluxations, dislocations and arthritis (except the scapulothoracic joint). These can be detected by tenderness on targeted palpation.

LABRAL INJURY

The glenoid labrum can be injured through repetitive overhead movements (e.g. ball throwing, tennis serving), or trauma (e.g. fall on outstretched arm). The superior labrum anterior to posterior (SLAP) lesion being the most common. The gold standard of diagnosis is by magnetic resonance arthrography. Treatment includes conservative and surgical repair. SLAP repairs are rare except in high performance throwing athletes, which are few in Australia.

LONG HEAD OF BICEP DYSFUNCTION

Long head of bicep tendinopathy is usually associated with RCD or labral injuries, caused by mechanical force and extreme load. It causes anterior shoulder pain and there is localised tenderness on palpation.

INFLAMMATORY JOINT DISEASE

These include rheumatoid arthritis, reactive arthritis/Reiter's syndrome and psoriatic arthritis. They are characterised by early morning stiffness and pain >30 minutes, where pain improves with activity and worsens during periods of inactivity. There may be polyarthropathies.

GOUT

Gout can affect any joints in the body. In acute gout, patients present with rapid onset of severe pain, swelling and erythema of the affected joint, tendon or bursa. Definitive diagnosis is by the presence of monosodium urate crystals in joint aspirations.

POLYMYALGIA RHEUMATICA

It presents with a symetrical bilateral hip and shoulder pain, weakness and reduced ROM, and prolonged morning stiffness. CRP and ESR are almost always elevated; in one study, it was found to be high in 72.2% and 83.3% of the patients with polymyalgia rheumatica, respectively.[133]

DISLOCATION

The majority (90%) of cases are traumatic anterior dislocation, when the patient's shoulder is forcefully abducted and externally rotated.[134] An MRI should be organised to assess the structural damages to formulate the management plan. Usually, if the patient is younger than 30, has complicated injuries, engaged in competitive sports or has recurrent re-dislocations, surgical repair should be considered. On the other hand, someone over 30 with uncomplicated injuries can be treated conservatively.[135]

METASTASIS

It is worth noting that the proximal humerus is a common site of metastasis, estimated at 7% of all metastatic sites.[136]

FROZEN SHOULDER (ADHESIVE CAPSULITIS)

Its etiology remains unclear but is thought to be due to an immune response. The pathology is thought to be inflamed and thickened glenohumeral joint capsule and synovium. Frozen shoulder follows the sequence of freezing, frozen and defrosting phases, typically lasting 18–30 months. A degree of residual dysfunction often remains after recovery.

History

Sometimes preceded by trauma or without any obvious cause. It is characterised by global and progressive restriction of range of movement (ROM), and night pain. It is more common in women over 40. Its incidence is much higher in diabetic patients. It is worth checking for diabetes in patients with frozen shoulder.

Examination

Restricted and painful movement in at least two planes, usually external rotation plus abduction and/or internal rotation. **The ROM is restricted in both active and passive movements,** whereas RCD is restricted only in active but not in passive movements. The patient would experience no pain within a certain limited ROM, but would have **'end range over pressure pain'.**

Investigations

Diagnosis is usually more clinical than radiological. A plain X-ray is advisable to exclude other pathologies. MRI is rarely required; it may show thickening of glenohumeral joint capsule and synovium.

Treatment

Treatment includes doing nothing, gentle mobilisation, oral prednisone, intra-articular corticosteroid injection, manipulation under anaesthesia, and open surgical or arthroscopic release; none of which have consistent success. Intensive physical treatments usually make the condition worse. Patients should be reassured that the condition will gradually improve with time, which is probably the best approach.

SUBACROMIAL BURSITIS

The subacromial bursa is situated between the acromion and the distal end of the supraspinatus. It can become inflamed and swollen when there is excessive movement and friction between the two, for example, sporting activities such as swimming or tennis, or any repetitive aggravation. Bursitis can occur with supraspinatus tendinitis and tears. Again, like other conditions such as OA or supraspinatus tears, imaging findings of bursitis do not necessarily indicate that the pain is due to it.

History

Trauma, onset and duration is important. Occupation and sporting activities also need to be noted.

Examination

Painful arc sign, Hawkins impingement sign and positive external rotation lag test together point to RCD.

Investigations

Investigations include a plain X-ray to exclude spurs, ultrasound will show bursitis or tendinopathy. Like RC tears, a high percentage of patients with imaging evidence of bursitis are asymptomatic. Therefore, **treat the patient, not the imaging findings.**

Treatment

Trial some gentle manual therapy and exercises first. If that fails, follow with a course of NSAIDs, then ultrasound-guided injection.

Cervical radiculopathy and cervical facet joint arthropathy can cause pain in the shoulder region as well. These will be discussed in the neck region.

The distribution of pain from myofascial trigger points from the neck/shoulder/arm region, cervical nerve root radiculopathies and cervical facet joint arthropathies can sometimes overlap. For example, a latissimus dorsi trigger point pain versus a C8 nerve root radiculopathy versus a lower cervical facet joint arthropathy. However, there are individual features that can differentiate them (see Table 1).

ROTATOR CUFF DISEASE

Of all musculoskeletal (MSK) presentations in general practice, shoulder problems are the third most common. Amongst shoulder problems, rotator cuff disease (RCD) is the most common.[137]

Rotator cuff muscles include:

S Supraspinatus (abduction of the arm)
I Infraspinatus (external rotation of the arm)
T Teres minor (external rotation of the arm)
S Subscapularis (internal rotation of the arm)

Posterior View

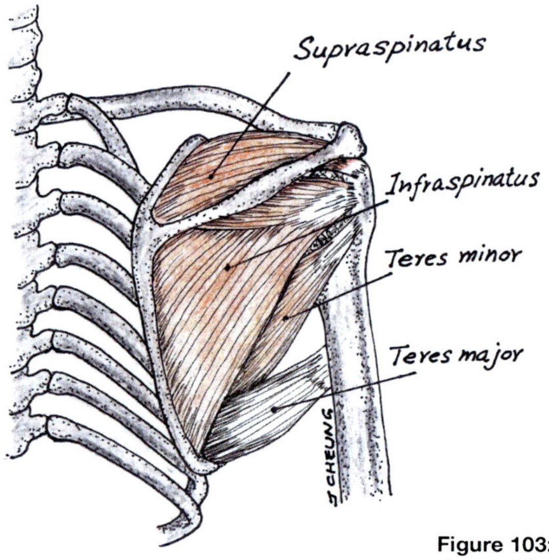

Figure 103: Posterior and anterior views of the rotator cuff muscles

Anterior View

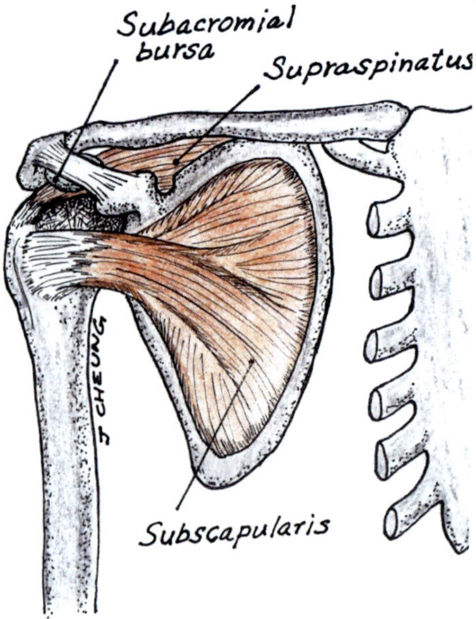

Rotator cuff disease includes

- RC muscle strain
- RC muscle tendinopathy
- RC muscle tears (partial or full thickness)

These can occur when:

1. the muscular contraction is restricted forcefully due to, for example, lifting a weight, a heavy shopping bag or falling on outstretched hands; or
2. repetitive strain from, for example, sporting or occupational activities.

In the older age group, when natural degeneration sets in, much less force is needed to cause a tear. In fact, often there are no obvious history of injuries. It is not uncommon to have tear progression after a partial tear – one study shows this to occur in 80% of cases after two years.[138]

History

Trauma, sporting and occupational activities, onset and duration and presence of constitutional symptoms would point to a different diagnosis. Pain level (visual analogue scale VAS), degree of disability and the biopsychosocial model should also be considered. One needs to exclude symptoms of referred pain from other shoulder muscles and the neck. Profession, handedness and sporting activities are important.

Examination

Look for RC muscle wasting. It is important to record the range of movement of the shoulder for future reassessment. The RC muscles can be palpated for tenderness and trigger points.

There are 21 clinical tests for RCD. Consensus agrees that painful arc sign, Hawkins impingement sign and positive external rotation lag test together point to RCD, but these tests cannot differentiate between RC strain, tendinosis, tears or subacromial bursitis. Painful arc sign, drop arm sign and positive external rotation lag test together point to a full thickness rotator cuff tear with high degree of likelihood ratio.[139,140] Weakness and pain in external rotation while the shoulder is in adduction is also one of the best signs of any rotator cuff pathologies. Like most MSK conditions, a cluster of tests is needed for diagnosis.

In RCD, the ROM is only restricted in active movements, not in passive movements. Whereas both are restricted in shoulder OA and frozen shoulder.

Some Shoulder Clinical Tests

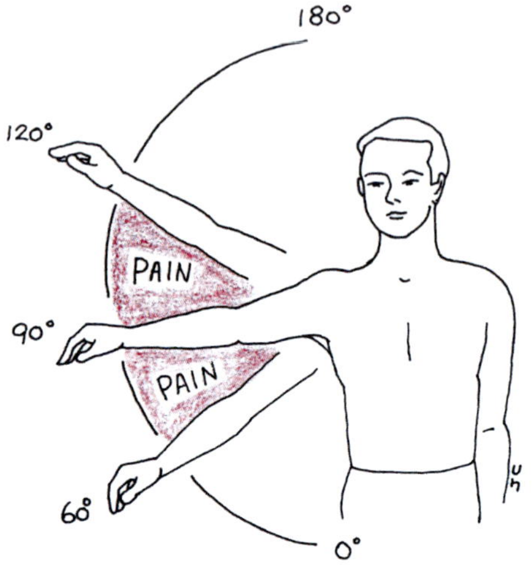

Figure 104: Painful Arc Test – Patient abducts arm from 0 to 180. Positive test: pain between 60 and 120 indicates subacromial or rotator cuff disorder.

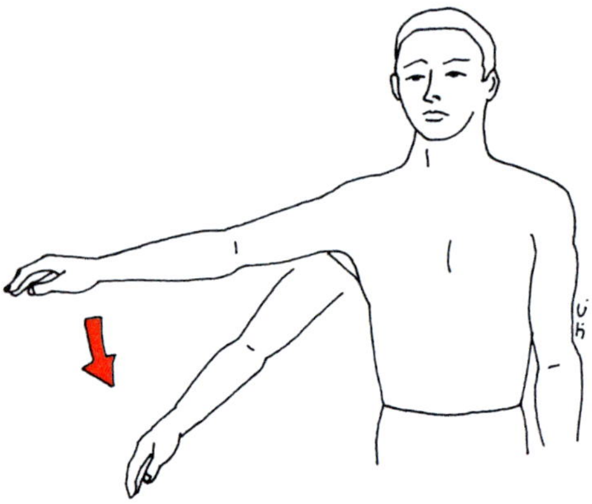

Figure 105: Drop Arm Test – Patient is asked to lower arm slowly from maximum abduction. Positive test: immediate drop of arm and pain.

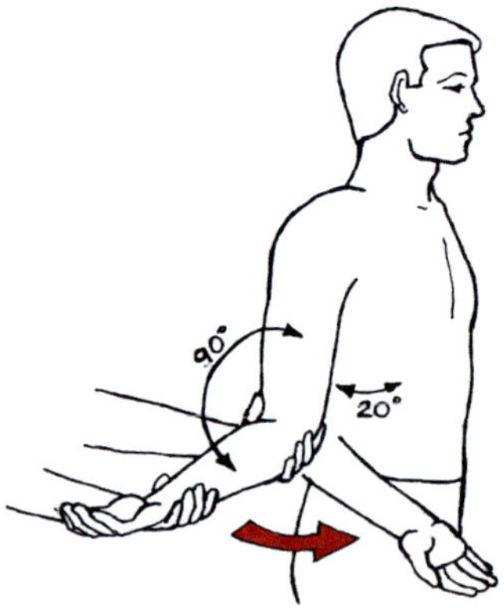

Figure 106: External Rotation Lag Test –

Examiner passively rotates the patient's arm into full external rotation and asks the patient to maintain that position.

Positive test: the patient is unable to maintain the position of full external rotation, and the arm swings back to a forward position.

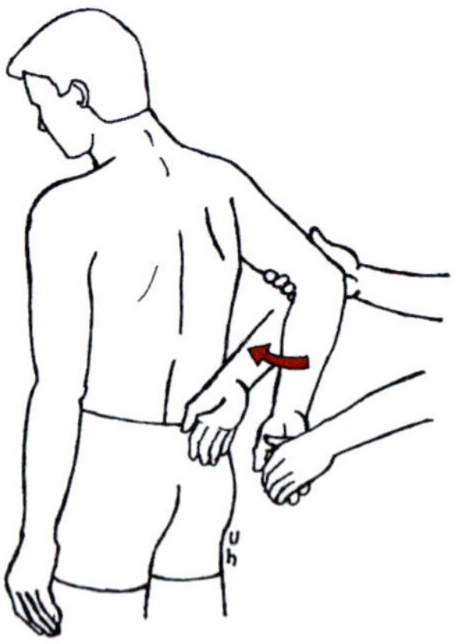

Figure 107: Internal Rotation Lag Test –

The hand is lifted off the back by the examiner and the patient is asked to maintain that position.

Positive test: the patient is unable to maintain the position, the arm just swings towards the back.

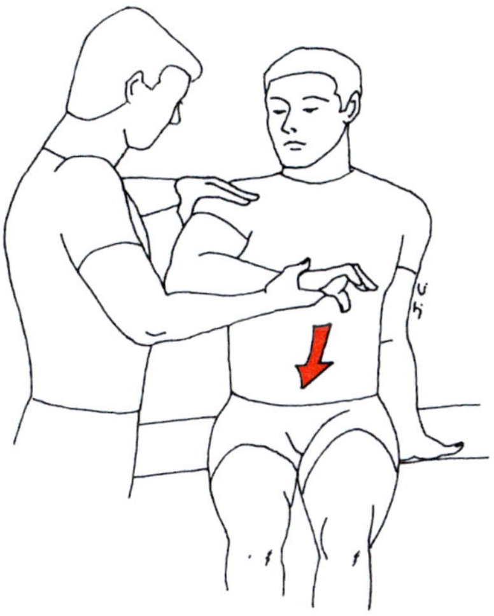

Figure 108: Hawkins Test –

Patient's elbow flexed to 90° and shoulder held at 90° flexion, the examiner internally rotates the shoulder.

Positive test: pain

Investigations

Plain X-ray to exclude OA, spurs, fractures, lytic and sclerotic lesions. If surgery is contemplated, MRI is necessary for diagnosis, as ultrasound on rotator tears are often inaccurate. One cannot assume that shoulder pain is from RC tear just because imaging shows it – as one study found that 65.3% of RC tears were asymptomatic.[141] Treat the patient, not the radiological findings.

OTHER SHOULDER MUSCLE PROBLEMS

The RC muscles are not the only muscles that can cause shoulder pain. I can count more than 10 other muscles attached to the shoulder area that can cause pain in the shoulder region.

My approach is that, for any shoulder pain, after excluding the red-flag diagnosis, it is worthwhile looking for any TrPs and treating them.

Basically, TrPs can result from either a traumatic injury to the muscle, constant contraction of the muscle due to repetitive activities, or continuing activation to protect a nearby painful joint or structure.

Finding trigger points (TrPs) and treating them successfully can

- **eradicate the pain completely (when the TrPs are the cause);**
- **improve some of the pain (as the TrPs cause some of the pain);**
- **exclude TrPs as the cause of the pain, then move on to consider other possible diagnoses; and**
- **often avoid expensive imaging or invasive treatments.**

Whatever the pathology may be, whether it is OA, muscular, ligamentous or cartilaginous tears, or bursitis, they can strain the numerous muscles in the area, thus, causing pain. These trigger-point pains can often become the dominant pain, over and above the original pathologies.

Treatment modalities of TrPs include various manual therapies, massages, exercises (for example yoga, designated stretches, strengthening, mobilising, neuromuscular programs), heat, older traditional methods (for example, acupuncture and cupping) and newer methods (for example, photobiomodulation/lower-level laser light therapy). Logically, these should be tried first before medications and invasive techniques.

Cervical radiculopathies and cervical facet joint arthropathies can cause pain in the shoulder region as well. This will be discussed in the neck segment.

FRAMEWORK OF QUESTIONING IN NECK PAIN SYNDROMES

A **framework of questions is useful** when approaching pain syndromes. With practice, a mental framework of questioning will become automatic.

1. Are there any **red flags?** e.g. unstable fractures, urgent neurological presentations, urgent vascular presentations, acute/serious infection and undiagnosed malignancies.
2. Any history of **trauma or sporting injuries?** Causing possible fractures, joint injuries, muscle and ligament injuries. Bear in mind that injuries can occur without any trauma in the older age group e.g. Falls and MVAs.
3. Could the patient's **employment, sports and activities** have contributed to the presenting problem? E.g. office worker who works long hours on the computer.
4. Is it **infective?** Unexplained pain with fever, abscess, septic arthritis, osteomyelitis.
5. Is it **osteoarthritis?** e.g. insidious in onset, 'I have had this neck pain for years', morning stiffness less than 30 minutes, pain worse with activities, improves with rest.
6. Is it an **inflammatory joint disease?** Typically, prolonged morning stiffness of greater than 30 minutes, pain worse with rest, improves with activities, other joint involvement.
7. Is it **gout?** Can affect joints and ligaments, thought to be underdiagnosed.[142,143]
8. Is it a **radiculopathy?** Pain fits the corresponding dermatomes, possible sensory and motor changes.
9. Is the pain from **muscle strain/myofascial trigger points?** This can give rise to referred pain.
10. Is it a **neuralgia?** e.g. neuralgia in the occipital nerves and post herpetic neuralgias.
11. Is it a **tumour (benign or malignant) or a cyst?** e.g. primary or metastatic cancer, synovial cysts.
12. Is the pain coming from **neighbouring structures?** e.g. neck pain from cervical lymphadenopathy.
13. Is the pain coming from **distal pathologies?** e.g. cervical spinal metastasis.

PAIN SYNDROMES OF THE NECK REGION AND CERVICOGENIC HEADACHES

Neck pain is the fourth leading cause of disability after back pain, depression and arthralgias. Approximately half of the population will have a clinically significant neck pain over their lifetime and annual prevalence is more than 30%.[144] Like lower back pain, most neck pains will resolve within a relatively short time. Doctors are likely to be presented with more severe cases or chronic ones.

OSTEOARTHRITIS OF THE NECK

It is a very common cause of neck pain, its incidence increasing with age and more so with previous injuries, such as whiplash accidents, falls and sporting injuries. Imaging of the neck after 40 years of age would invariably show evidence of OA, however, it does not mean that any neck pain is caused by it. As mentioned earlier, the severity of OA on imaging has a poor correlation to the degree of pain or, indeed, whether it is the cause of the pain. **There are far too many instances when patients are given a diagnosis of OA for their neck pain simply due to the imaging findings.**

Most clinicians would agree that the pain and dysfunction of an arthritic joint deteriorates very gradually. Consequently, if a patient presents with a relatively sudden onset of pain or a sudden increase of pre-existing pain, with or without a history of injury, we cannot just assume it is from OA. Muscle and ligamentous injury and strain must also be considered. Only after the **soft tissue causes of neck pain** have been addressed can OA be considered as the cause.

Symptoms

Patients describe a gradual deterioration of dull neck pain, restricted and painful ROM of the neck. It is worse in the morning, settling somewhat under 30 minutes – except for inflammatory joint disease, which usually takes more than 30 minutes). Movements of the neck, such as turning to reverse the car or looking up, can cause pain. The pain has often been present for years and is gradually getting worse. If arthritis in the facet joints is the cause of the pain, there may be pain in the occipital area, neck and upper back, but not adhering to any dermatomal distributions. Other joints in the same patient may have some arthritis.

Examination and Diagnosis

There may be a reduction of ROM, pain on movement, tenderness on palpation over the facet joints or overlying deep paravertebral muscles. Heberden's nodes and signs of other OA joints would add to the diagnosis. Examination and clinical tests excluding other conditions.

Tests

Imaging includes X-ray, CT scan and MRI.

Treatment

Start off with stretching, loosening exercises and manual therapies. Pharmaceutically, paracetamol, topical NSAIDs and/or oral NSAIDs can be tried. Facet joints, if implicated, can be treated with intra-articular corticosteroid injections, medial branch blocks and ablations (see next section). If the pain is mainly arising from inflammation in the intervertebral joints, these invasive treatments are ineffective. Opioids are not recommended as treatment for OA.

CERVICAL RADICULOPATHY

The pathology is compression or irritation of the nerve root caused by a disc bulge or herniation, ligamentum flavum hypertrophy and any causes leading to a narrowing of the neural foramina or lateral recesses, such as a disc height reduction, vertebral osteophytic encroachment, facet joint arthritis, facet joint synovial cyst or tumours. Incidence ranges between 0.832 and 1.79 per 1000-person year from two high-quality studies and one low-quality study.[145]

Symptoms

Neuropathic pain and/or parathaesia radiation in dermatomal distribution, with or without muscle weakness. Muscle weakness may involve the shoulder, elbow movements, supination, pronation and grip.

In radiculopathy, when the nervous tissue is irritated by firm structures such as the disc, osteophyte, cyst or ligamentum flavum, the pain tends to be more constant and severe than a myofascial pain referred from a nearby muscle e.g. latissimus dorsi (see Table 1).

Examination

Muscle weakness, reflex changes and sensation changes.

Table 4: The Most Common Vertebral Levels Affected in Cervical Radiculopathies

	Muscle Weakness	**Reflex Changes**
C4 (<10%)	None	Biceps, brachioradialis
C5 (10%)	Shoulder abduction, elbow flexion	Biceps, brachioradialis
C6 (20–25%)	Biceps, brachioradialis	Triceps
C7 (45–60%)	Elbow extension, wrist flexion	Triceps
C8 (10%)	Finger grip	Triceps

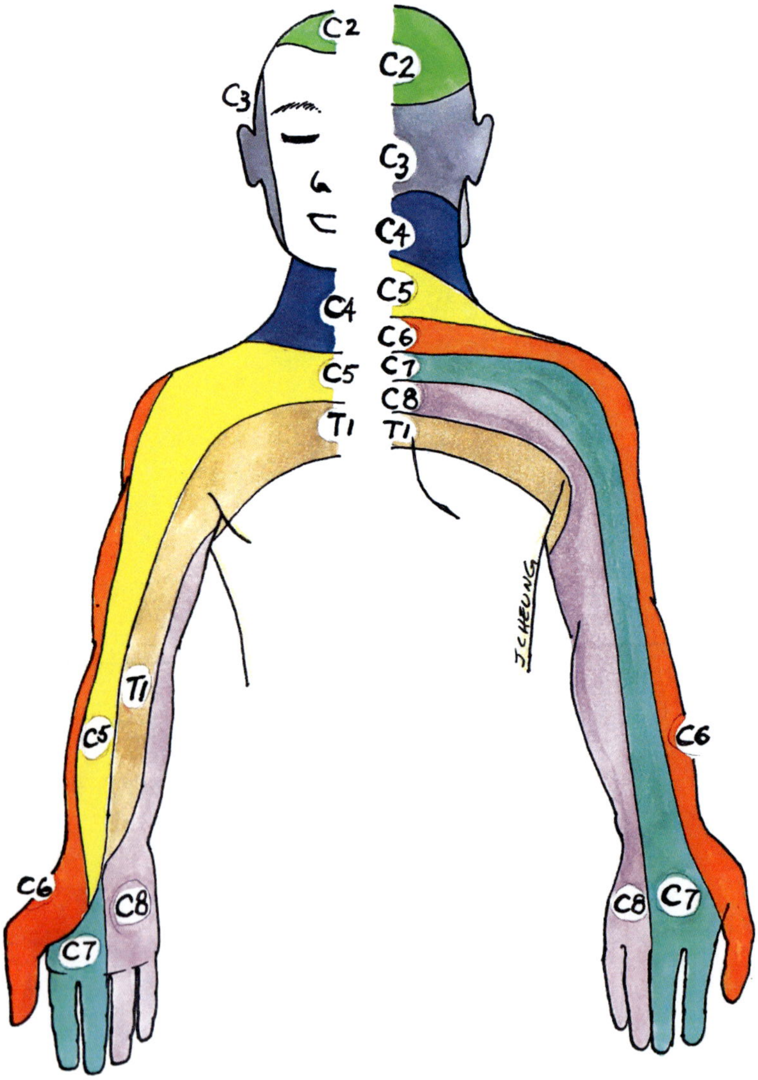

Figure 109: Cervical nerve dermatomes

Table 5: One Simple Way to Remember Reflexes

Ankle	S	1
Knee	L	2, 3, 4
Biceps	C	5, 6
Triceps	C	7, 8

Investigations and Diagnosis

MRI provides the most accurate assessment. However, unless findings in CT and MRIs are significant and obvious, they may not be conclusive. Imaging often includes multiple probable sites of impingements, and one still needs to rely on pain distributions and physical examination findings to confirm the exact causative site.

The pain distributions of cervical radiculopathies, myofascial trigger points in the neck and shoulder and lower cervical facet joint pain can sometimes overlap. However, there are features that can differentiate them (see Table 1).

Treatment

Conservative measures should be trialled first. Unless there are indications for prompt surgical intervention, such as:

1. dysfunction of bowel and bladder control (in myelopathy);
2. significant and progressive muscle weakness; and/or
3. prolonged periods of severe intractable pain despite optimal therapeutic treatments.

A course of NSAIDs can be tried, which may reduce the oedema of an inflamed and swollen facet joint impinging on the nerve root. Paracetamol may help the pain. Manual therapies and massages may loosen tight shoulder and neck muscles, thus, reducing the traction on nerves and thereby easing the irritation at the nerve root. The next step would be a targeted CT-guided injection whether it is intra-facet, peri-foraminal or epidural. This can be both therapeutic and diagnostic, to determine whether the targeted injection at the specific level relieves the pain. It is usually performed by an interventional radiologist who specialises in such procedures. It is a safe procedure, however, the risks are more substantial for patients on anticoagulants.

As in the lumbar radiculopathy, surgical intervention is superior to conservative treatment in pain relief and restoring function in the short and medium term but is no different in the long term.[146]

CERVICAL FACET JOINT ARTHROPATHY

Cervical facet joints have been well established in the literature as a common source of axial neck pain, with an estimated prevalence of 25–66%.[147]

It can be degenerative or traumatic. In one study, cervical facet joint pain is estimated to be the cause in 54–60% of neck pain following whiplash injuries.[148] It is estimated that the joint space capacity is 1–2 ml. Its innervation comes from the medial branch of the posterior rami of the spinal nerve. Each facet joint has a dual nerve supply from the spinal nerve at the same level and the level above.

Symptoms

Pain distributions are different to that of the cervical nerve dermatomes, where facet joint pain tends to be more axial in distribution and rarely extends past the elbow. They do not usually have associated sensations of numbness as in radiculopathies. There is no muscle weakness or clumsiness in the arm or finger activities (see Table 1).

NB. The pain distribution of intervertebral arthropathies and injuries are thought to be similar to that of the facet joints of the same levels.

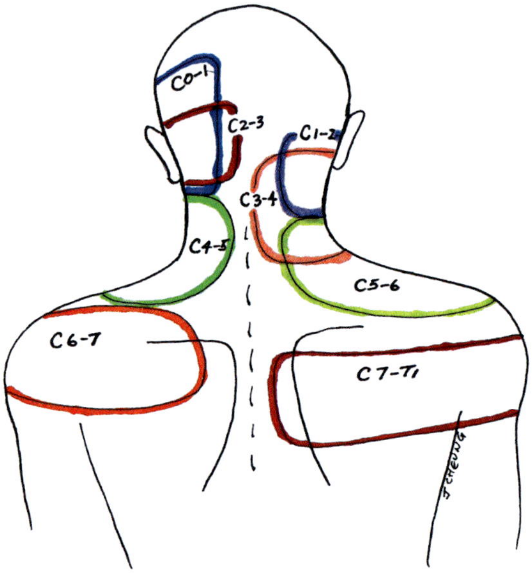

Figure 110: Patterns of referred pain from cervical facet joints

Examination

1. ROM may be reduced
2. Extension-rotation test: with the neck fully extended, rotate the neck to both sides (thus loading the facet joints), the test is positive if pain is exacerbated
3. With the patient prone, localised pain when pressing on the articular pillars from C2-3 to C6-7, points to facet joint arthropathies,
4. With the patient prone, palpate for tenderness of segmental muscles overlying the facet joints; these muscles share the same nerve supply as the facet joints

Investigations

Plain X-ray, CT, MRI and bone scan. In many instances, X-ray, CT or MRI would show multiple-level facet joint arthropathy, making it difficult to determine which one is causing the pain. If a CT-guided facet joint injection is contemplated, a bone scan with single photon emission computed tomography (SPECT) would help to clarify which facet joint(s) are 'hot' to inject (by detecting dynamic osteoblastic activities that are active with inflammation).

Treatment

Again, conservative measures should be trialled first. Topical NSAIDs, a course of paracetamol or oral NSAIDs can be used. Manual therapies, massage therapies, stretching and loosening exercises can be employed as well, to cover the possibility that the pain may have been muscular rather than acetogenic in the first place.

If pain persists and is significant, and a bone scan with SPECT can identify a likely facet joint to target, a CT-guided intra-articular corticosteroid/LA injection can be administered. However, even with a favorable outcome, pain can recur some time after the successful injection. For a more lasting effect, radiofrequency medial branch ablation or medial branch cryoablation can be performed, preceded by a testing medial branch block. Systemic review of radiofrequency medial branch ablation in treating chronic neck pain has level two evidence in efficacy.[149,150,151]

Cervical radiculopathy, osteoarthritis and muscular strain (trigger points). These three conditions share some common features in that the pain can be in the head, neck and shoulder regions; and can radiate down the arm. However, there are clinical features that can help us to differentiate them. Please refer to Table 1.

While OA, radiculopathy, trigger points and neuralgias share some common features, they can be differentiated (see Table 1).

Table 1: Different Neuromuscular Pains

	Nerve root impingement	**Peripheral nerve entrapment**	**Facet joint arthropathy**	**Muscular myofascial trigger points**
Distribution of pain	Fits the dermatomes, tends to include the extremities in distribution	Area innervated by the nerve, can radiate along the course of the nerve	Fits the facet joint pain distributions, tends to be more axial in distribution, rarely passes the elbow or knees	The affected muscles, their attachment sites and adjacent areas (these can overlap with other causes of pain e.g. TrPs in Latissimus dorsi overlapping with C8 radiculopathy)
Nature of pain	Tends to be more constant, tends to be severe	Tends to be more constant, tends to be severe	Worse on movements, especially in extension and rotation (when the facet joints are loaded)	Tends to be intermittent, tends to be less severe, pain can be aggravated by certain movements when the affected muscles are activated
Numbness	Possible	Possible	Usually not	Possible
Muscle weakness and associated clumsy movements	Possible	Possible	Nil	Nil
Reflex changes	Possible	Rarely	Nil	Nil
Tenderness on palpation on the painful area	Nil	Can be tender at the site of impingement	Can be tender on the facet joint and the overlying intervertebral muscles	Tender trigger points of the relevant muscles
Useful clinical examination/ tests	Reflexes, power, sensation	Reflexes, power, sensation	Localised tenderness on palpating over the facet joints, extension – rotation test	Palpation of all the muscles in the painful area and adjacent muscles

Dr Joe Cheung

NB. The pain distribution of intervertebral joints/discs degeneration and injury is thought to be similar to that of facet joint arthropathy.

THORACIC OUTLET SYNDROME (TOS)

The incidence is 2–3/100,000 per year.[152] It consists of neurogenic, venous and arterial types. Neurogenic TOS accounts for more than 90% of all TOS cases.[153] Typically, TOS occurs in the 20–50- age group and more often in females. It is an impingement of the thoracic nerves (comprising of C5 to T1 nerve root) passing through the thoracic outlet. It can be caused by trauma (e.g. motor vehicle accident, fractured mid clavicle or whiplash injuries), repetitive injury, anatomical variations (e.g. cervical rib) or malignancy (e.g. compression effect).[154,155]

Symptoms

Upper limb and extremities heaviness, parathaesia with above-the-shoulder activities. There can also be associated pain in the neck, shoulder, arm, supraclavicular area, chest and occipital headaches.

Examination

There may be wasting of abductor pollicis brevis, hypothenar and interossei muscles. Clinical tests include Adson's test, upper limb tension tests (ULTTs) and elevated arm stress tests (EASTs). For EAST, the arms are placed in the surrender position, shoulder abducted to 90 degrees and in external rotation with the elbow flexed at 90 degrees. The patient slowly opens and closes their hands for three minutes. A positive test results in precipitation of heaviness, parathaesia, pain or weakness.[156]

Investigations

Investigations include:

- Imaging (CT, MRI, Ultrasound) which will identify cervical ribs, callus in previous clavicular fractures;
- nerve conduction studies;
- local anaethestic injection into anterior scalene muscle (to see if it abolishes symptoms).

Treatment

Conservative treatment of stretching, postural exercises and a muscle-strengthening regime should be trialled first. Injections of LA, steroids or Botox into anterior scalene and pectoralis muscle should be trialled before surgical options.

CERVICAL MYELOPATHY

The prototypical spinal cord injury is still commonly viewed as traumatic cord injury. However, the leading cause is actually degenerative cervical myelopathy (DCM). This is caused by age-related degenerative conditions such as disc herniation, spondylosis, osteophytic encroachment or posterior longitudinal ligament hypertrophy when the spinal cord is compressed. The incidence of DCM is estimated to be six in a million in Australia and rising as the age of the population increases.[157] In the early phases, the presentation is quite non-specific, making diagnosis difficult. It is rare but important to have a high level of suspicion for this condition, as early diagnosis and appropriate treatment gives a much better outcome. Other causes of cervical myelopathy include trauma and inflammation (myelitis).

Synptoms

- Neck pain
- Upper limb radicular pain
- Parathaesia in one or more extremities
- Unsteady gait
- Clumsiness with fine motor activities e.g. doing up buttons or writing
- Bowel and bladder control dysfunction (in very late stage)[158]

Examination

Gait imbalance, hand clumsiness, numbness and weakness. Fine motor dysfunction of hands, hyperreflexia, clonus and spasticity. Positive Babinski sign, positive Hoffman's sign (flexion of the thumb and index upon flicking the nail of the middle or ring fingers), positive Spurling's test (with the neck in extension, lateral flexion, axial compression reproduces symptoms in the extremities).

Investigations

MRI gives a definitive diagnosis. In early cases, a common differential diagnosis is carpal tunnel syndrome, when a nerve conduction study can differentiate the two.

Treatment

Depending on the causes and severity, DCM can be treated conservatively or surgically.

AUTOIMMUNE CAUSES OF NECK PAIN

There are a number of autoimmune diseases that can cause neck pain:

- Rheumatoid arthritis (RA) – cervical spine involvement is the second-most common features of RA, affecting more than half of all cases.[159,160]
- Axial spondyloarthritis (ankylosing spondylitis) – where neck pain and neck involvement are common
- Reactive arthritis (Reiter's syndrome) – occurs after a digestive or genital chlamydia infection. Typically, it involves an acute asymmetrical oligoarthritis of the large joints of the lower limb. Axial arthritis can occur at the cervical, thoracic and lumbosacral spine as well as sacroiliitis
- Scleroderma
- Myositis
- Psoriatic arthritis

Symptoms such as significant and prolonged morning stiffness, joint pain in areas other than the neck, and general mobility dysfunction help to diagnose autoimmune diseases. Blood tests may confirm the diagnosis.

GOUT

Axial gout has been estimated to affect 14–35% of patients with gouty arthritis.[161,162] In one study, it affected the cervical spine in 29% of the axial gout cases.[163] Symptoms include neck pain, back pain and radiculopathy. Imaging includes CT-scan evidence of erosions in the facet joints and/or tophi. It is thought to be under-diagnosed.

NECK MUSCULAR STRAIN

This entity will be covered in the cervicogenic headache section. Besides causing cervicogenic headaches, **I believe neck muscular strain is the most common cause of neck pain.**

OTHER NECK STRUCTURES GIVING NECK PAIN

Besides musculoskeletal causes, other causes include soft tissue trauma, various infections, lymphadenopathies, benign or malignant tumors, thyroid pathologies, upper GIT pathologies and oral dental problems.

RED FLAGS IN HEADACHES

Headaches have many causes, but before we look at cervicogenic headaches, we need to rule out any red flags (see Table 6).

Table 6: Headache Red Flags[164]

Sign or Symptom	Related Secondary Headaches
Systemic symptoms including fever	Headache attributed to infection or nonvascular intracranial disorders, carcinoid or pheochromocytoma
Neoplasm in history	Neoplasms of the brain; metastasis
Neurologic deficit or dysfunction (including decreased consciousness)	Headaches attributed to vascular, nonvascular intracranial disorders; brain abscess and other infections
Onset of headache is sudden or abrupt	Subarachnoid haemorrhage and other nonvascular intracranial disorders
Older age (after 50 years)	Giant cell arteritis and other headache attributed to cranial or cervical vascular disorders; neoplasms and other nonvascular intracranial disorders
Pattern change or recent onset of headache	Neoplasms, headaches attributed to vascular, nonvascular intracranial disorders
Positional headache	Intracranial hypertension or hypotension
Precipitated by sneezing, coughing, or exercise	Posterior fossa malformations; Chiari malformation
Papilledema	Neoplasms and other nonvascular intracranial disorders; intracranial hypertension
Progressive headache and atypical presentations	Neoplasms and other nonvascular intracranial disorders
Pregnancy or puerperium	Headaches attributed to cranial or cervical vascular disorders; postdural puncture headache; hypertension-related disorders (e.g. preeclampsia); cerebral sinus thrombosis; hypothyroidism; anaemia; diabetes
Painful eye with autonomic features	Pathology in posterior fossa, pituitary region, or cavernous sinus; Tolosa-Hunt syndrome; ophthalmic causes
Post-traumatic onset of headache	Acute and chronic post-traumatic headache; subdural haematoma and other headache attributed to vascular disorders
Pathology of the immune system such as HIV	Opportunistic infections
Painkiller overuse or new drug at onset of headache	Medication overuse headache; drug incompatibility

CERVICOGENIC HEADACHES (CH)

Neck problems are commonly overlooked as a potential cause of headaches. If you ask any 'hands on' health practitioners such as physiotherapists, osteopaths, massage therapists and beauticians who perform lots of facial massages, they will say that the neck has everything to do with headaches. If we all look out for neck injuries in the history and palpate the neck area diligently, doctors would come to that same realisation, especially in frequently recurring or continuous headaches.

It is of interest that a significant percentage of patients with marked abnormal physical findings in the neck (reduced ROM, tender muscle spasms) are unaware that they have any neck issues until it is demonstrated to them.

A lot of neck pathologies can cause headaches, e.g. trauma to the neck, cervical arthropathies including osteoarthritis, inflammatory joint diseases, cervical radiculopathies etc. These have been covered previously. I would now like to concentrate on cervicogenic headaches caused by TrPs (CHs – T) in the neck region.

I would like to classify CHs – T into two types:

1. **Mild and recent onset:** Without a significant trauma, more recent onset – probably caused by simple muscular strain resulting from sports, lying on the lounge watching TV, lengthy time spent on the laptop or the phone, or a restless night in bed.
2. **Severe and chronic:** With a history of significant trauma, for example, a serious car accident or a very bad fall **(recent or long ago)** – these headaches are **frequent, recurring or even continuous.** The headaches may have been going on for a while, even years. A minor aggravation of the neck has often preceded the onset of the headaches, with the patient unable to recall the original injury from long ago.

Symptoms

Often these patients do not have a past history of headaches at all, or may have had infrequent headaches or periodic classical migraines. Then, **suddenly, frequent or continuous headaches** begin. For patients with past history of classical migraines, these constant headaches from CHs – T are often unlike their typical migraines. Most 'tension headaches' develop well into the day and subside after a good sleep. CHs – T patients, however, tend to wake up with a headache, and episodes can last for days. CHs – T are typically suboccipital, radiating to the temporal and retro-orbital regions. Sometimes a newly acquired neck problem will trigger migraines from infrequent to frequent occurrence.

Examination

A targeted examination seals the diagnosis. The ROM is key and it is important to measure and record neck rotations, forward flexion, extension and side flexions. An asymmetrical ROM is important to note but not specific to CHs – T. Typically, the most common causative TrPs are found in the levator scapulae, trapezius (the section above the scapular spine), the sternocleidomastoid, the suboccipital muscle groups and the deeper posterior cervical muscles. Almost always, the TrPs are more prominent on one side, usually the side of the headaches. Often there are related TrPs in the supraspinatus, rhomboid and pectoralis major (clavicular section). They should all be noted and targeted for treatment.

Investigations

The diagnosis of CHs – T is usually clinical.

Treatment

Cervicogenic Headaches (Mild and Recent Onset) Most of these would probably resolve by themselves with time. Targeted trigger-point soft-tissue massages, stretching and loosening exercises (Fig. 176) would facilitate recovery. If recurrence occurs, encourage the patient to do daily neck stretching exercises. Sometimes these headaches can be caused by a reversible 'subluxed, jammed' facet joint, in which case a measured spinal adjustment or manipulation may be required by a manipulative physiotherapist or a trusted osteopath/chiropractor to treat the problem.

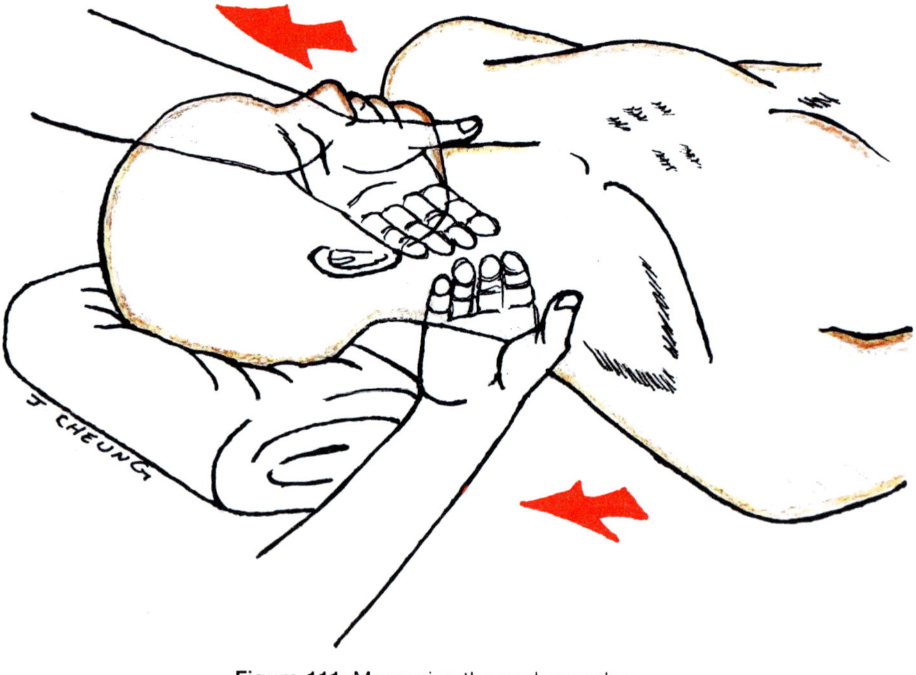

Figure 111: Massaging the neck muscles

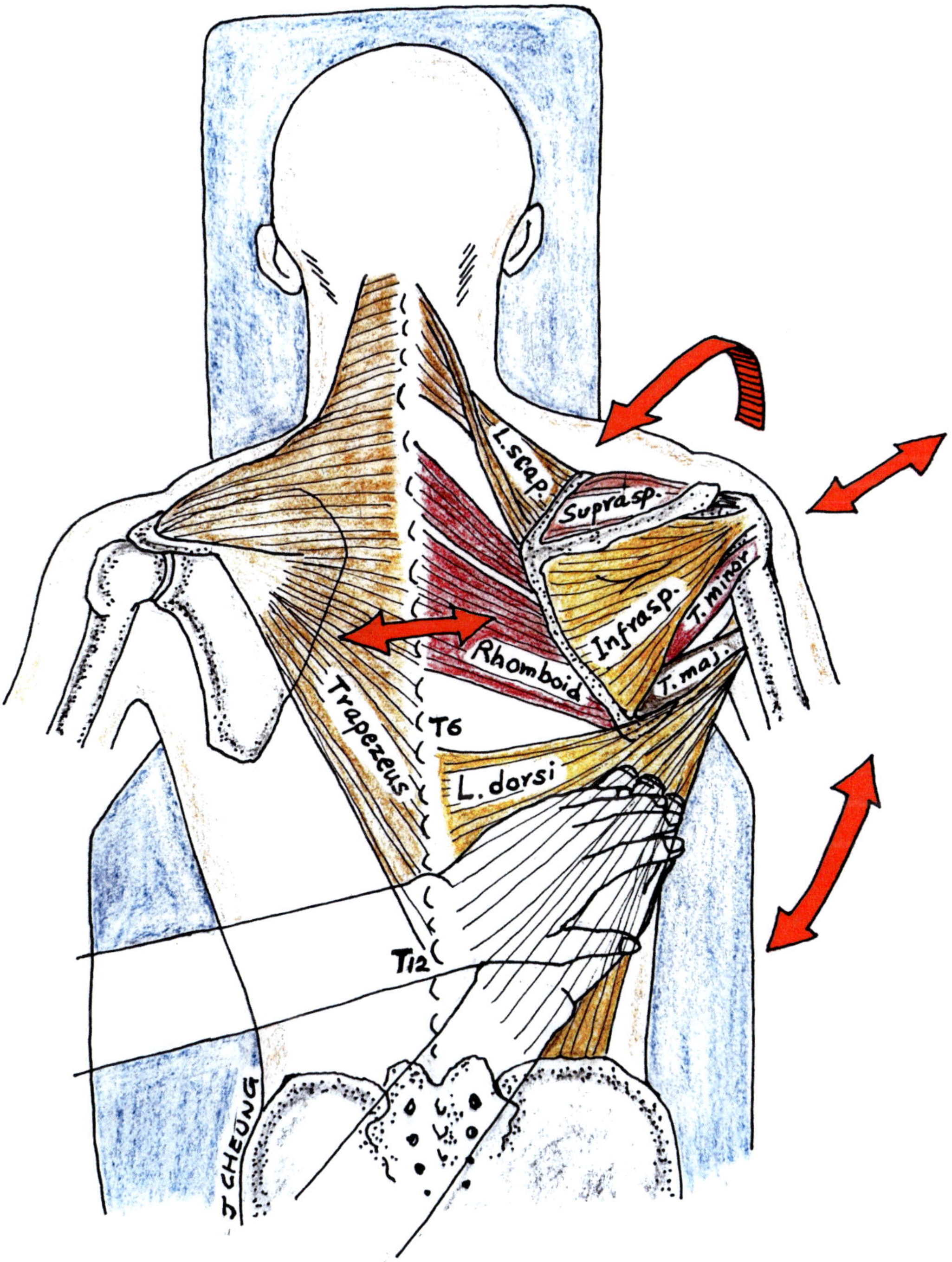

Figure 112: Massaging the shoulder and neck muscles

Cervicogenic Headaches (Severe and Chronic) These are very resistant to treatment. In one study, chronic cervicogenic headaches (CH) accounted for 33% of patients attending a pain clinic.[165] The majority of these patients have a serious whiplash injury or a significant head and neck trauma as the cause of the CH.

Various modalities are used: manual therapies, exercises, stretching programs, yoga, differentials, TENs, low-level laser therapies, acupuncture, 'dry needling', cupping, heat packs, tractions, intensive education program and psychological techniques. Pharmacologically, paracetamol, NSAIDs, muscle relaxants, opioids, antidepressants (tricyclics and SSRIs), anti-epileptics and anti-migraine medications can be trialled. Facet joints are treated with corticosteroid injections, medial branch blocks and ablations. Trigger points are injected with saline, hypertonic dextrose solutions, LA, corticosteroid, and three monthly multiple Botox injections (the PREEMPT protocol). The sheer number of different modalities implies that none are consistently effective.

There exists a complex relationship between chronic CH and migraines. First, the two can coexist. Neck dysfunction is a common trigger for migraines; long periods of sleep and bedrest with a migraine can aggravate the neck, and CH can be mistaken for migraines. Most clinicians who recognise the significance of CH would agree that any improvement on existing neck dysfunction would benefit the recurrence rate and severity of migraines.

A new treatment for chronic frequent migraines has become available through the PBS. After 40 years of research, Calcitonin gene-related peptide (CGRP) monoclonal antibodies have made a significant impact on patients with frequent migraines. It targets the CGRP that causes the headaches. These treatments can reduce the number of migraine days per month by half. Available through the PBS are erenumab, fremanezumab and galcanezumab.[166] However, these treatments are not curative, given by injection subcutaneously every month and the long-term side effect profiles are still uncertain.

The solution remains elusive for clinicians treating chronic, frequent CH who recognise the key is to eradicate the TrPs. For example, in a patient with chronic, frequent CH, some of these TrPs may have been there for 30–40 years. These TrPs are solid, hard 'lumps' up to the size of half a squash ball and resistant to all the above-mentioned treatments.

As indicated later on, I have found the YNSA treatment to be very effective in improving and often eradicating these cervicogenic headaches and the TrPs that cause them.

SOME FACIAL MUSCLES THAT CAN CAUSE HEADACHES

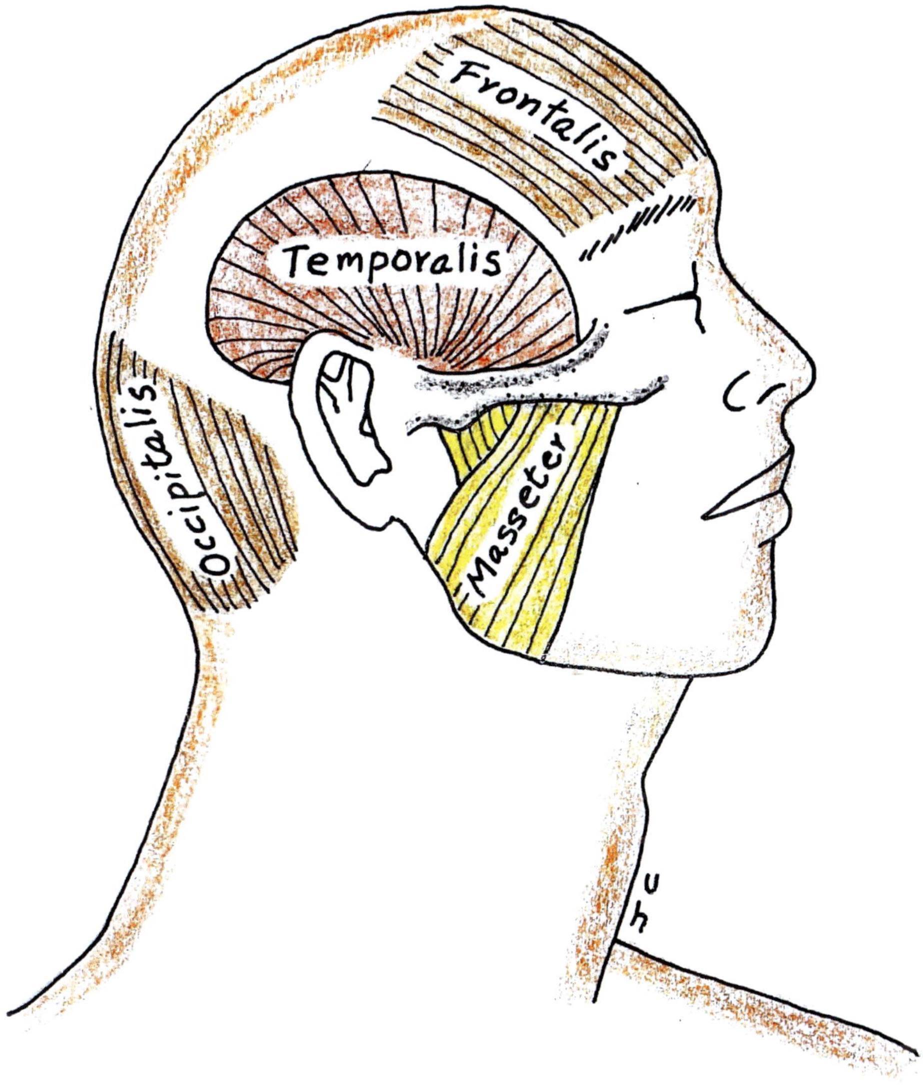

Figure 113: Diagram of common facial muscles that can cause headaches

POSITION OF THE PATIENT AND EXAMINER WHEN PALPATING THE SHOULDER AND NECK REGIONS

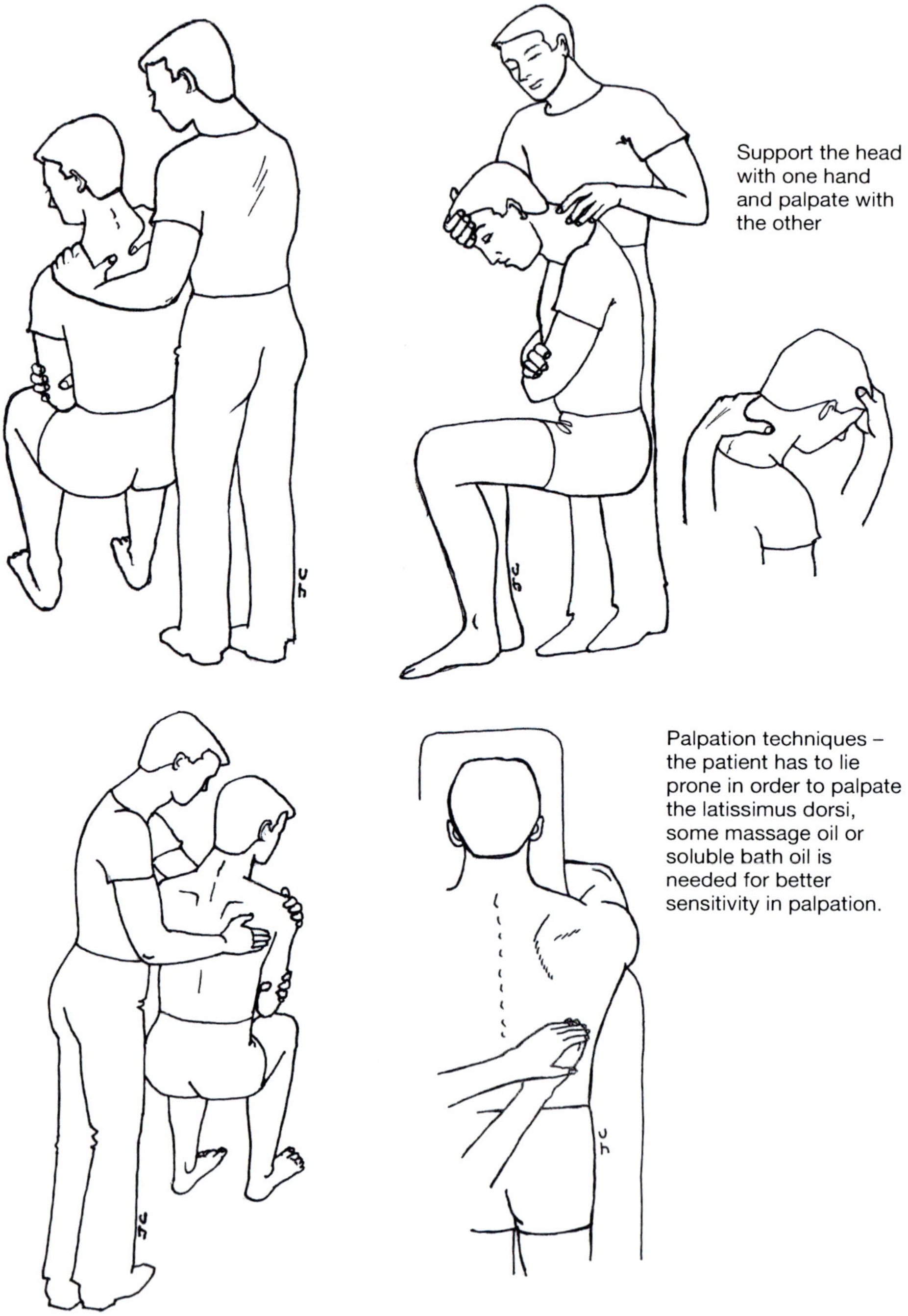

Figure 114: Palpation diagrams for examining the shoulder and neck

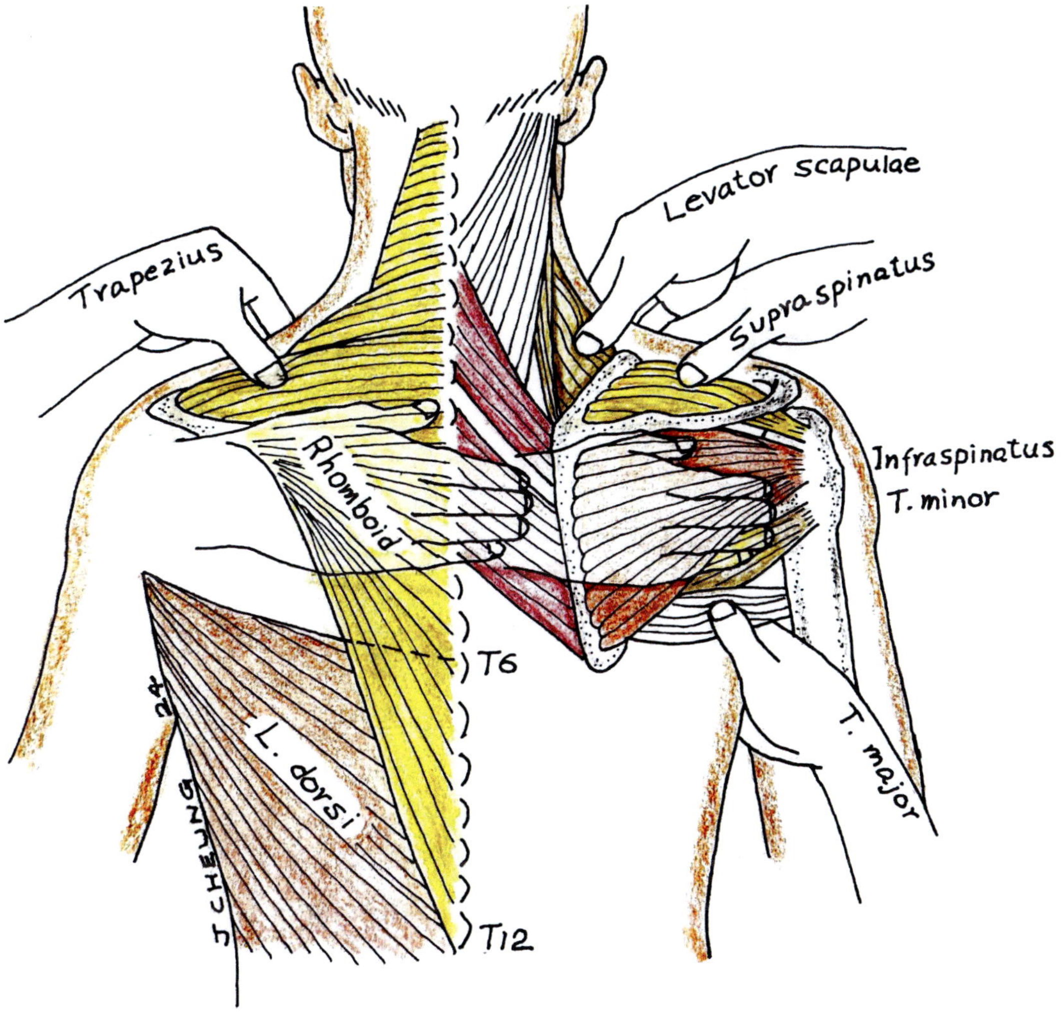

Figure 115: Palpation diagram for the TrPs in the shoulder and neck region

NB. Three short videos on TrP palpation techniques for the knee, lower back, neck/ shoulder regions are available on YouTube under joecheungYNSA, or visit http://www.joecheung.com.au

CASE STUDIES ON SHOULDER AND NECK PAIN

Most of the case studies (with some exceptions) utilise the modality of YNSA for treatment. This is only intended for readers who are interested in or practise the modality of acupuncture.

THE SUPRASPINATUS AND ITS TrPs

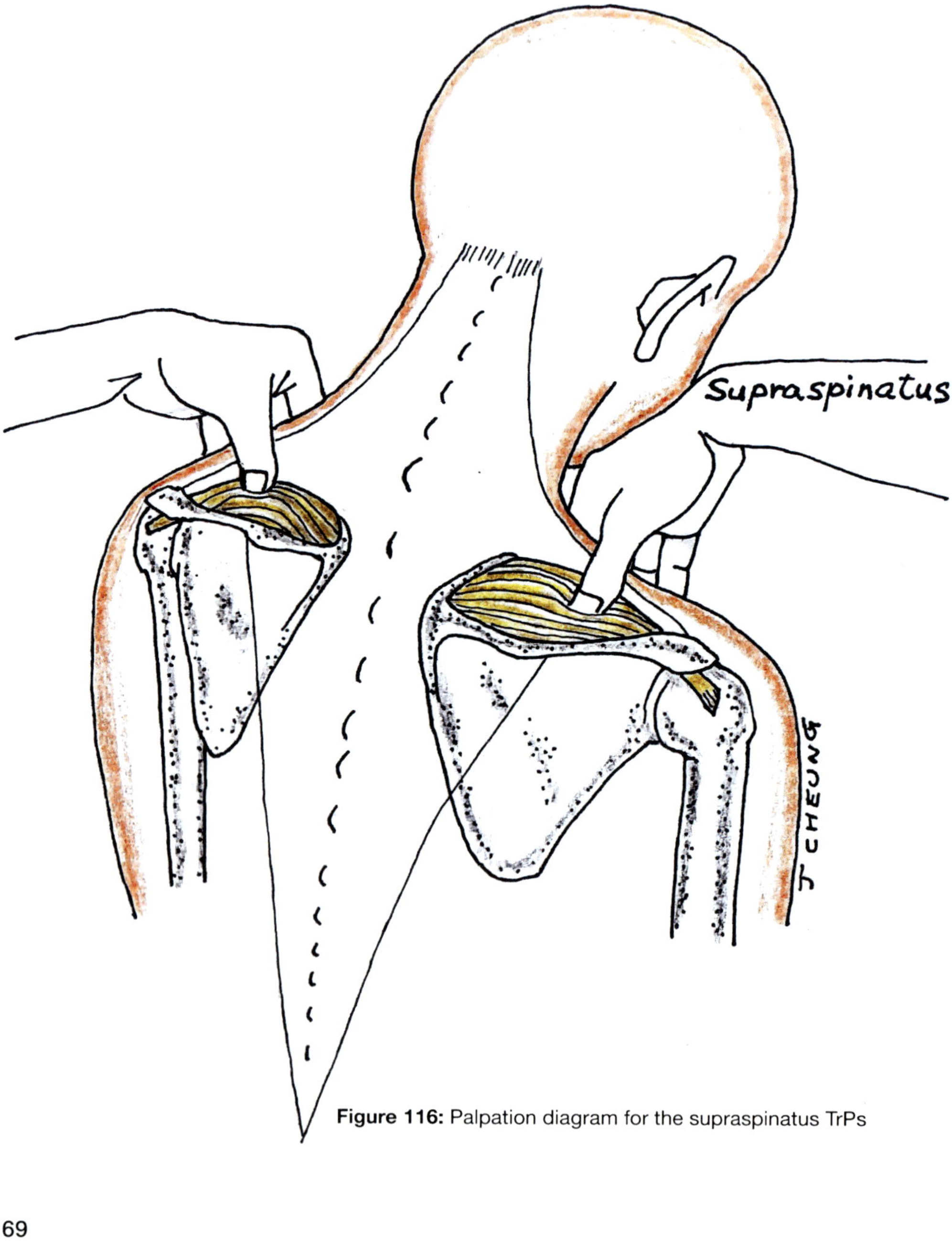

Figure 116: Palpation diagram for the supraspinatus TrPs

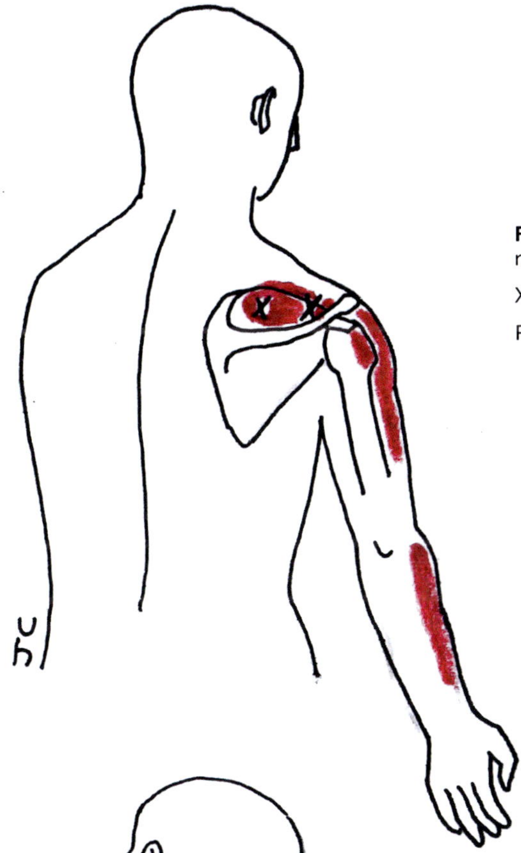

Figure 117: Supraspinatus TrPs and their referred pain pattern

X = TrPs

Red area = the referred pain

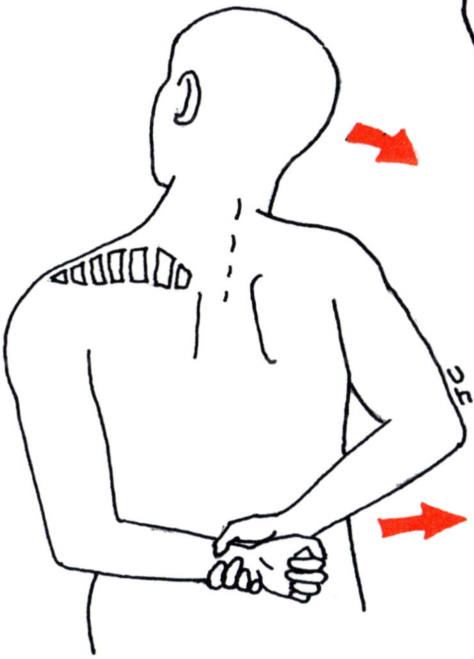

Figure 118: Useful stretch for the supraspinatus

THE INFRASPINATUS, TERES MINOR, TERES MAJOR AND RHOMBOID AND THEIR TrPs

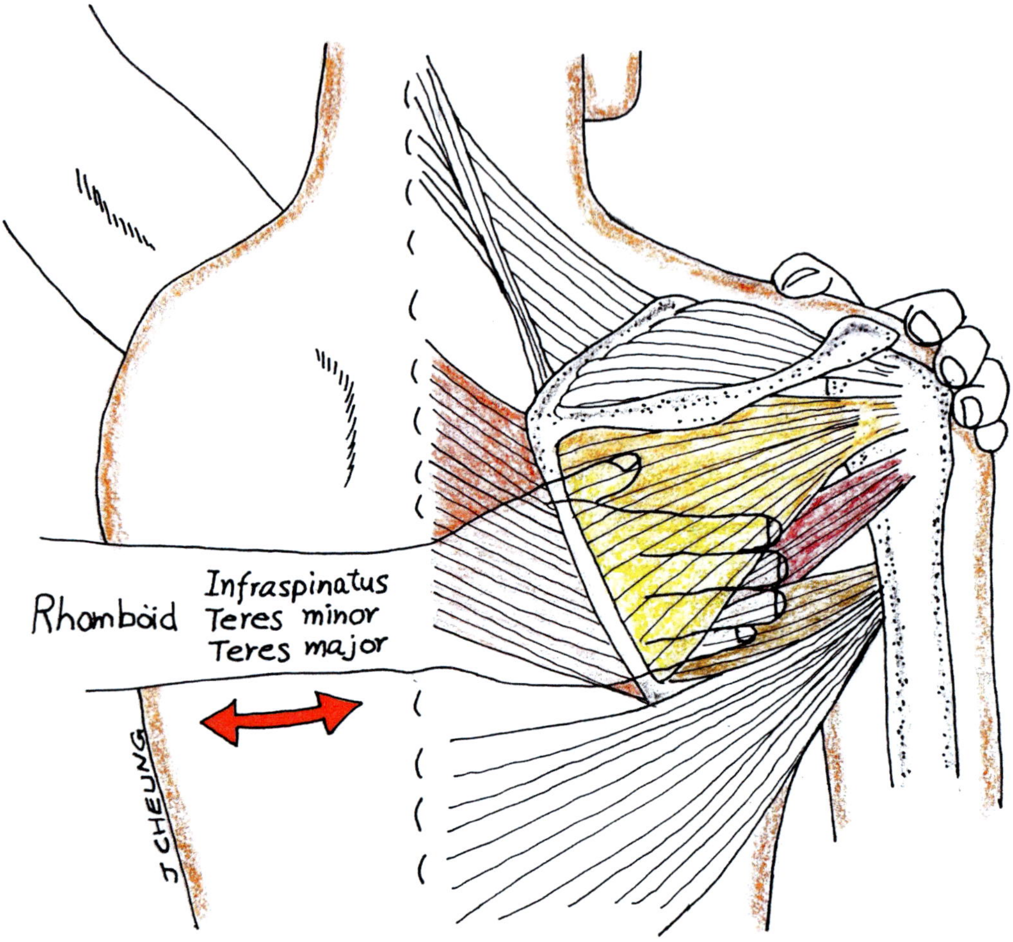

Figure 119: Palpation diagram for the infraspinatus, teres minor, teres major and rhomboid TrPs

NB. For any shoulder pain syndromes, it is important to palpate for TrPs in all the relevant muscles and eradicate them.

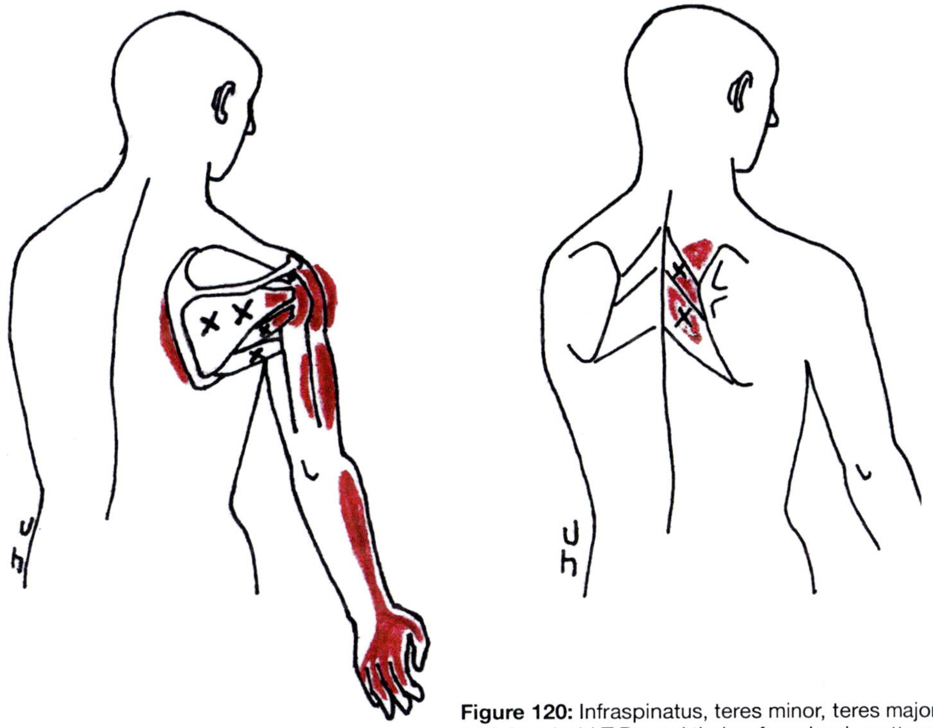

Figure 120: Infraspinatus, teres minor, teres major and rhomboid TrPs and their referred pain pattern

X = TrPs

Red area = the referred pain

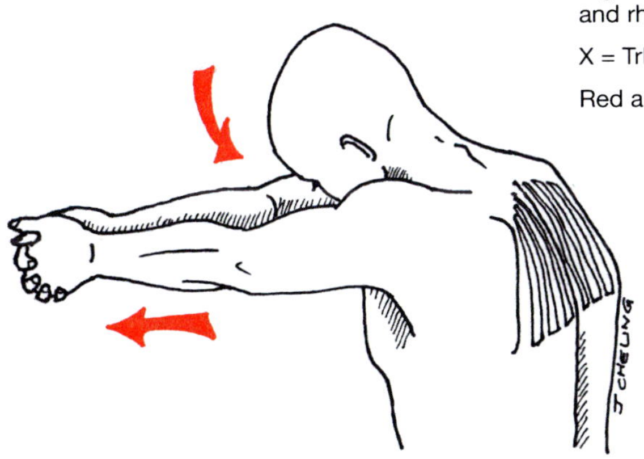

Figure 121: A useful stretch for the rhomboid

Figure 122: Loosening exercises for the internal and external rotators, using the unaffected arm to move the injured arm

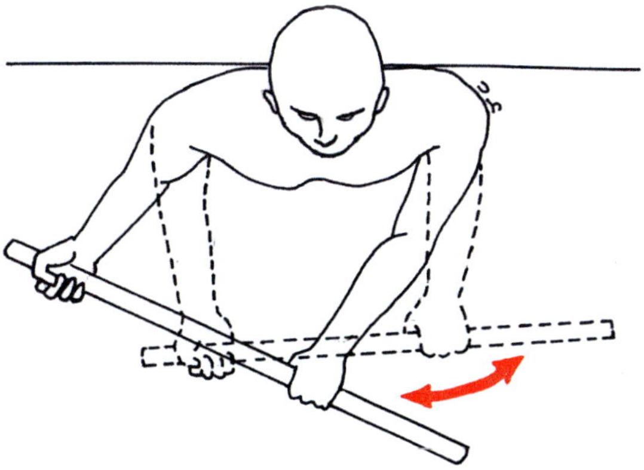

CASE STUDY 23 (left shoulder pain – left supraspinatus, infraspinatus, teres major, levator scapulae, rhomboid and the clavicular section of the pectoralis major TrPs, treated with YNSA)

HISTORY: A 55-year-old female office worker presented with a six-month history of moderate 4/10 left shoulder pain. She did not recall any specific injury. Shoulder movements were painful but she could hang clothes on the line and fasten her bra with some difficulty. The pain centred in the left shoulder, radiating down the outer border of the upper arm and at times the forearm. There was no parathaesia or weakness. She did not have any prolonged morning stiffness.

Her BMD was 29 and she was prediabetic, on HRT for menopausal symptoms, and had no other significant medical problems. X-ray showed minor arthritic changes and the ultrasound showed subacromial bursitis. Diclofenac helped the pain moderately when used but only for that day. Her GP referred her for a guided bursitis injection, which did not work. Her GP suggested a repeat injection in a few weeks. She was concerned about repeated corticosteroid injections that may trigger off the onset of diabetes and presented for a second opinion.

REASONING: With her age group and being prediabetic, frozen shoulder had to be considered. However, it was unlikely as the restricted ROM of a frozen shoulder tends to be progressive, and the patient's ROM had not changed in six months. The pain was not very aggressive and the absence of prolonged morning stiffness made inflammatory joint disease also unlikely. As her pain and limitation of movement were not significant, her history pointed to either a minor RCD, a bursitis (the corticosteroid injection might have failed) or TrPs. OA was also a potential cause of her pain.

EXAMINATION: Painful arc test was negative. She had full forward flexion and full abduction, but it was painful at the end of the range. Her external shoulder rotation was quite painful at the end of the range, which indicated possible dysfunction in the infraspinatus and teres minor. Internal rotation was normal. Targeted palpation was made for all the shoulder muscles and tender TrPs were found on the left supraspinatus, infraspinatus, teres major, levator scapulae, rhomboid and the pectoralis (clavicular section).

DIAGNOSIS: The pain was most likely caused by TrPs of the left supraspinatus, infraspinatus, teres major, levator scapulae, rhomboid and the pectoralis (clavicular section). The aim was to clear the TrPs first, before considering OA or a bursitis as a cause.

INVESTIGATIONS: None necessary.

TREATMENT: A press needle was placed on the left shoulder point of the chest somatotope (Fig. 123-125) with immediate improvement in the ROM and pain (estimated to be about 10%). The active points of the left supraspinatus, infraspinatus, teres major, levator scapulae, rhomboid in the K somatotope plus the active point of the pectoralis in the J somatotope were needled with further 10% improvement.

THE CHEST SOMATOTOPE

This is another somatotope discovered by Dr Yamamoto. From my experience, it is very effective in treating any neck, shoulder and elbow conditions. The active acupuncture points are located just below the costochondral joints, at the first, second and third intercostal space respectively, as shown in the diagram below. The active points are identified as a tiny palpable nodule and intensely tender to the patient. It has to be located precisely and a 'press needle' applied. It is important to note that an acupuncture needle should NEVER be used on the chest, as it may puncture the lung. The press needle can be left in situ for several days.

Figure 123: The location of the neck, shoulder and elbow points in the chest somatotope

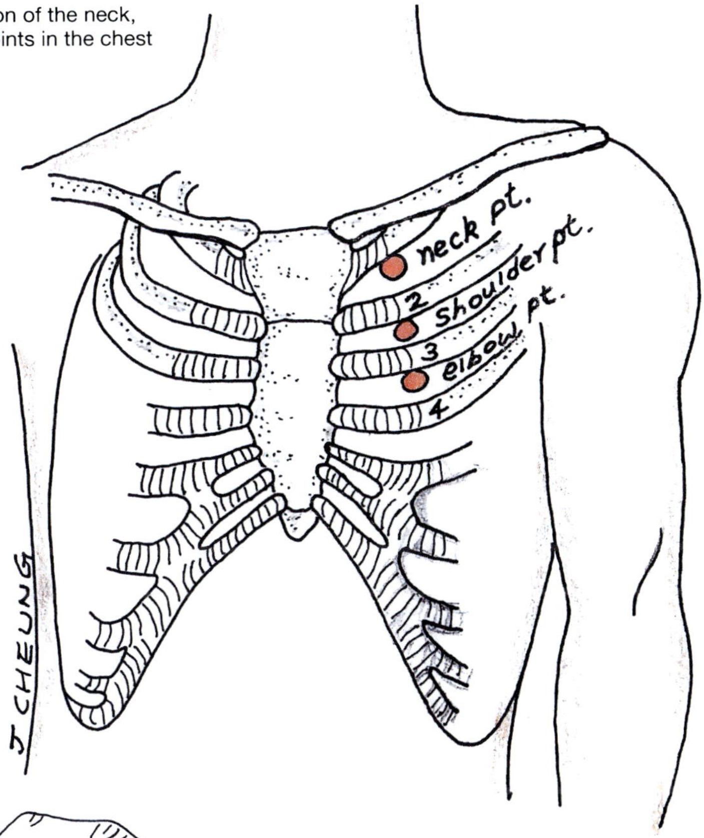

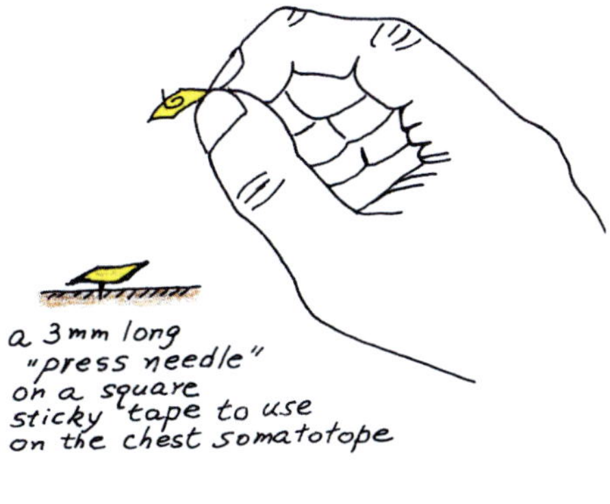

Figure 124: Method of applying a press needle onto an active point

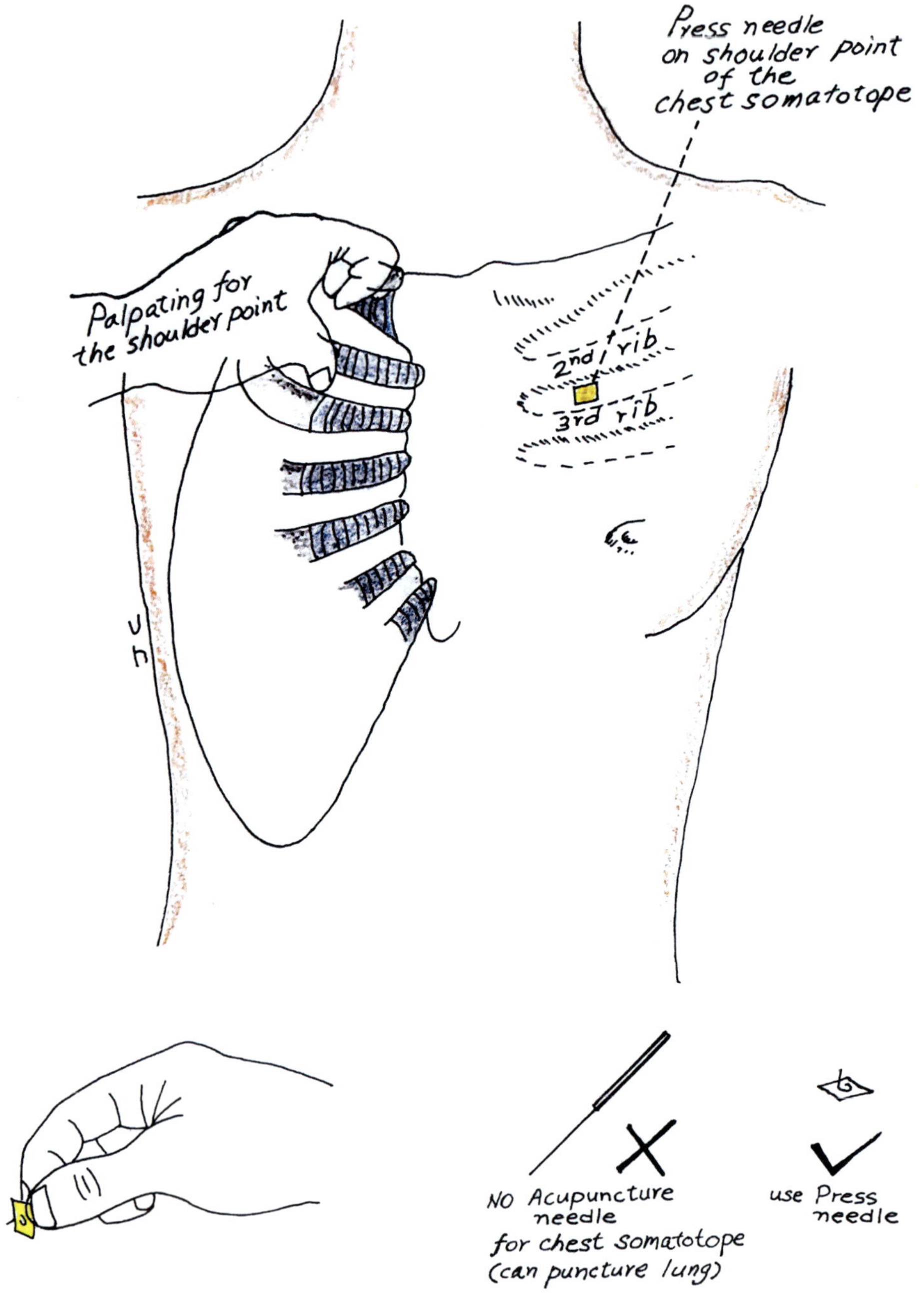

Figure 125: Palpating for an active point in the chest somatotope and applying the press needle

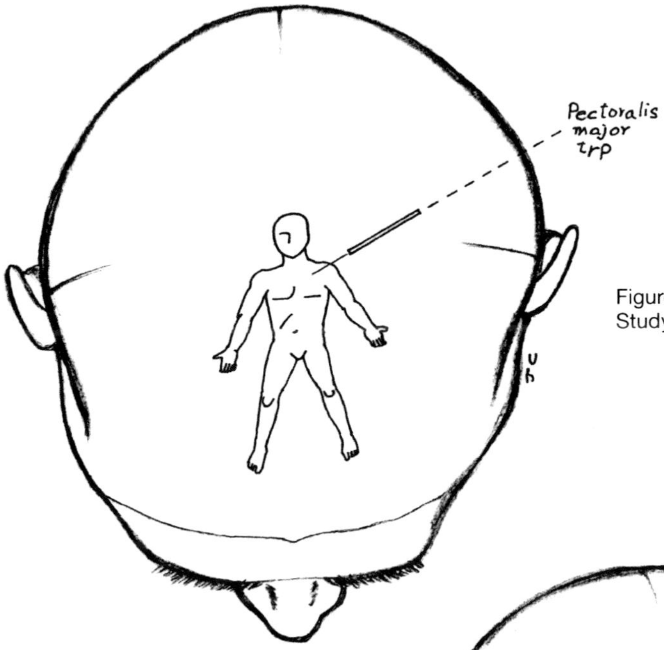

Figure 126: TrPs treatment for Case Study 23 (J Somatotope)

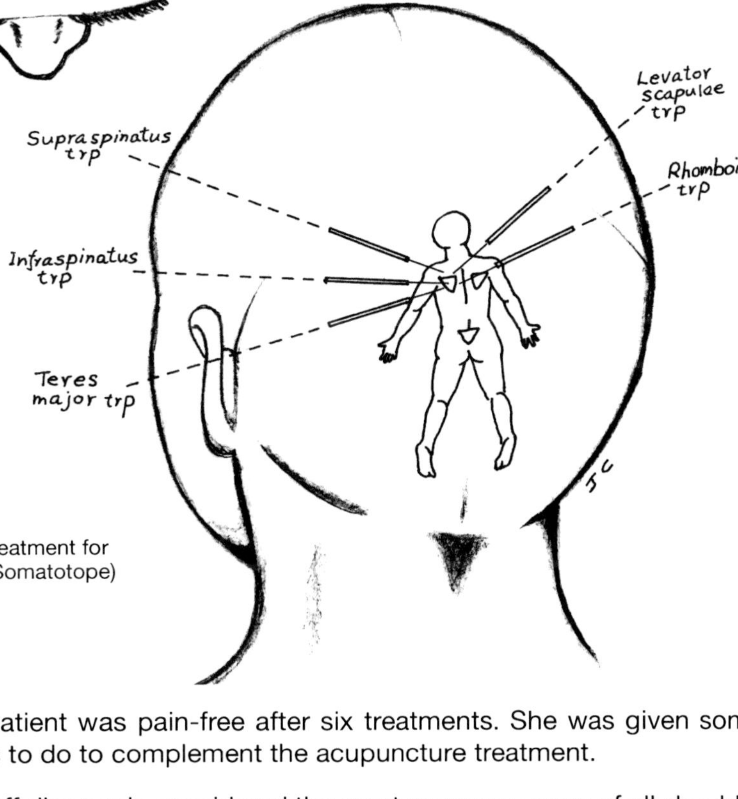

Figure 127: TrPs treatment for Case Study 23 (K Somatotope)

OUTCOME: The patient was pain-free after six treatments. She was given some stretching exercises to do to complement the acupuncture treatment.

NB. While rotator cuff disease is considered the most common cause of all shoulder problem presentations, there are more than 10 other muscles in the shoulder region that can cause shoulder pain and dysfunction. I believe they must all be assessed and treated, if necessary, in order to address any shoulder problems.

CASE STUDY 24 (left shoulder/deltoid pain – left levator scapulae, rhomboid, supraspinatus, infraspinatus and clavicular head of pectoralis TrPs, treated with YNSA)

HISTORY: A 69-year-old, female office worker presented with a two-month history of left shoulder pain around the deltoid area. Pain was quite severe, up to 8/10. Pain was present most of the time and radiated down to the elbow area, waking the patient up at night multiple times. There were no parathaesia nor weakness. The patient could hang clothes on the line and fasten her bra. She denied prolonged morning stiffness. There was a long history of moderate neck OA and several years of finger joint pains and bilateral big toe MTPJ pain. She had a right mastectomy five years prior and was almost due for her annual breast check. She had osteopenia, controlled hypertension, and her vitamin D and calcium levels were satisfactory.

It was reassuring that she did have a shoulder X-ray to rule out lytic and sclerotic lesion. The X-ray also reported moderate OA at the glenohumeral joint and the acromioclavicular (AC) joint. Her GP referred her to have some physiotherapy treatment, but the therapy was too painful for her to persevere and she did not feel comfortable taking strong medication. As her daughter experienced success with acupuncture, she presented for treatment.

REASONING: After an in-depth history was taken, inflammatory joint disease and frozen shoulder were unlikely. She had some pain on shoulder movement, so RCD and other shoulder muscle strains were possible. The pain did not radiate further down from the deltoid area and there was no parathaesia and muscle weakness, which rendered cervical radiculopathy unlikely albeit still possible. C6, C7 facet joint arthropathy can refer pain to the deltoid area (Fig. 110).

EXAMINATION: Painful arc, shoulder extension lag test and shoulder internal lag test were all negative, but there was pain at the end of full abduction and external rotation. C5,6,7 sensation, bicep and tricep reflexes were normal; shoulder flexion and abduction, elbow flexion and extension, wrist flexion and extension were all normal. The cervical extension/rotation test was positive for facet joint arthropathy.

There were TrPs at the left levator scapulae, rhomboid, supraspinatus, infraspinatus and clavicular head of pectoralis. Specifically, the deltoid was non-tender. Examination of the neck showed localised marked tenderness over the left C6 facet joint.

DIAGNOSIS: The diagnosis was left C6 facet joint arthritis, referring the pain to the deltoid area. As some of her pain may have been due to the multiple muscular TrPs, a decision was made to treat these TrPs first.

INVESTIGATION: As the pain was severe, an MRI of the cervical spine could help the treatment plan.

TREATMENT: A press needle was placed on the shoulder point on the chest somatotope (Fig. 123-125), and the K and J points for the abovementioned TrPs were needled, resulting in immediate improvement in discomfort on abduction and external rotation. However, the deltoid area pain remained and was exacerbated every time she extended her neck.

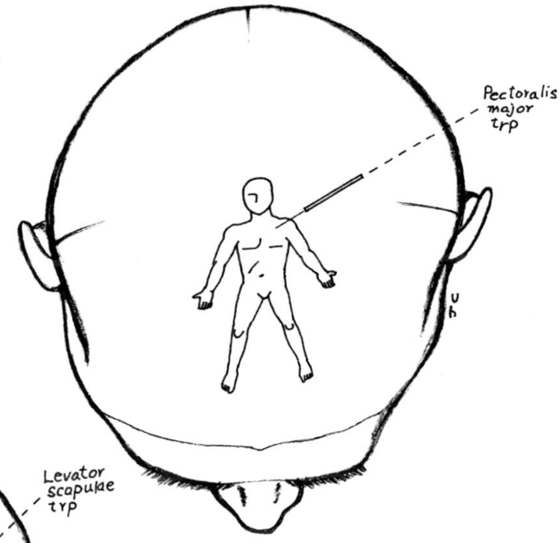

Figure 128: TrPs treatment for Case Study 24 (J Somatotope)

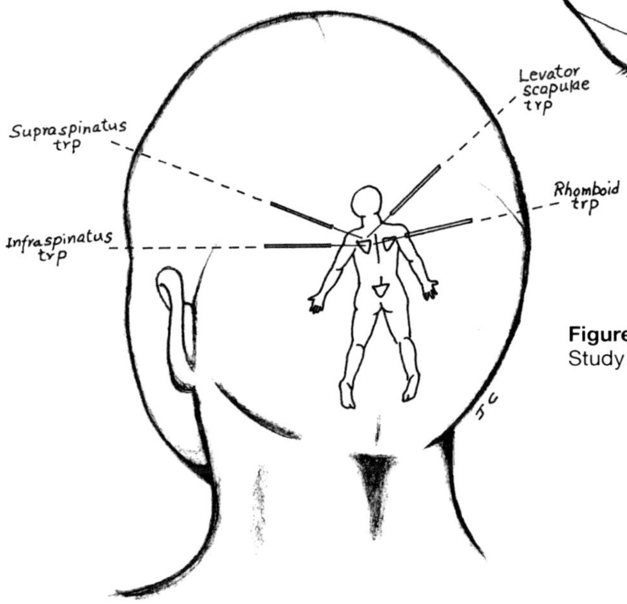

Figure 129: TrPs treatment for Case Study 24 (K Somatotope)

OUTCOME: The patient rang me after three treatments, wanting to terminate acupuncture treatments as it did not help the deltoid area pain, she said her GP had organised a cervical MRI for her. She had not tried NSAIDs consistently before, so I suggested she try daily NSAID for two weeks in the meantime. Her MRI showed multiple-level facet joint arthropathy and multiple levels of possible nerve route impingement but not conclusively at the left C5,6,7 levels. Interestingly, her pain disappeared several weeks after our conversation and she remained pain-free two months later. In hindsight, the cause of her deltoid area pain was most likely due to OA of the left C6 facet joint, and the two weeks of NSAID had successfully helped the pain.

NB. Pectoralis major (clavicular section) TrPs often result from neck and shoulder problems, as it balances the tight posterior muscles. It is important to treat it as well.

CASE STUDY 25 (right shoulder pain – supraspinatus, levator scapulae, infraspinatus, teres minor, SCM, anterior deltoid and clavicular section of the pectoralis major TrPs, treated with YNSA)

HISTORY: A 27-year-old female, a recently arrived refugee, presented with at least a 10-year history of chronic right shoulder pain. It was rated at 6/10 most of the time. She recalled having twice dislocated her shoulder as a child. Her shoulder joint appeared to be stable, with no further dislocations since age 10. She could hang clothes on the clothesline and fasten her bra, but shoulder movement was painful and weak. The pain did not radiate and there were no parathaesia. She had previous psychological trauma, was anaemic with low iron, insufficient calcium and low vitamin B12 from including very little meat in her diet. She also had low vitamin D from being covered from head to toe traditionally. Her GP ordered an X-ray and an ultrasound, which ruled out OA but identified thickening of the subacromial subdeltoid bursae and possible impingement during abduction. No muscle tears were reported.

REASONING: It was good there was no recurrent dislocation and the history did not point to any nerve damage. It was likely the shoulder pain was due to TrPs, which would hopefully still be treatable after so many years. OA was possible.

INVESTIGATIONS: None necessary.

EXAMINATION: Shoulder flexion at 140 degrees, abduction at 170 degrees. External rotation was weak and painful, pointing to an infraspinatus and teres minor dysfunction. There were significant TrPs at the right infraspinatus, teres minor, supraspinatus, levator scapulae, rhomboid, SCM, anterior deltoid and the clavicular section of the pectoralis major.

DIAGNOSIS: The dysfunction was due to the above TrPs.

TREATMENT: The patient was treated with YNSA, with the active points above needled as well as the shoulder point in the chest somatotope.

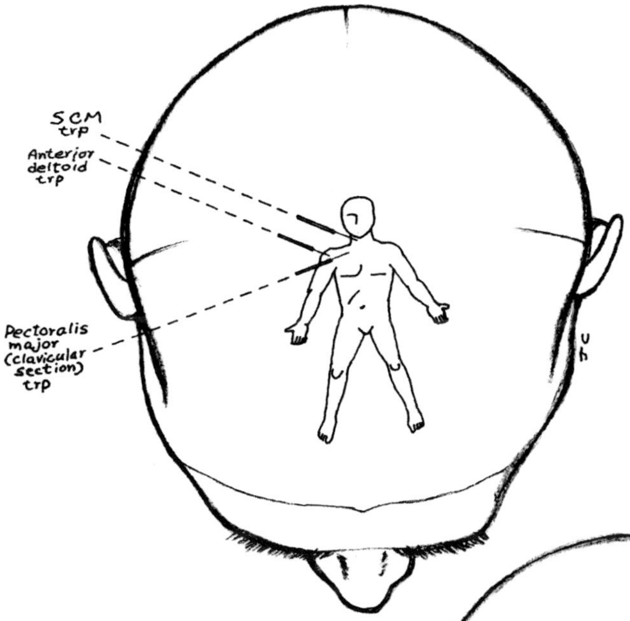

Figure 130: TrPs treatment for Case Study 25 (J Somatotope)

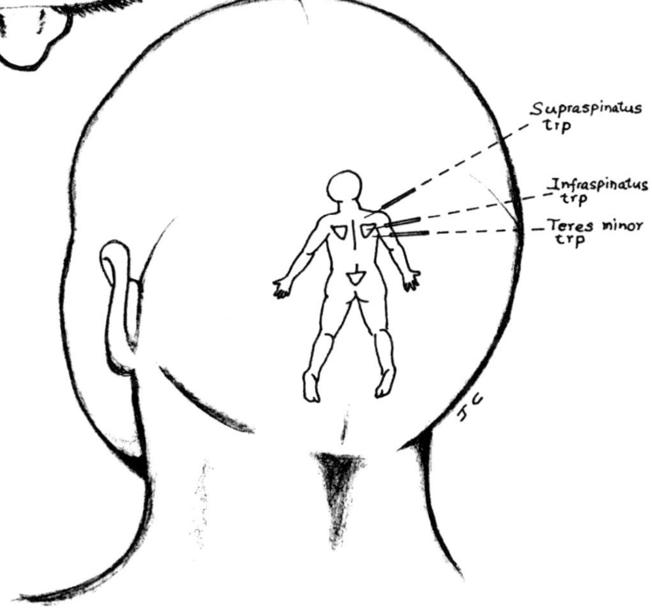

Figure 131: TrPs treatment for Case Study 25 (K Somatotope)

OUTCOME: There was immediate improvement with each needle insertion. The patient had full ROM after the first two treatments and the strength of her internal rotation improved with each treatment. Stretching and strengthening exercises were gradually added. She was pain-free and the shoulder strength normalised after six treatments. It was a very pleasant surprise for the patient and myself.

NB. From my experience, the YNSA system can be very effective in eradicating hard, sizable TrPs that have been present for many years. I have used manual therapies for such TrPs many, many times without any improvements. I have also injected them with LA and corticosteroid without success.

CASE STUDY 26 (right posterior scapular pain – rhomboid TrPs, treated with YNSA)

HISTORY: A 44-year-old female IT worker presented with a five-month history of pain in the right posterior scapular area. It had been there intermittently for about three years, but five months ago she aggravated it swimming against a strong current and made it worse. After this last injury, she experienced three weeks of sharp, severe pain, which settled into a constant, low-grade 4/10 pain. She observed that reaching the right arm forwards aggravated it and lying supine relieved it. Neck movement did not aggravate the pain. There was no pain or parathaesia down the arm, nor were there any arm or hand weakness. She did have a four-year history of low-grade, right neck pain after a whiplash sustained in a car accident 20 years before. She said the neck pain usually only occurred in long car trips and did not bother her too much. She had no other significant medical problems.

REASONING: Cervical radiculopathy was possible for C7 or C8. However, the pain did not radiate down to the fingers, which made it less likely. C7 facet joint arthropathy could give pain in the scapular area as well. As the pain was aggravated by arm movement, TrPs appeared to be the most likely cause.

EXAMINATION: The patient had full shoulder ROM, but any shoulder movement would aggravate her posterior shoulder pain. Neck rotation to the right was reduced to 60 degrees versus 65 degrees to the left. The extension-rotation test for facet joint arthropathy did not aggravate her right shoulder pain. Her upper-limb sensation, power and reflexes were normal. On palpation, her pain was precisely localised to the rhomboid minor, when the patient said, 'That's the pain I was telling you about!' There were also minor TrPs in both trapezii, SCM and right pectoralis major (clavicular section). Very localised tenderness was found over the right C6 facet joint.

DIAGNOSIS:

1. Right rhomboid injury
2. Right C6 facet joint OA from the car accident 20 years ago

INVESTIGATIONS: No imaging was planned as it would not have changed the treatment plan.

TREATMENT: A decision was made for a trial of YNSA. Active points at the K somatotope for bilateral trapezius, right rhomboid and right C6 paravertebral muscles were needled, as well the J somatotope for right pectoralis and bilateral SCM (multiple TrPs).

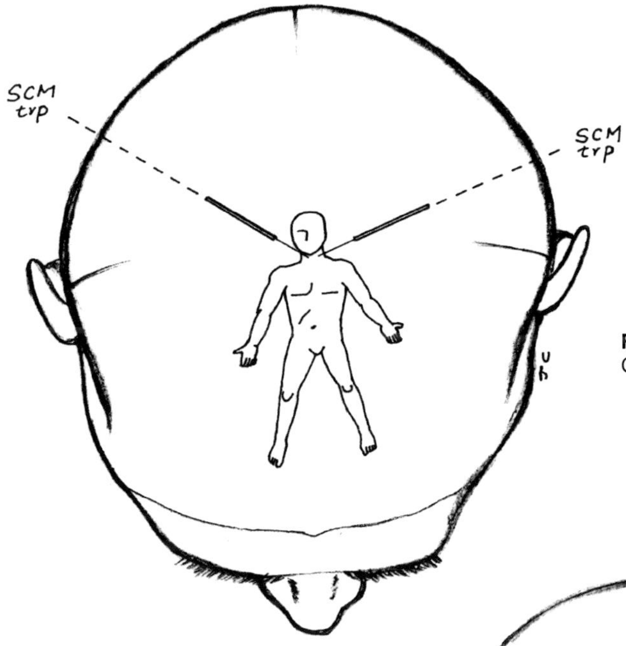

Figure 132: TrPs treatment for Case Study 26 (J Somatotope)

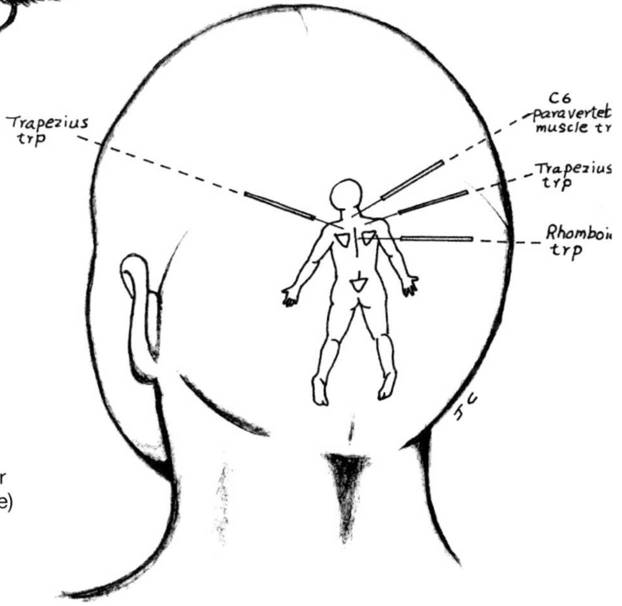

Figure 133: TrPs treatment for Case Study 26 (K Somatotope)

OUTCOME: Her rhomboid TrPs cleared completely as well as her posterior shoulder pain after seven treatments, confirming the pain was from an injured right rhomboid. The acupuncture treatment was accompanied by stretching and strengthening exercises. Her minor neck pain did not improve within the seven treatments, neither did the restricted ROM of the neck and the C6 tenderness. It is my belief that, while acupuncture can help the muscle TrPs around the joint and the associated inflammation, it cannot reverse degenerated joint surfaces. With the popularity of gym and weight training, it is not uncommon to see rhomboid injuries and, from my experience, they are often very responsive to YNSA treatments.

THE TRAPEZIUS AND ITS TrPs

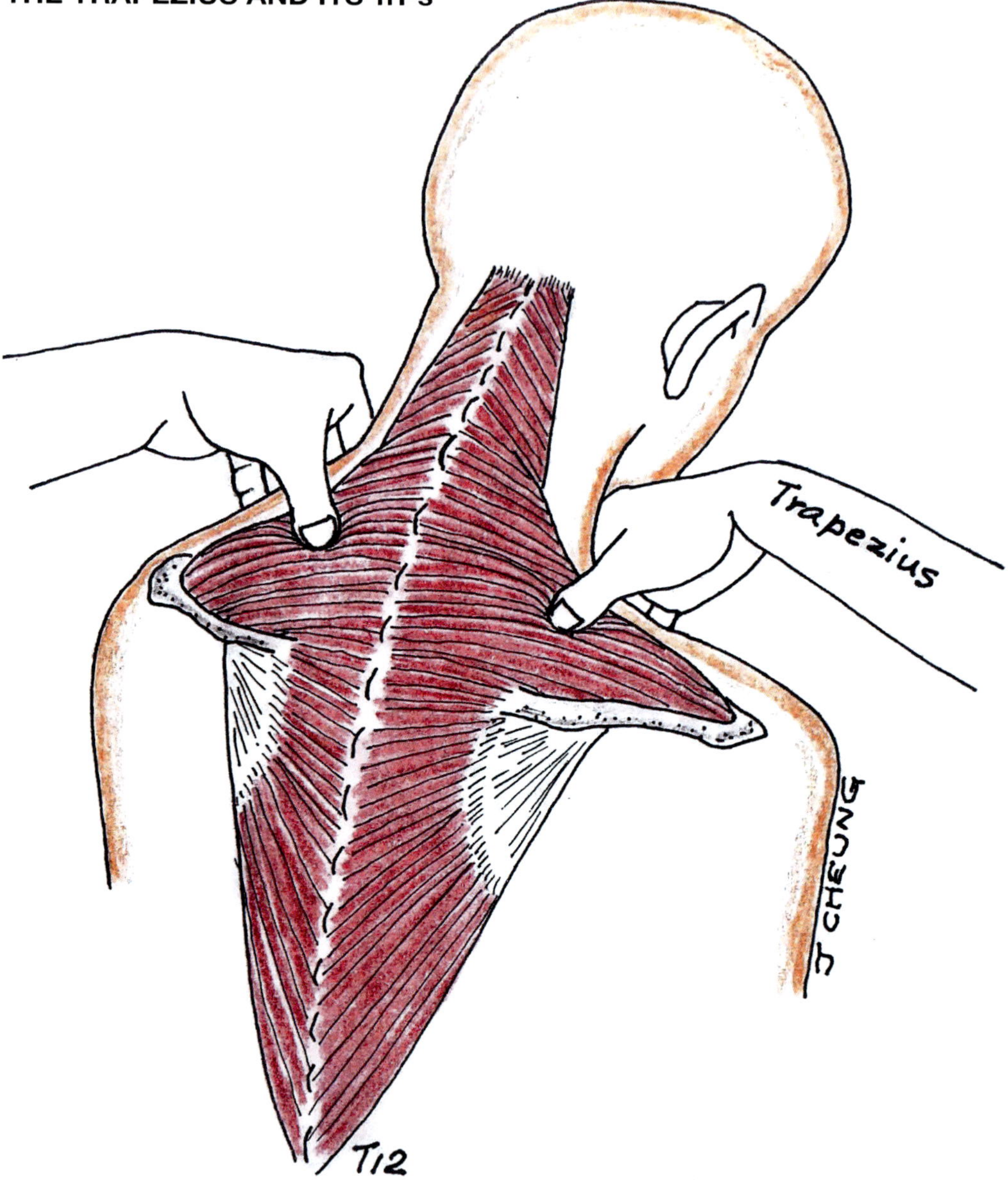

Figure 134: Palpation diagram for the Trapezius TrPs

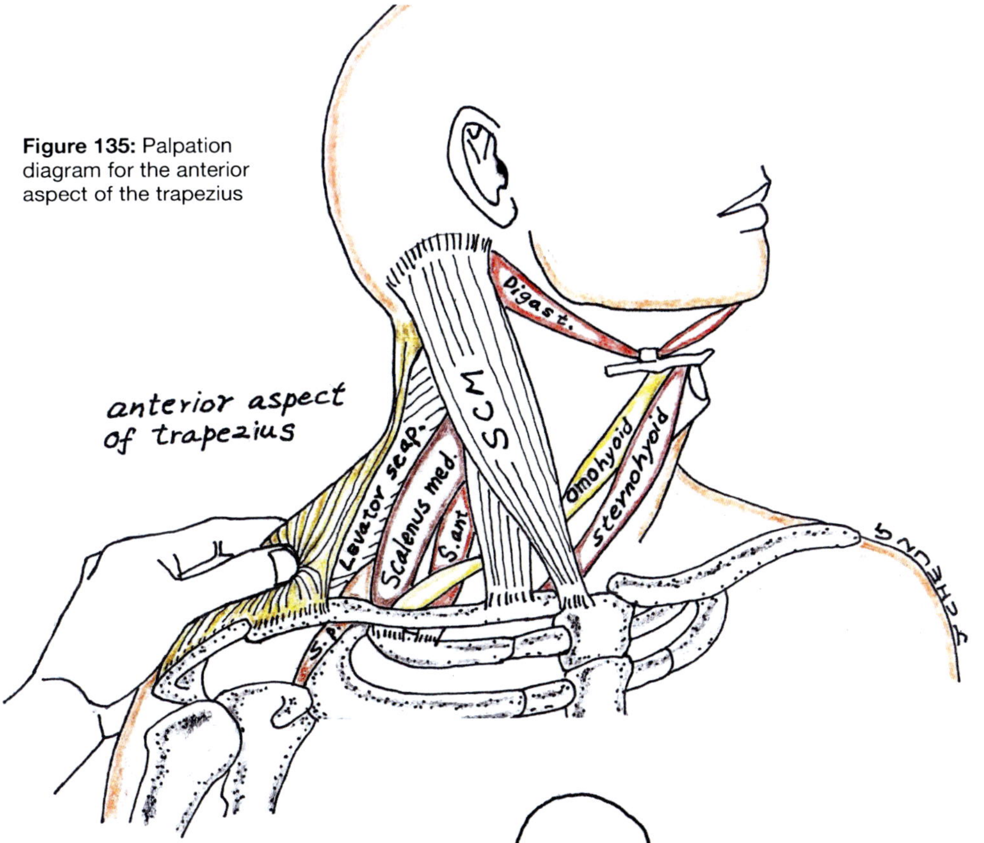

Figure 135: Palpation diagram for the anterior aspect of the trapezius

NB. Often, trapezius TrPs are one of the main causes of a cervicogenic headache. We need to palpate for both the TrPs in the posterior aspect and the anterior aspect of the muscle and treat both in the K and J somatotopes respectively.

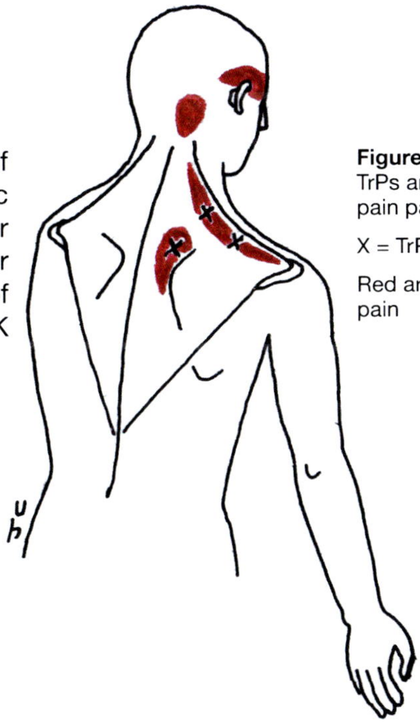

Figure 136: Trapezius TrPs and their referred pain pattern

X = TrPs

Red area = the referred pain

THE LEVATOR SCAPULAE AND ITS TrPs

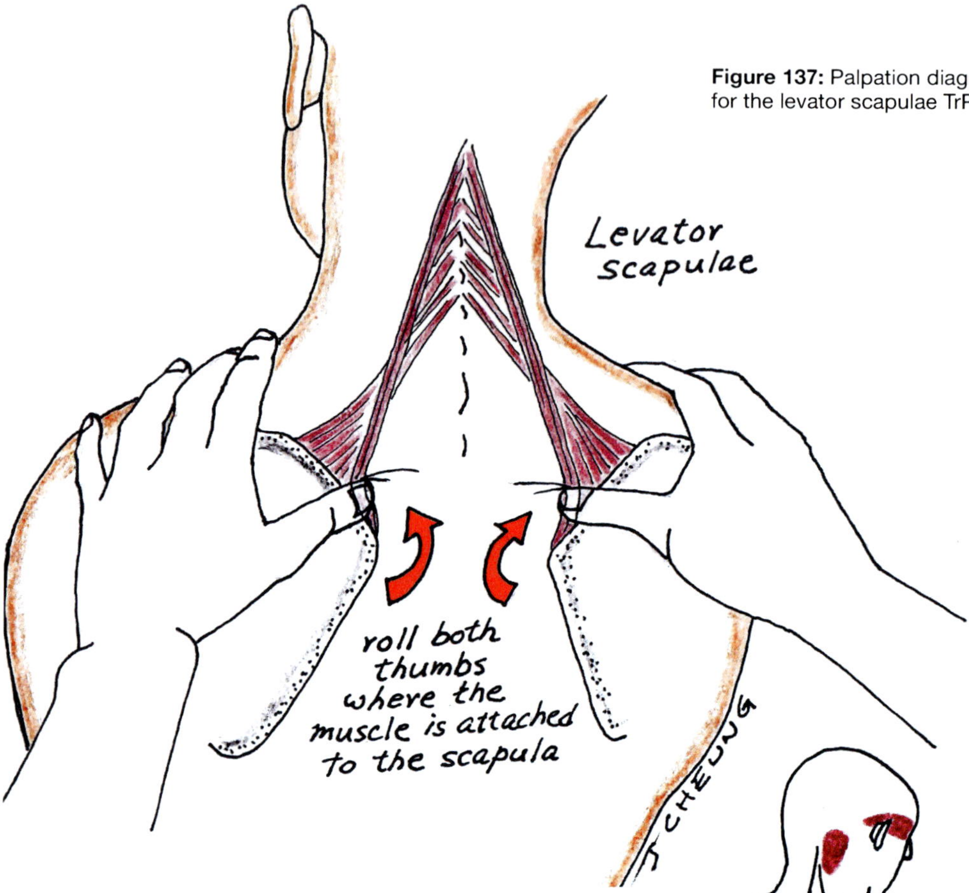

Figure 137: Palpation diagram for the levator scapulae TrPs

NB. From my experience, TrPs in the levator scapulae are almost always involved in any shoulder pain, neck pain and cervicogenic headaches. They must be eradicated in order to resolve these conditions

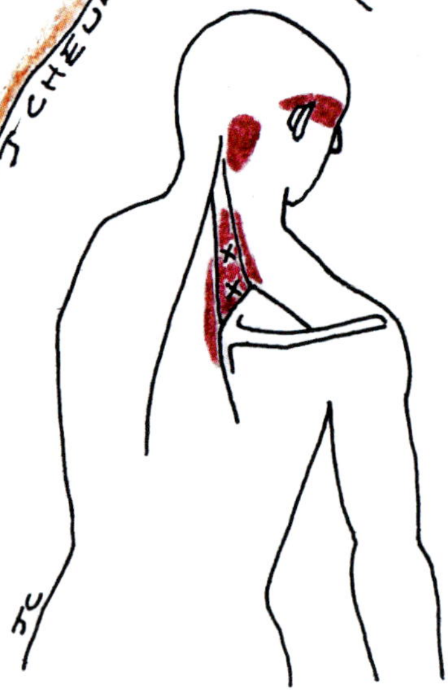

Figure 138: Levator scapulae TrPs and their referred pain pattern

X = TrPs

Red area = the referred pain

THE SUBOCCIPITAL MUSCLES AND POSTERIOR CERVICAL MUSCLES AND THEIR TrPs

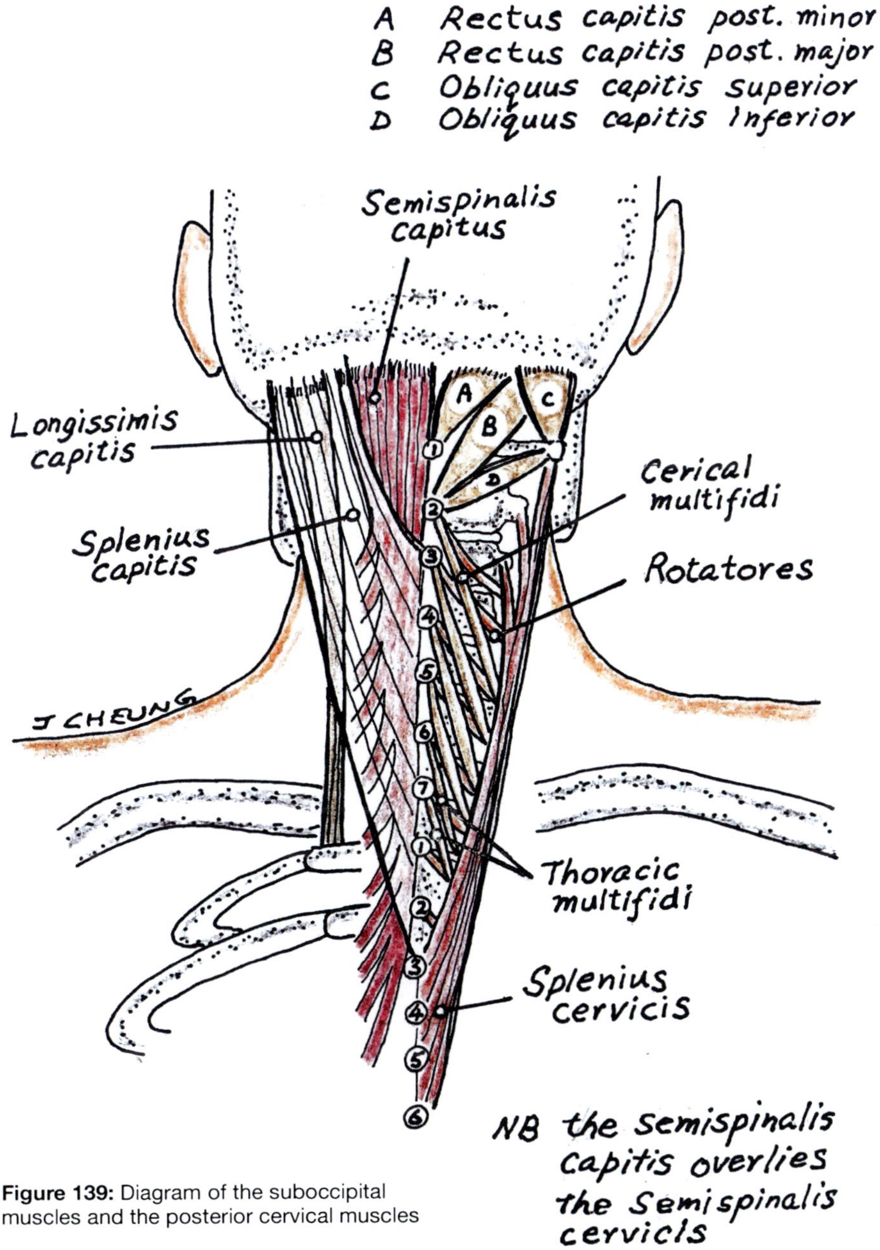

Figure 139: Diagram of the suboccipital muscles and the posterior cervical muscles

NB. While the semispinalis capitis overlies the semispinalis cervicis, the latter is not shown in this drawing.

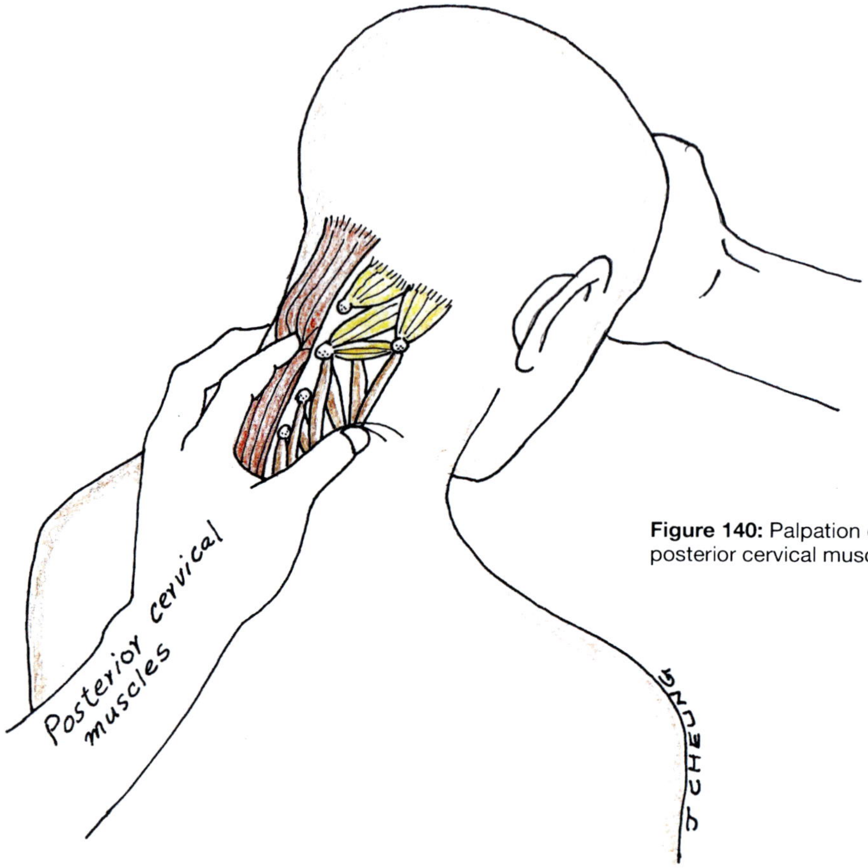

Figure 140: Palpation diagram for the posterior cervical muscles TrPs

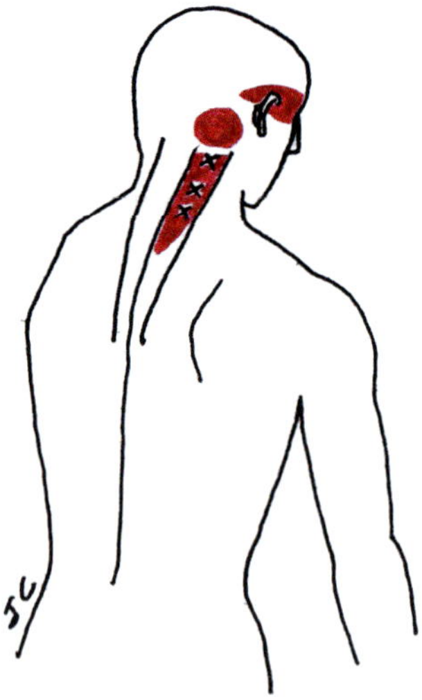

Figure 141: Suboccipital muscles and posterior cervical muscles TrPs and their referred pain pattern

X = TrPs

Red area = the referred pain

NB. In cervicogenic headaches, we need to palpate for all the TrPs in the suboccipital muscles and posterior cervical muscles, and eradicate them.

CASE STUDY 27 (cervical spine OA, treated with physiotherapy, CT-guided injections and NSAIDs)

HISTORY: A 60-year-old male presented with a long history of neck pain and stiffness. He had three significant surfing injuries when he was 'dumped' headfirst in his 20s. The constant pain had been there for at least 30 years and was gradually worsening in the last 12 months. The pain was generally around the mid neck to lower neck and the left shoulder region, aggravated by neck movements. There was no radiation of pain to any dermatome distribution, no parathaesia, no muscle weakness and no other significant joint problems. The pain used to be a fairly constant 3/10 ache and he would take diclofenac 50mg every third day or so, controlling the pain quite well. However, it had gradually become a constant 7/10. He had tried physiotherapy treatments over the years and some short-acting slow-release oxycodone but did not find the effect any better than the diclofenac.

REASONING: The gradual increase in pain pointed to a deteriorating OA. In the older age group, imaging is necessary to exclude lytic and sclerotic lesions as well as osteoporotic fractures.

EXAMINATION: He was fit and lean, sharp and positive in his attitude. His ROM was restricted, bilateral neck rotation was only 45 degrees to the right and 55 degrees to the left, and painful towards the end of the range. There were trigger points in his trapezius, left scapulae and rhomboids bilaterally – the left more so than the right. On deeper palpation, there was localised tenderness over the left C3/4 and C6/7 facet joints. Muscle power was normal, bicep and triceps reflex normal. When the patient was asked to extend and rotate his neck, the pain was exacerbated (the extension-rotation test was positive).

DIAGNOSIS: The diagnosis was that of OA, which was probably worse on the left C3/4 and C6/7, as the pain distribution pointed to those facet joints. As facet joint injections were a possibility, an MRI was ordered. It confirmed widespread OA changes in all the facet joints, probable neural foraminal narrowing at multiple levels and significant intervertebral OA changes. There were trigger points in the muscles mentioned, which were worthwhile treating before any invasive interventions.

TREATMENT: The patient did not feel comfortable with acupuncture, so we formulated a plan:

1. In the first instance, before any pharmaceutical or invasive measures, weekly physiotherapy manual therapies were started, targeting the trigger points of muscles mentioned, alongside daily stretching and loosening exercises.
2. There was some improvement in ROM and a slight change in the pain level. Topical diclofenac was trialled without success and adding paracetamol did not help either.
3. A bone scan with SPECT was then ordered to look for facet joints to inject. Subsequently, left C3/4 and C6/7 intra-articular corticosteroid and LA were performed. Unfortunately, this made no difference to the pain.
4. Arrangements were made to perform medial branch block to the two facet joints, again with no significant improvement either.

INVESTIGATIONS: As above.

OUTCOME: In hindsight, perhaps the patient's main pain came from the OA in the intervertebral joints, making these interventions ineffective. Ultimately, the only effective treatment was taking a diclofenac 50mg daily, which reduced the pain from 7/10 to 3/10. He continued to do stretching and loosening exercises every morning, which helped the pain, and applying heatpacks at night also helped. He attempted to not take the diclofenac daily; unfortunately, the pain would return to 7/10 on those days. Taking the diclofenac daily came with the possible side effects of GIT bleed and CV events but there was no alternative. He was sensible in that he would not let the pain rule his life, he continued to work part-time, involve himself with voluntary work and play golf. Opioids were not indicated in treating chronic pain or OA.

THE STERNOCLEIDOMASTOID AND ITS TrPs

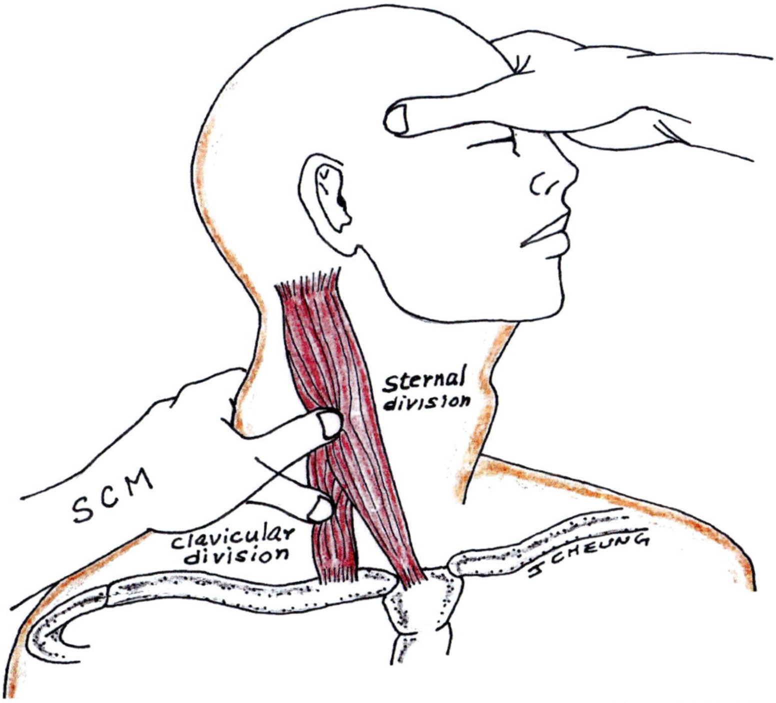

Figure 142: Palpation diagram for the sternocleidomastoid TrPs

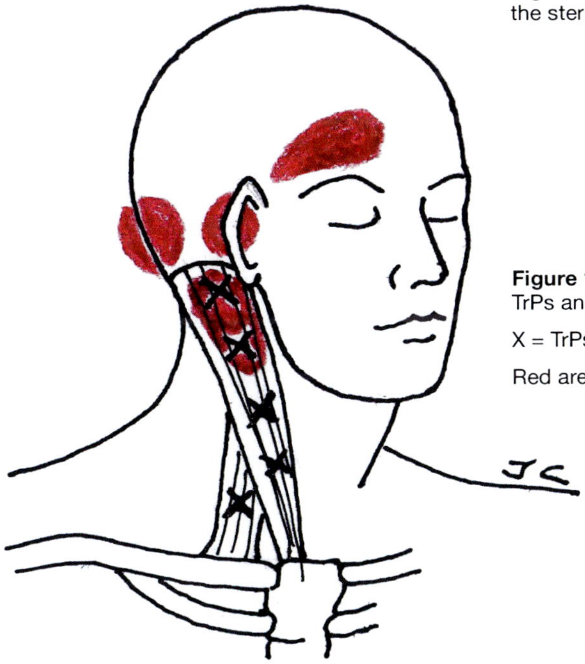

Figure 143: Sternocleidomastoid TrPs and their referred pain pattern

X = TrPs

Red area = the referred pain

NB. I believe that in treating cervicogenic headaches and shoulder problems, **eradicating ALL the SCM TrPs is very important.** Usually there are multiple TrPs in the SCM, in both the sternal and clavicular divisions. When using YNSA, the active acupuncture points are found in the J somatotope, often in multiple numbers and close to each other. These TrPs need to be eradicated one by one with due patience in order to succeed. At times, we see patients with an earache, when the history and examination make both otitis media or otitis externa unlikely, palpate the proximal attachment of the SCM, as a TrP there can cause an earache.

NB. In very complicated neck presentations, besides using the J and K somatotopes, adding the Ypsilon points guided by palpating the YNSA neck diagnostic zone would improve the results further.

Tips

Acupuncturists often have difficulties locating the active points on the scalp somatotopes. My suggestion:

1. Use anatomical knowledge to work out proportionately where a trigger point could be (Fig. 23 and 24).
2. Hopefully, you have a strong intention to heal – you must trust that.
3. Give up the desire to control the outcome, and the points often will then come to you.
4. If the desired result does not eventuate, reposition the needle and try again.

- There is a way to confirm the accuracy of a selected point on the scalp before needling. While applying very firm pressure on the point with your palpating fingertip, re-palpate the TrP for an improvement or ask the patient to move the painful and/or restricted body part (e.g. neck or shoulder). If there is a definite improvement, one is then reassured the point is correct and can insert the needle with confidence.
- Practitioners often complain that they find it hard to master YNSA or that, in their hands, YNSA is not very effective. Having given a number of YNSA workshops, my assessment is as follows. The somatotopes are quite small, for example, the J and K somatotopes to my estimation measure only about 6cm in length each. It is quite easy to locate the active point incorrectly or miss the point when needling, thereby not getting a positive result. In order to be sure that the needle insertion is accurate, we must confirm it by re-palpating the TrPs straight after each needle insertion, ensuring that a 15–20% improvement has been achieved, otherwise re-palpate and re-insert the needle until that has been achieved. I often have to re-locate the needle several times.

CASE STUDY 28 (acute stiff neck – bilateral levator scapulae, bilateral SCM, right trapezius and posterior cervical TrPs, treated with YNSA)

HISTORY: A 58-year-old female retiree presented with a three-day history of acute stiff neck. Any attempt to rotate the neck was extremely painful. There had been family stress at home and, as a result, poor quality of sleep. There was no trauma or infection. There was no radiation of pain, no parathaesia and no muscle weakness. A recent X-ray revealed generalised moderate OA. There had been similar episodes before, with spontaneous recovery within a short time. Her past history included breast cancer six years ago and her recent breast check was normal.

REASONING: With a past history of breast cancer, imaging was necessary to rule out lytic and sclerotic lesions. Otherwise, the history pointed to a mechanical cause.

EXAMINATION: Rotation of the neck was restricted to 35 degrees bilaterally. On palpation, there were bilateral levator scapulae, bilateral SCM, right trapezius and posterior cervical TrPs.

INVESTIGATIONS: An X-ray was performed recently.

TREATMENT: YNSA was used, and active points on the J and K somatotopes of bilateral levator scapulae, bilateral SCM, right trapezius and posterior cervical muscles were needled, with immediate resolution of the restricted ROM. Only one treatment was needed.

OUTCOME: The patient's stiff neck cleared after one treatment only. She was instructed to do regular neck stretching exercises to prevent recurrences.

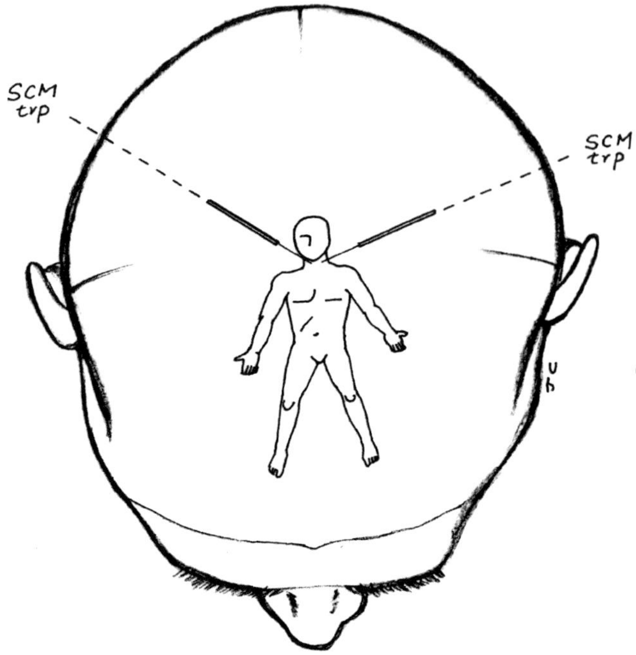

Figure 144: TrPs treatment for Case Study 28 (J Somatotope)

Figure 145: TrPs treatment for Case Study 28 (K Somatotope)

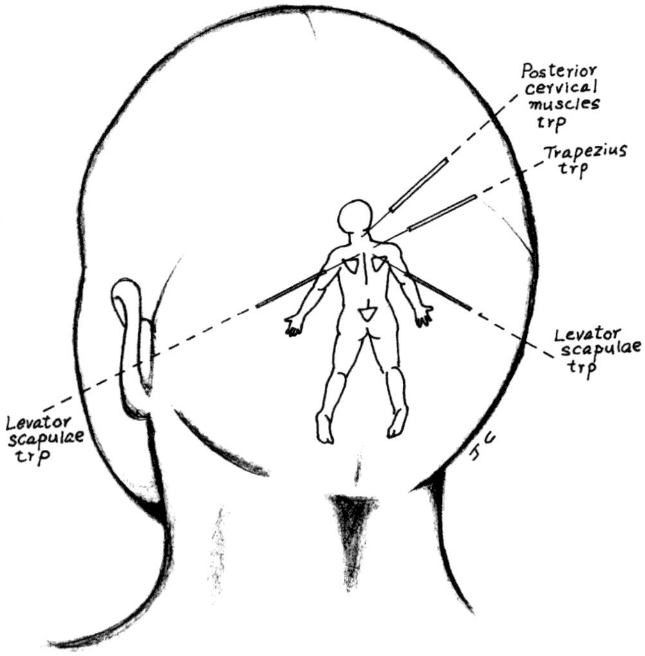

CASE STUDY 29 (C5,6 radiculopathy, treated with cervical discectomy and fusion)

HISTORY: A 56-year-old, female, part-time office worker, presented with a three day history of significant weakness in the right (dominant) upper limb. She was unable to hold a cup of coffee without dropping it. She experienced 5/10 pain over the anterolateral border of the right arm. She had recurrent low-grade neck pain for at least five years. There was no history of trauma. She had no significant past medical history, had regular breast checks, screening colonoscopy and BMD tests. Vitamin D and calcium levels were normal.

REASONING: The symptoms pointed to radiculopathy.

EXAMINATION: Right shoulder abduction, elbow flexion and wrist extension were weaker than the left and the bicep jerk was diminished. There were no obvious sensory changes.

INVESTIGATIONS: MRI showed severe degeneration at C4/5, C5/6 and C6/7 levels. There were multiple bilateral neuroforaminal stenosis, most marked at right C5/6 and C6/7 levels, and the foramina were almost obliterated at those levels.

DIAGNOSIS: These findings pointed to C5 and C6 radiculopathy, as the muscle weaknesses were significant and appeared to be progressive, and an urgent appointment was arranged with a neurosurgeon.

TREATMENT: A C4/5 and C5/6 anterior cervical discectomy and fusion was performed.

OUTCOME: The patient reported instant relief from the pain down their arm as well as the post-operative restoration of muscle strength.

CASE STUDY 30 (whiplash – multiple neck TrPs, treated with YNSA)

HISTORY: A 25-year-old female presented with a one-day history of constant neck discomfort (6/10 on VAS), dizziness and a heavy feeling in the head. She was driving the day before and had been forced to brake abruptly when the car in front stopped unexpectedly, causing her neck to jar. The symptoms developed gradually later that day. She had no symptoms of any viral illness and system review was normal. She had no significant PH and no previous history of headaches or neck problems.

REASONING: This is a classical presentation of a moderate whiplash injury. However, it was prudent to exclude red-flag conditions for headaches, such as infection, fractures and head injuries.

EXAMINATION: Afebrile, neck ROM was full, except that there was pain at the end of left rotation and left lateral flexion. Very tender muscle spasms (TrPs) were found over the left trapezius, left levator scapulae, left rhomboid, left pectoralis and mid paravertebral muscles on the right. The patient reported significant pain on palpating these TrPs. There was no localised tenderness on the cervical spine to indicate a fracture.

DIAGNOSIS: The history was very typical of a whiplash injury, and examination and palpations confirmed the diagnosis. The ROM was full in this patient, however, in more severe cases, it would have been restricted. A mild whiplash injury with less severe symptoms would probably recover without intervention. Moderate and severe cases would usually take a long period to recover, even with appropriate treatments. A lot of severe cases would proceed to have chronic neck pain or recurrent headaches, as in the next case study.

INVESTIGATIONS: If the headache and neck pain persisted, imaging of the cervical spine and cerebral MRI may be indicated.

TREATMENT: In this case, the patient was treated with YNSA, which from my experience, yields excellent results for whiplash injuries. The active points of the left trapezius, left levator scapulae, left rhomboid, left pectoralis and mid paravertebral muscles on the right were needled at the J and K somatotope with immediate results. A press needle was applied to the neck point in the chest somatotope with further improvement. Objectively, straight after the needle insertion, the TrPs softened significantly and the pain at the end of ROM subsided. The acupuncture needles remained in situ for 20 minutes before removal. The patient subjectively rated a 70% improvement in neck pain, head dullness and dizziness.

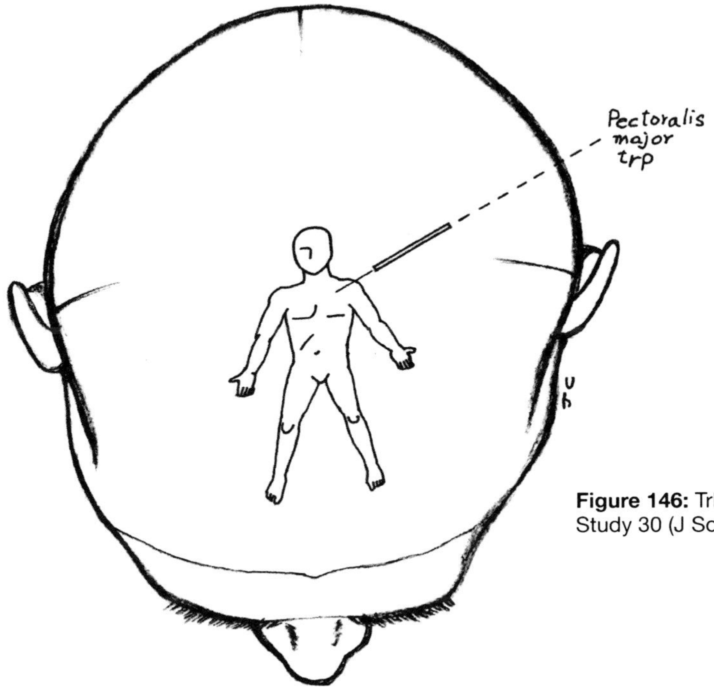

Figure 146: TrPs treatment for Case Study 30 (J Somatotope)

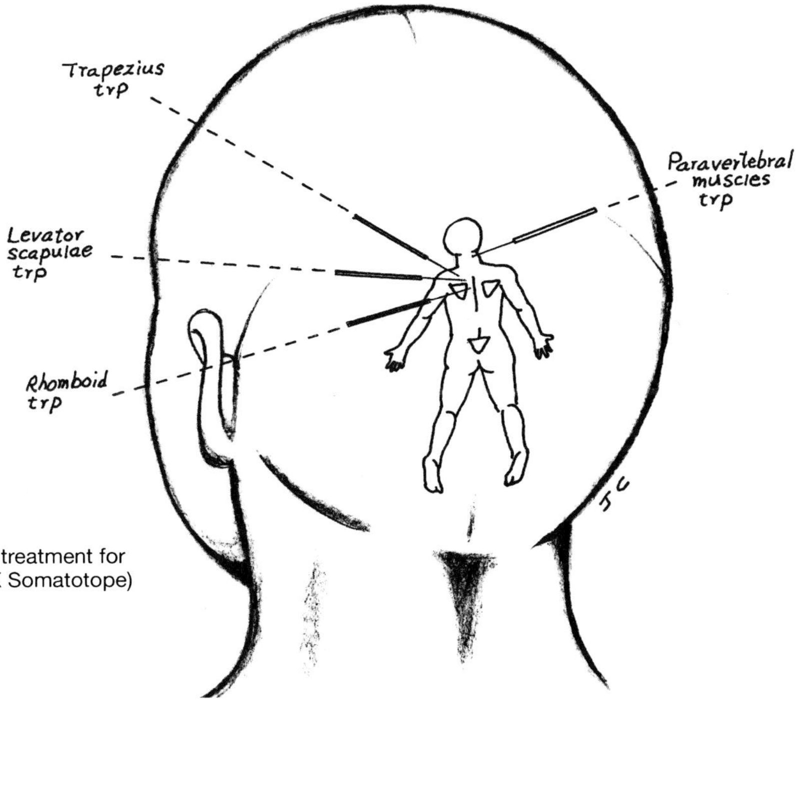

Figure 147: TrPs treatment for Case Study 30 (K Somatotope)

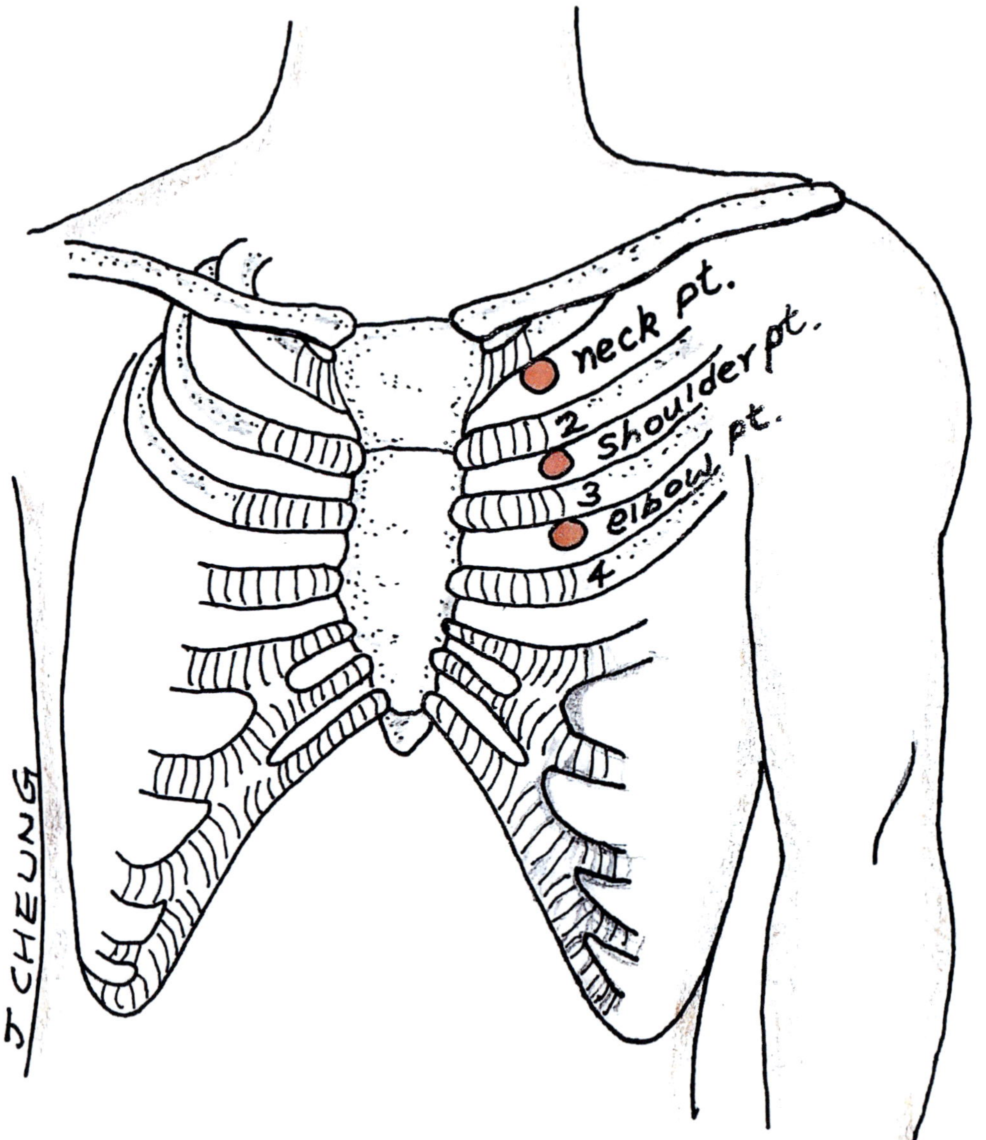

Figure 148: The location of the neck, shoulder and elbow points in the chest somatotope

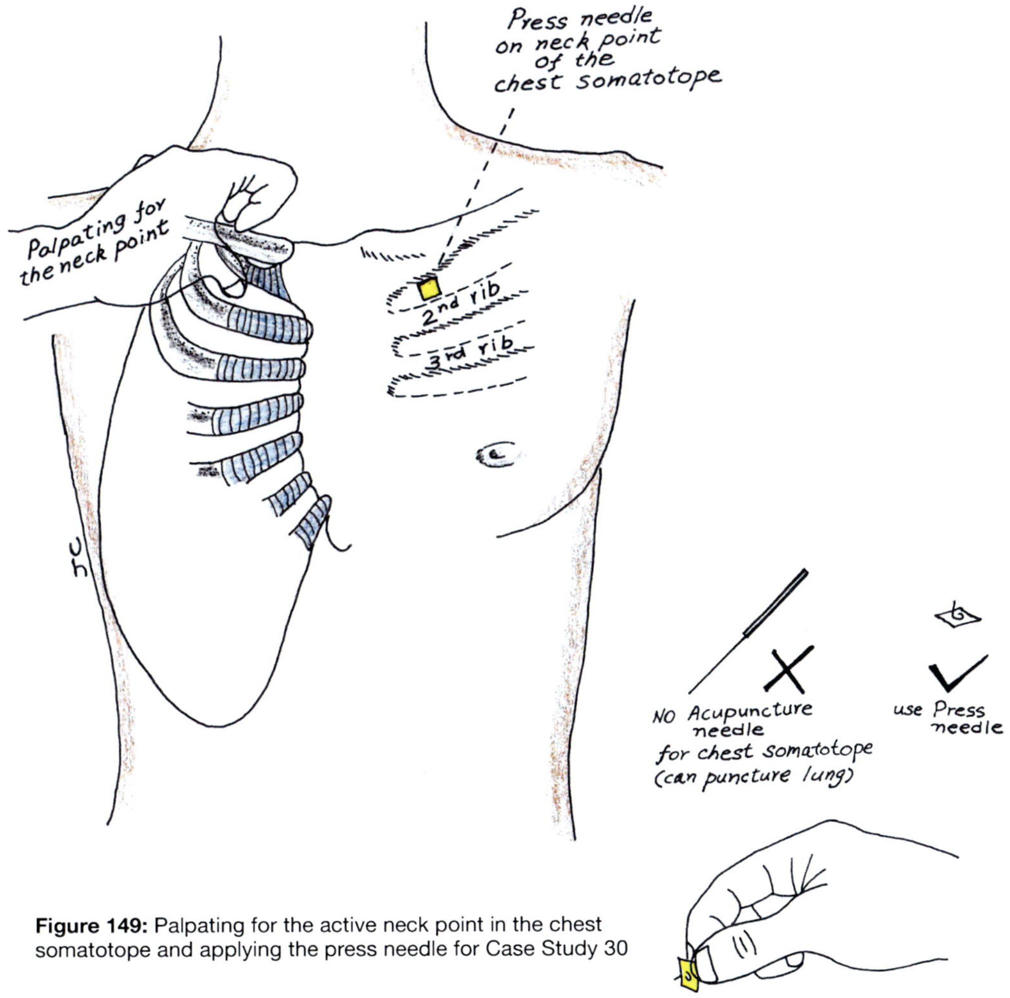

Figure 149: Palpating for the active neck point in the chest somatotope and applying the press needle for Case Study 30

OUTCOME: This treatment was repeated two days later and at the following week's review, she had fully recovered.

NB. The aetiology of whiplash injury probably involves micro-tears in the neck muscles, ligaments, joint capsule fibres and joint oedema. It is notoriously difficult to treat. Initially, it is too painful to do manual treatments of massage or mobilisations. Rest and a trial of NSAIDs and /or paracetamol may be used for several days to try to reduce the inflammation first. After that, a combination of gentle manual therapies, stretching and loosening exercises should be prescribed. Immobilisation with a neck brace may help the pain initially, but prolonged usage would add to a severe restriction of movement later. From my experience, YNSA is ideally suited in treating whiplash injuries. The earlier the treatment is initiated, the quicker the recovery. Even in severe chronic cases, the patient usually improves by 10–15% in each treatment, with an average of eight to ten treatments.

CASE STUDY 31 (cervicogenic headache – multiple neck TrPs, treated with YNSA)

HISTORY: A 47 year-old female office worker presented with a 10-month history of neck stiffness and severe right suboccipital headache radiating to her right jaw. The headaches were occurring every two weeks; VAS was at 10/10. However, in the two weeks before presenting, the headaches became constant. The headaches started after she was bedridden for a week with a debilitating viral illness. The headaches were not characteristic of migraines as there was no aura, no nausea, vomiting or photophobia. She did have PH of migraines with aura but only every 18 months or so. She had not suffered any neck problems before, no history of trauma, head injury or whiplash. At the time of presentation, she had no fever, infection or eye symptoms. She was seen by a neurologist, and a cerebral MRI and cervical CT scan were normal. A diagnosis of trigeminal neuralgia was made and the doctor offered her oral analgesics. Nurofen, codeine and pregabalin helped only slightly. She tried some massages with no success. There was no medical history of significance.

REASONING: Red-flag diagnoses were ruled out. In patients with very frequent or constant headaches, neck and shoulder TrPs are usually involved.

EXAMINATION: The patient had a severe 10/10 headache at the time. She was afebrile, a neurological examination was normal, her fundi were normal. Neck rotation was 45 degrees bilaterally and painful, side flexion was only 20 degrees and even more painful. Very tender TrPs were found on her right trapezius, right suboccipital muscles, bilateral SCM (multiple) and paravertebral muscles of her neck, with the right greater than the left.

DIAGNOSIS: The diagnosis was that of cervicogenic headache caused by the TrPs.

TREATMENT: She was treated with YNSA, active points of her right suboccipital muscles, bilateral cervical para-vertebral muscles, right trapezius in the K somatotope and bilateral SCM in the J somatotope. In addition, a press needle was applied to the right neck point of the chest somatotope. As soon as the needles were inserted into the relevant points, significant improvements occurred both objectively and subjectively. Her neck rotation improved from 45 to 60 degrees bilaterally and lateral flexion improved from 20 to 30 degrees, with much less pain. The TrPs were much improved as well. The patient's face lit up and, once the needles were removed after 20 minutes, she rated her headache as 4/10.

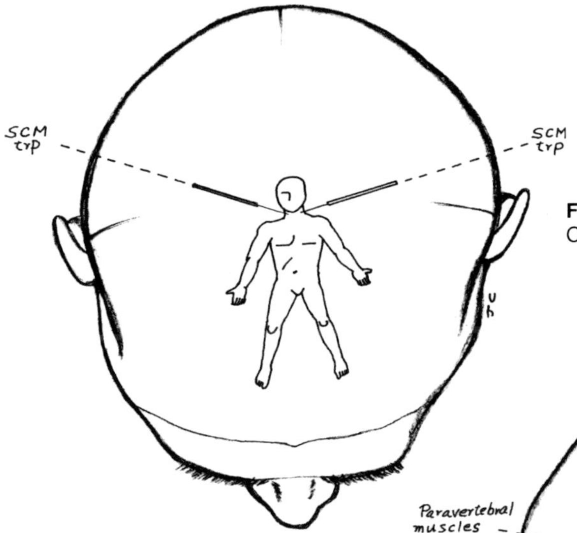

Figure 150: TrPs treatment for Case Study 31 (J somatotope)

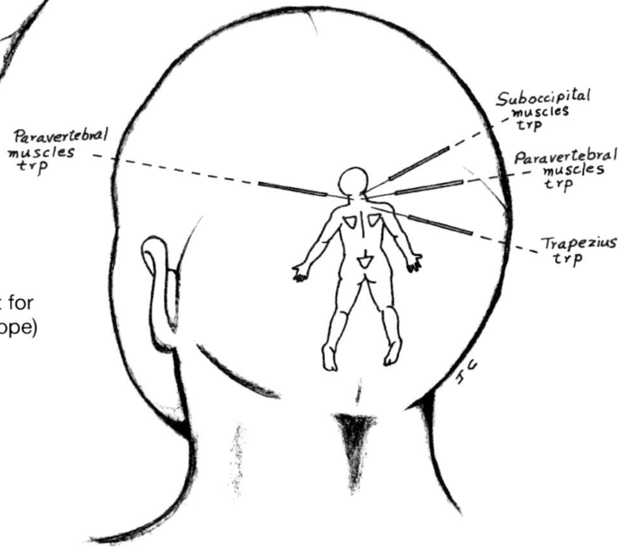

Figure 151: TrPs treatment for Case Study 31 (K somatotope)

OUTCOME: The patient continued to improve with each treatment and, after eight treatments, reported no headaches at all.

NB. The majority of patients with severe and frequent cervicogenic headaches have a past history of head and neck injuries. Such as: whiplash injuries from a MVA (usually being hit by another car from behind), surfing accidents, falls where the patient hits their head, being hit by a soccer ball and other sporting head trauma, and so on. Sometimes the injuries would have occurred a long time ago, but a recent minor accident can trigger severe and more constant headaches. At times, these headaches can also start after a prolonged period of being bedridden with a severe illness, with detrimental and prolonged sleeping positions causing the neck to strain. Typically, the sites of the pain are unilateral, sub-occipital, temporal or retro-orbital. Patients often wake up with a headache that lasts for days. There may be past history of infrequent migraines, but these recurrent ones are not of the migraine category. From my experience, once the TrPs are cleared, they will not return. With the clearance of these TrPs, the headaches tend to reduce in intensity and frequency, and sometimes cease completely.

CASE STUDY 32 (chronic cervicogenic headache – multiple neck TrPs, treated with YNSA)

HISTORY: A 43-year-old female office worker presented with severe recurrent headaches she'd been having since she was 20. The headache had increased in frequency in the last four years or so. It was occurring two to five times per week, often lasting up to two to three days. The centre of the headaches was around the left mastoid process area, radiating to the suboccipital and temporal area. She denied any dental problems. These headaches did not fit the criteria of migraines as there was no aura, no photophobia and no vomiting. She noted that stress, exercises, alcohol and poor sleeping positions would often precede the headaches. On a VAS, she rated them as 6–8/10. Cerebral MRI was normal.

She recalled two significant childhood falls. The patient did not remember whether she had injured her head or neck at the time. She was being managed by a neurologist and a recent cerebral MRI was normal. She had tried numerous medications, including betablockers, antidepressants, topiramate and sumatriptan, all of which were not helpful. She was treated with eptinezumab infusion every three months, which helped the headaches significantly. However, she decided against continuing due to the side effects. Up to this point, neck dysfunction had not been considered as a cause of her headaches.

REASONING: The site of the headaches pointed to the possibility of the SCM dysfunction, and the childhood falls could have contributed to a neck problem. It would be beneficial to target the SCM in the examination.

EXAMINATION: The patient had an 8/10 headache at the time. A neurological examination was carried out and was normal. Tinel's sign was negative for occipital nerve neuralgia. Neck rotation was normal at 75 degrees to the right but only 60 degrees to the left. Very tender TrPs were found at the left trapezius (at least three in number) and the clavicular section of the left pectoralis major. The most significant TrPs were at the proximal end of the left SCM and the muscle was very, very tender all along its length. The patient exclaimed, 'How did you know it was there? That's the centre of my headache!'

DIAGNOSIS: It was very likely that the chronic SCM TrPs had contributed to her headaches, and it was worthwhile to try to eradicate it and see how it would affect her headaches.

INVESTIGATIONS: None necessary.

TREATMENT: The patient was treated with YNSA. Active points of the left trapezius in the K somatotope, the active points of the left SCM (multiple points) and the pectoralis in the J somatotope were needled. The left neck point in the chest somatotope was also treated with a press needle. Even after the first treatment, there was instant improvement in the ROM and the TrPs.

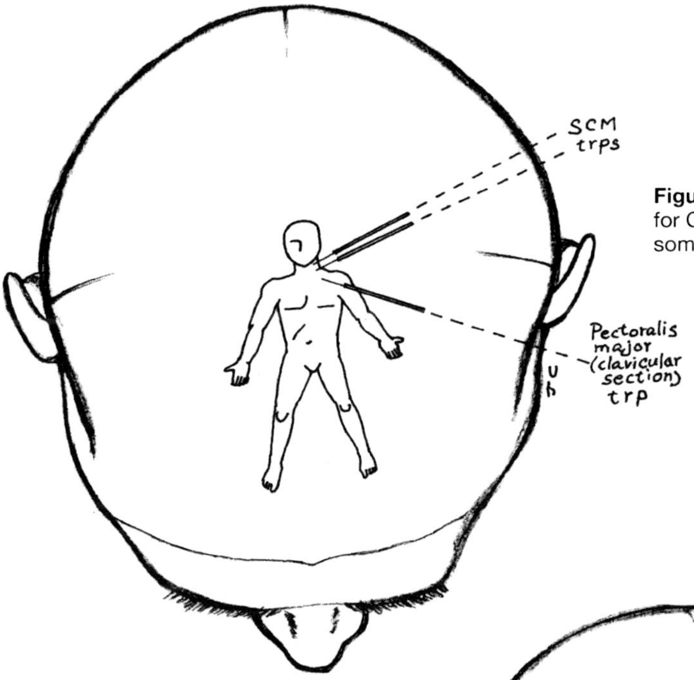

Figure 152: TrPs treatment for Case Study 32 (J somatotope)

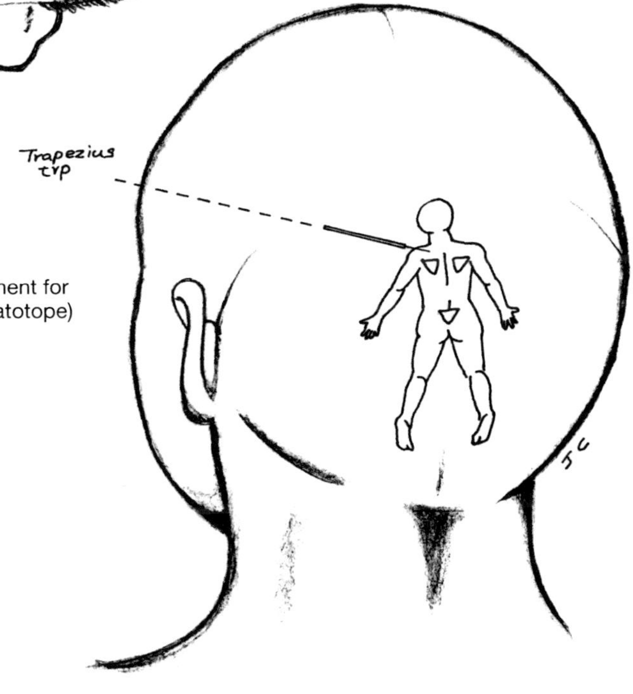

Figure 153: TrPs treatment for Case Study 32 (K somatotope)

OUTCOME: There was about a 10% improvement with each treatment. The patient had to travel interstate frequently, so there were often gaps in her weekly visits. It took four months for the treatment program to complete, after which she happily reported no headaches at all.

CASE STUDY 33 (C6 radiculopathy – multiple neck TrPs, treated with YNSA)

HISTORY: A 48-year-old female presented with a one-week history of left shoulder area pain associated with parathaesia, which radiated down her arm to her first two fingers. She rated the pain in the VAS as 6/10 and fairly constant. She reported no arm weakness and shoulder movements did not aggravate the pain. There was no history of trauma or shoulder problems. Her history included chronic mild neck stiffness and discomfort and severe recurrent migraines, successfully treated by YNSA over three months. In her opinion, the migraines had improved by about 80%.

REASONING: This appeared to be consistent with a cervical radiculopathy in the C6 distribution. Cervical facet joint arthropathy can refer pain to the shoulder but usually not down to the fingers. Pain from TrPs in the shoulder region can radiate down the arm but would be aggravated by shoulder movements (see Table 1).

EXAMINATION: Shoulder ROM was full and not painful, which ruled out rotator cuff diseases or muscle strain as a cause. She had a pre-existing reduction in the neck rotation to the left. Her sensation was normal, but her bicep strength was slightly weaker (which is not definitive as she was right-handed). The extension-rotation test for facet joint arthropathy was negative (as C5, C6 and C7 facet joint arthropathies can refer pain to the shoulder area). Reduced bicep and brachioradialis jerks sealed the diagnosis.

DIAGNOSIS: The diagnosis was a left C6 radiculopathy, subsequently confirmed by a cervical spine MRI.

TREATMENT: Dr Yamamoto, who discovered the YNSA system, had a very keen interest in neurology. Besides mapping out the many scalp somatotopes, he also found acupuncture points for all the cranial, cervical, thoracic and lumbar nerves as well (Fig. 154). He used these acupuncture points to treat neurological conditions such as radiculopathies, post herpetic neuralgias and CVAs. After ruling out red flags that require prompt surgical intervention, we can trial YNSA treatment on radiculopathies. I have had many successes with minor radiculopathies, when there is no red-flag criteria for urgent surgical intervention.

The treatment includes targeting:

1. the specific spinal nerve points in the A, E and D points (Fig. 154);
2. the neck point in the chest somatotope (Fig. 148 and 149) for cervical radiculopathies;
3. any TrPs in the region e.g. for a minor lumbar radiculopathy, loosening tight muscles in the piriformis, gluteals and hamstrings may take some tension off the nerve roots;
4. the painful region in the J and K somatotope.

In this case study, the patient was treated with YNSA targeting:

1. the left A6 point;
2. the left neck point in the chest somatotope;
3. TrPs for the left trapezius and SCM (multiple TrPs there);
4. the painful region – anterior aspect of the left shoulder, arm and finger area.

THE A, E, D POINTS AND THE CRANIAL NERVE POINTS

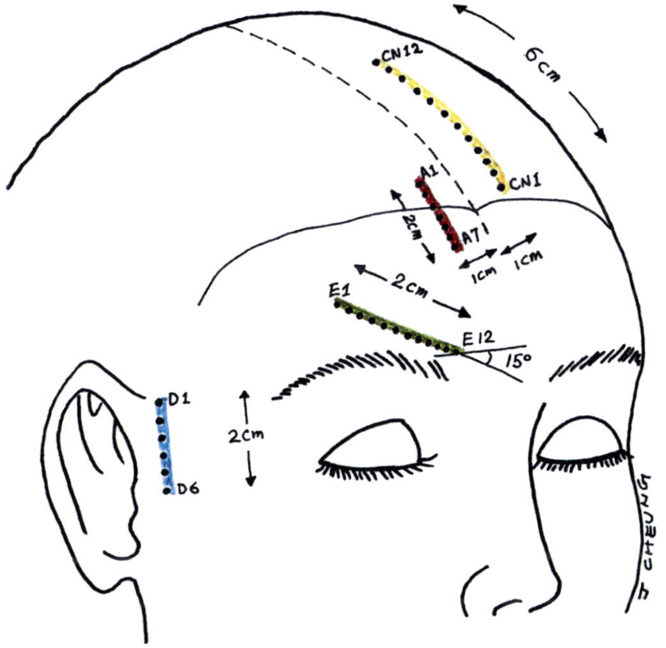

Figure 154: A, E, D and cranial nerve (CN) points in the YNSA system

- The A1 to A7 represent cervical nerves 1 to 7, with the A3 situated at the hairline. The E1 to E12 represent thoracic nerves 1 to 12.
- The D1 to D6 represent lumbar nerve 1 to sacral nerve 1.
- The CN1 to CN12 represent cranial nerve 1 to 12. (CN1 is located just posterior to the hairline, 1cm lateral to the midline.)

Their locations are found by palpating for a tiny, depressed spot (at times a raised spot), correlating to a very painful sensation experienced by the patient. A needle is then inserted in the active point.

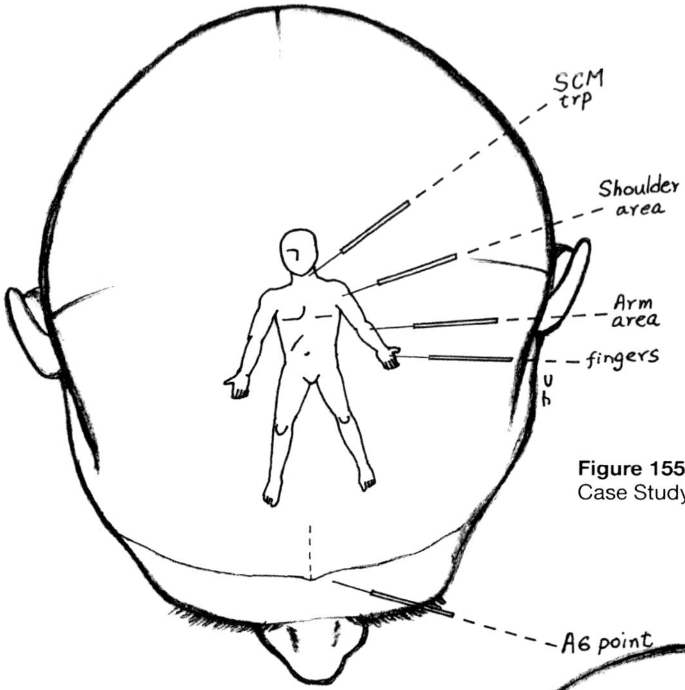

Figure 155: TrPs treatment for Case Study 33 (J somatotope)

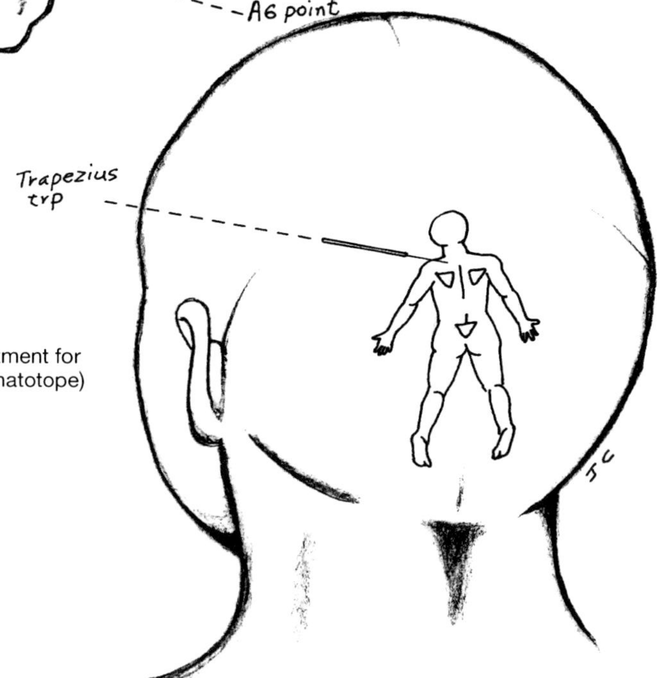

Figure 156: TrPs treatment for Case Study 33 (K somatotope)

OUTCOME: The patient made progressive improvements and, after eight treatments, was completely pain-free and her reflexes normalised.

THE SCALENE MUSCLES AND THEIR TrPs

Caution: Palpate very gently in this region, as there are a lot of important structures here, including the cervical plexus.

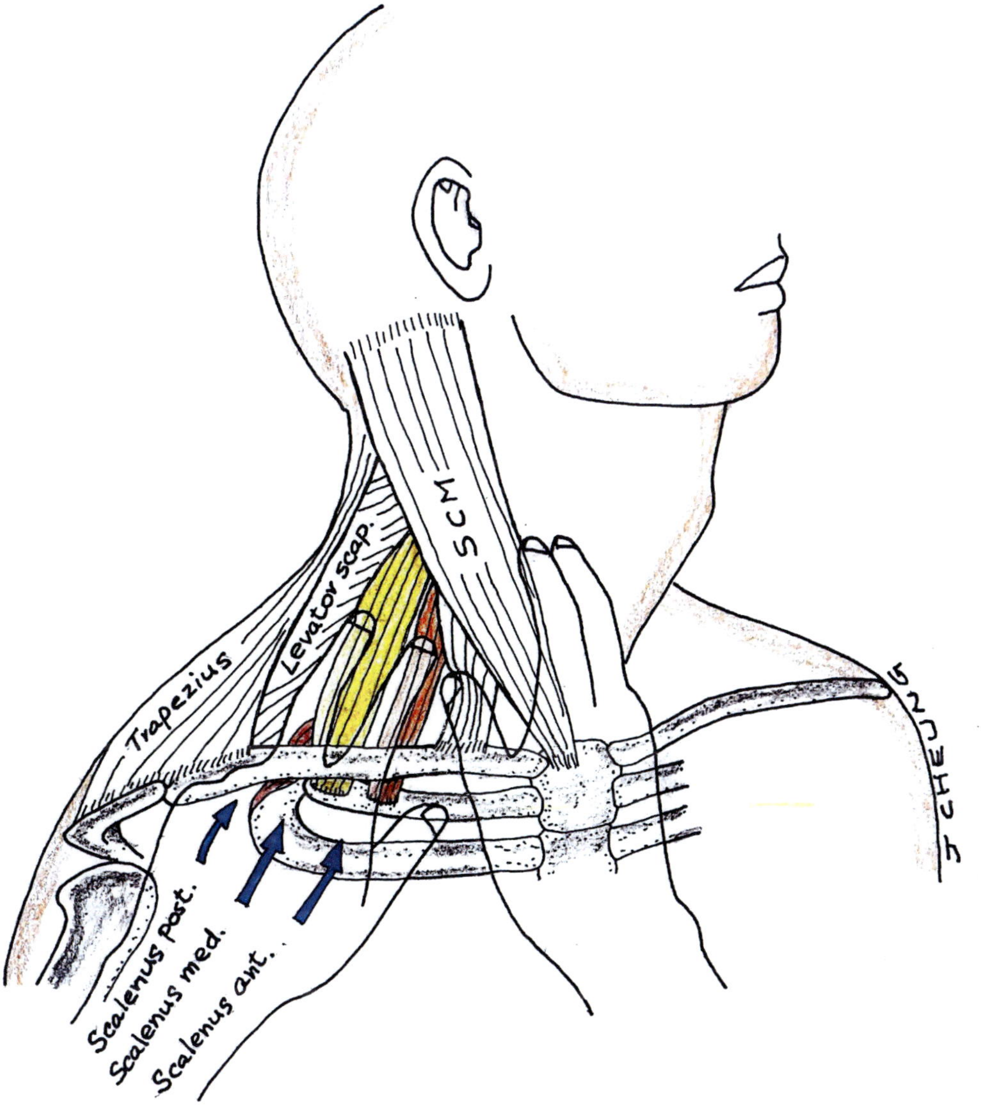

Figure 157: Palpation diagram for the scalene muscles TrPs

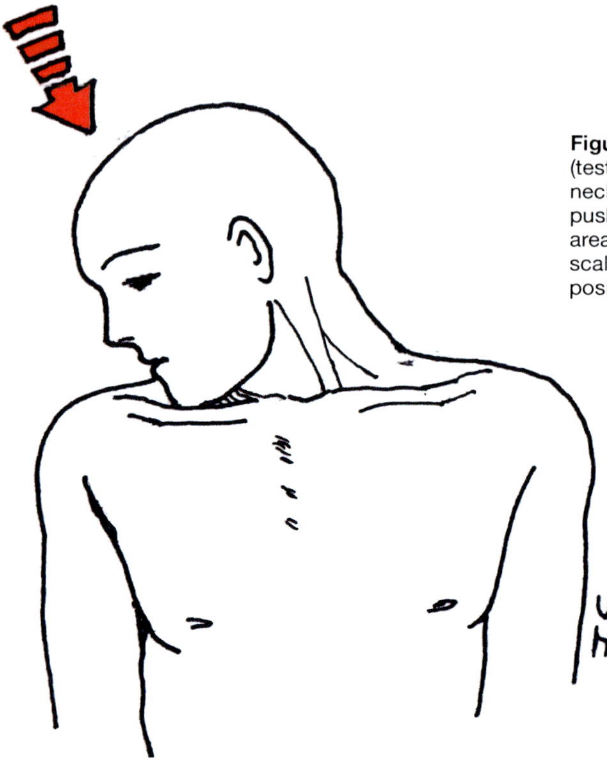

Figure 158: Scalene Cramp Test (testing the right side): Rotate the neck towards the painful side and push the chin into the clavicular area. An increase in pain in the scalene muscles means the test is positive.

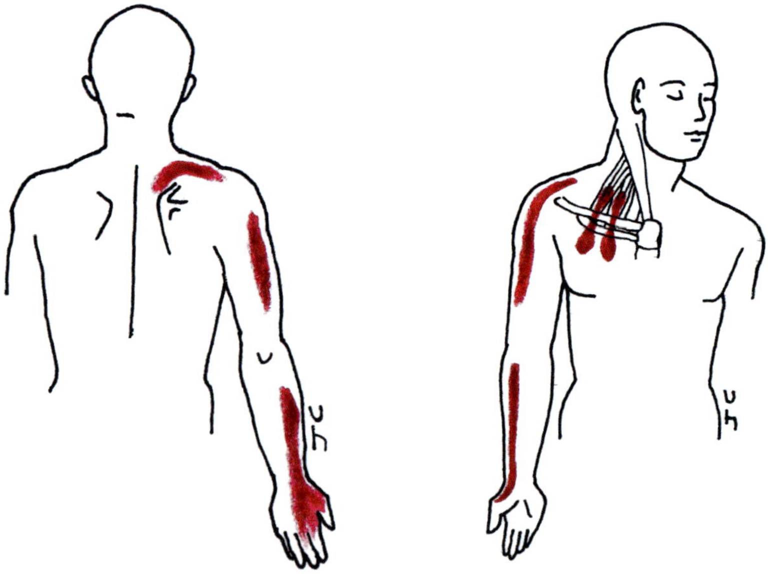

Figure 159: Scalenus TrPs and their referred pain pattern

X = TrPs

Red area = the referred pain

THE LATISSIMUS DORSI AND ITS TrPs

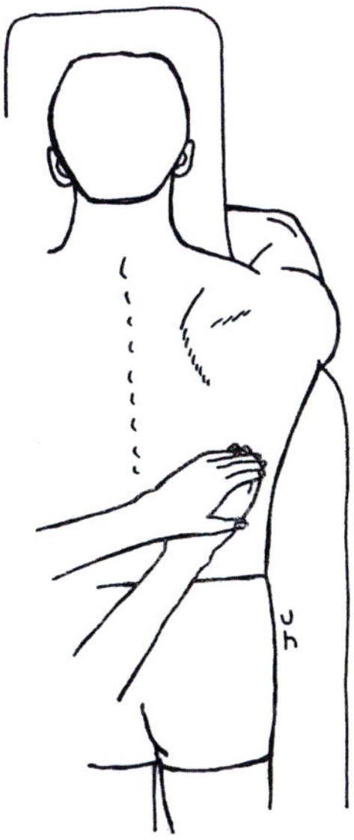

Figure 160: The position to palpate for the latissimus dorsi TrPs

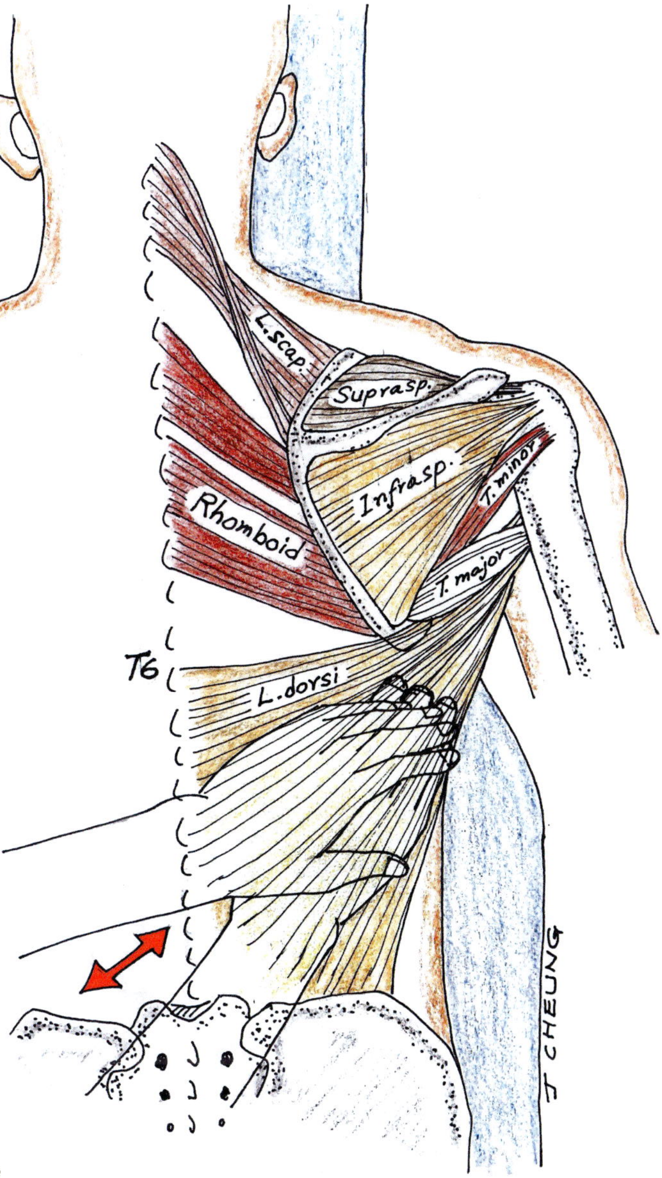

Figure 161: Palpation diagram for the latissimus dorsi TrPs

NB. The latissimus dorsi is a big muscle, and in order to palpate for its TrPs or to massage it, the patient needs to be lying prone (Fig. 160 and 161). A small amount of massage oil or soluble bath oil is necessary for the palpation.

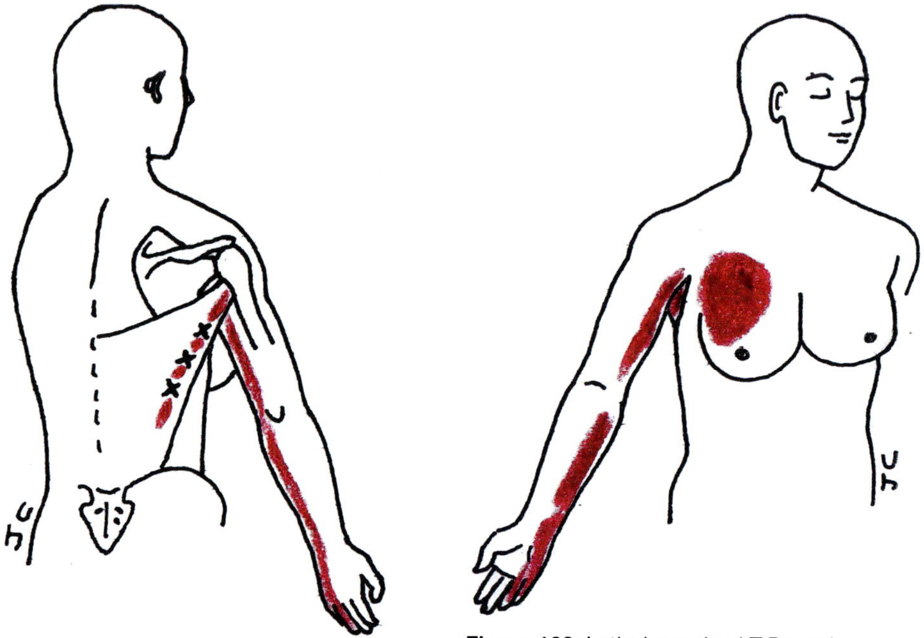

Figure 162: Latissimus dorsi TrPs and their referred pain pattern

X = TrPs

Red area = the referred pain

NB. The pain distribution from latissimus dorsi TrPs often mimics angina, breast pain, axilla pain, shoulder or chest pathologies.

CASE STUDY 34 (left shoulder pain – latissimus dorsi TrPs, treated with YNSA)

HISTORY: A 22-year-old female presented with a two-month history of intermittent sharp pain and tingling in the left scapular, axillary area, radiating down the inner arm to her last two fingers. There was no history of trauma. She did, however, regularly train with weights. The patient also swam regularly and had found it aggravated the pain so much that she had to stop. She indicated that she could hang clothes on the line and fasten her bra with slight discomfort. She was diagnosed with possible C8 radiculopathy by her GP and an MRI was ordered.

REASONING: Pain distribution was consistent with C8 radiculopathy, however, radiculopathy tends to be more constant in nature and not aggravated by very specific arm movements. Latissimus dorsi strain and TrPs would be more likely, as its referred pain pattern can also radiate down the inner arm to the last two fingers. Other shoulder muscle strains were also possible (see Table 1).

EXAMINATION: The patient had full ROM in the shoulder, but the pain was intensified on shoulder adduction and flexion. The painful arc test was negative.

Sensation in the C8 distribution, triceps reflex and finger grip were all normal. On muscle palpation, there were very tender TrPs along the lateral border of the latissimus dorsi, which, when pressed, recreated her pain.

TREATMENT: Her condition would have been suitable for YNSA treatment, however, she lived too far away. I advised her to see a physiotherapist for appropriate manual treatment.

OUTCOME: Six weeks later, she was pain-free.

NB. The Latissimus dorsi extends the arm at the shoulder and is used in swimming (just look at how well the muscle is developed in Olympic swimmers) and weight training. It also adducts the arm while retracting the scapular – the exact action in computer work – which probably explains why it is often strained for those using laptops a lot.

CASE STUDY 35 (left anterior chest pain – latissimus dorsi, levator scapulae, rhomboid, infraspinatus, pectoralis major and cervical paravertebral muscles TrPs, treated with YNSA)

HISTORY: A 22-year-old female presented with a five-hour history of 7/10 left-anterior upper-chest pain, radiating down the inner aspect of her left arm. The pain extended to her last two fingers. She was not short of breath and did not have any nausea. She had a very strong family history of ischaemic heart disease, although had no previous heart problems or any other health issues herself. While undergoing home renovations, she had been carrying building materials up and down two flights of stairs, including a large glass pane that morning. She avoided moving the left arm as it was very painful.

REASONING: Angina for five hours sounded unlikely. The symptoms pointed more to a muscular strain. A lot of shoulder muscle dysfunction can give shoulder, chest and axillary pain, and some can have radiation down the arm. However, care must be taken to ensure that it is not ischaemic before treating it as a muscular problem.

EXAMINATION: A physical examination was carried out. She was afebrile, BP was normal, lung and heart auscultation were normal. ECG was normal. She had full ROM in her left shoulder, but movements were uncomfortable, and the painful arc test was negative. Shoulder external rotation was painful, pointing to dysfunction in the infraspinatus and teres minor. On palpation, there were tender TrPs in her left levator scapulae, rhomboid, infraspinatus, paravertebral muscles, pectoralis major (clavicular head) and, most markedly, her latissimus dorsi.

INVESTIGATIONS: None necessary.

TREATMENT: She was treated with YNSA at the above points in the K somatotope and J somatotope. With every successful needle insertion, the TrPs improved.

After the first treatment, her pain was much better. However, the pain returned to the same severity 24 hours later. Most of the TrPs were much improved, except for the left infraspinatus, which was probably missed at the first treatment. At the second treatment, all the points were needled, including the infraspinatus.

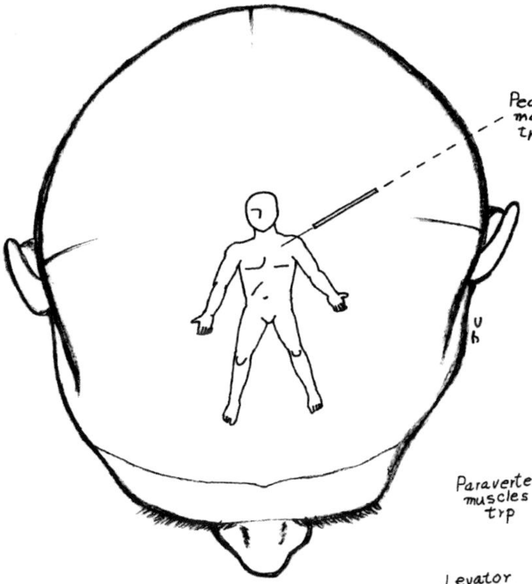

Figure 163: TrP treatment for Case Study 35 (J Somatotope)

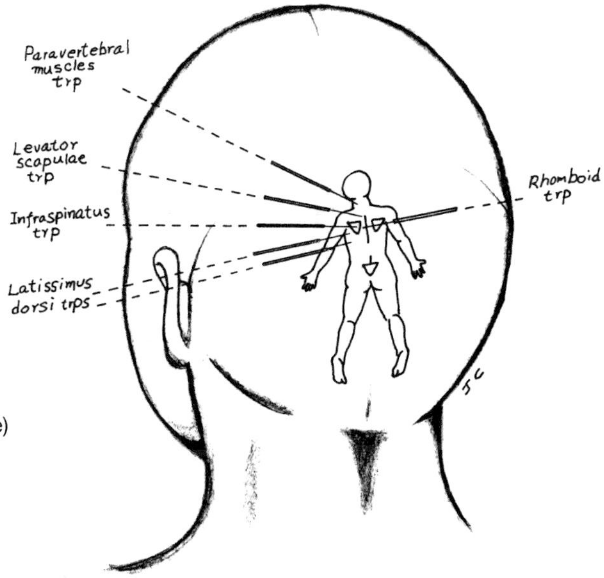

Figure 164: TrP treatment for Case Study 35 (K Somatotope)

OUTCOME: The patient was pain-free after four treatments.

NB. This case showed muscular TrPs can certainly mimic angina, however, care must be taken to exclude it first before treating it as a muscular problem. At times, patients with chest pain are investigated with a coronary angiogram, only to be told that the angiogram is normal and that the chest pain is probably muscular in nature. A lot of shoulder muscle dysfunction can give shoulder, chest and axillary pain, and some can have radiation down the arm e.g. scalene muscles, pectoralis, coracobrachialis, supraspinatus, infraspinatus, teres minor, teres major, rhomboid, subscapularis, triceps and especially the latissimus dorsi. An examination targeting these muscles with palpation would help to make the diagnosis, and with practice, it should take less than two minutes (Fig. 172).

However, care must be taken in assessing patients in this setting, as angina and muscular pain can co-exist and angina can also cause chest-wall muscle spasms.

THE PECTORALIS MAJOR AND ITS TrPs

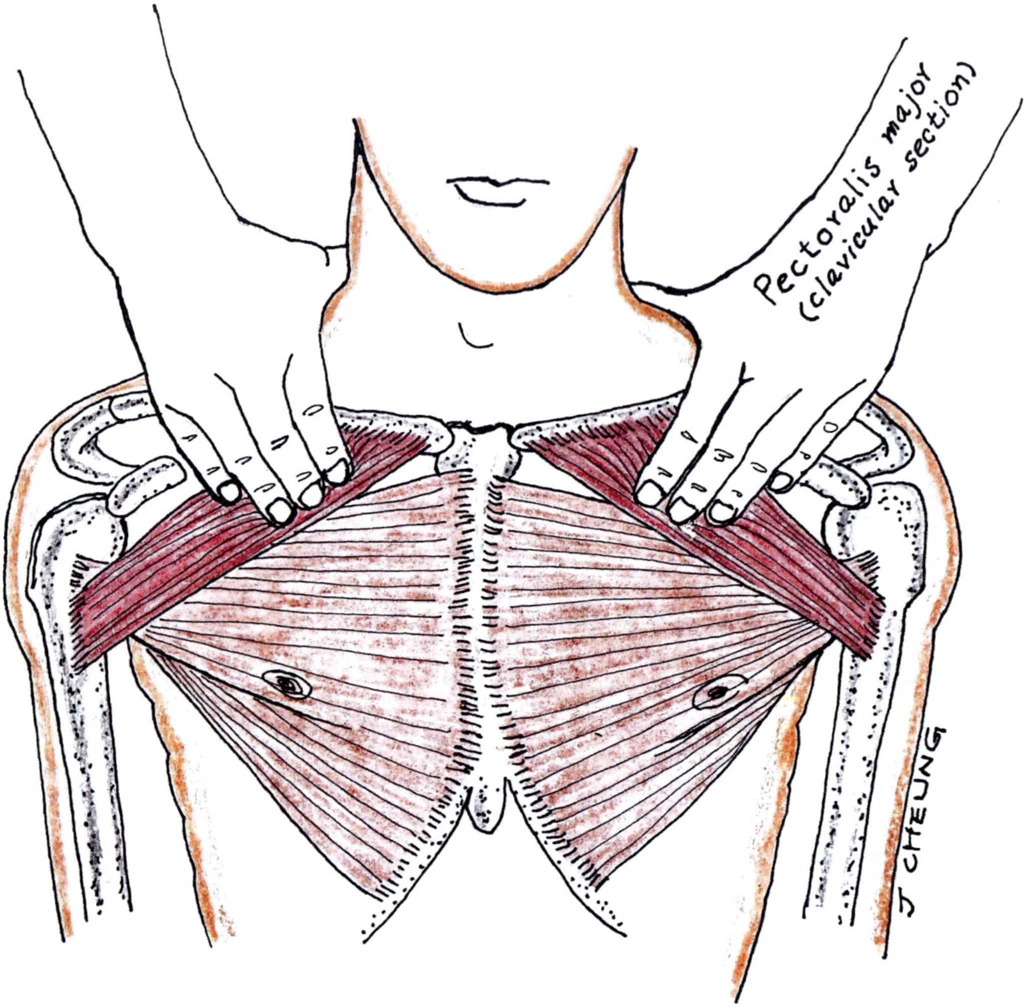

Figure 165: Palpation diagram for the pectoralis major TrPs

NB. Pectoralis major (clavicular section) TrPs often result from neck and shoulder problems, as it balances the tight posterior muscles. In these conditions, it is important to treat it as well.

THE CORACOBRACHIALIS AND ITS TrPs

Figure 166: Palpation diagram for the coracobrachialis TrPs

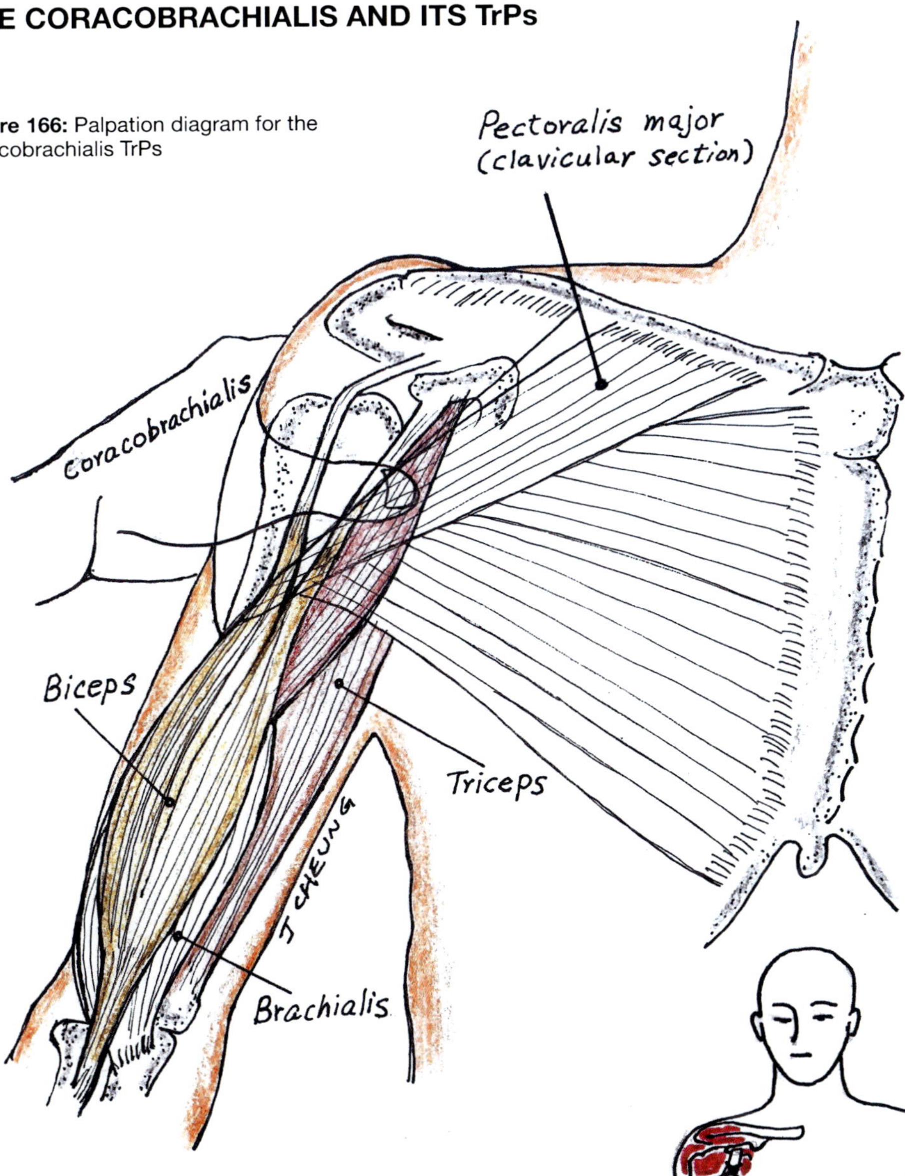

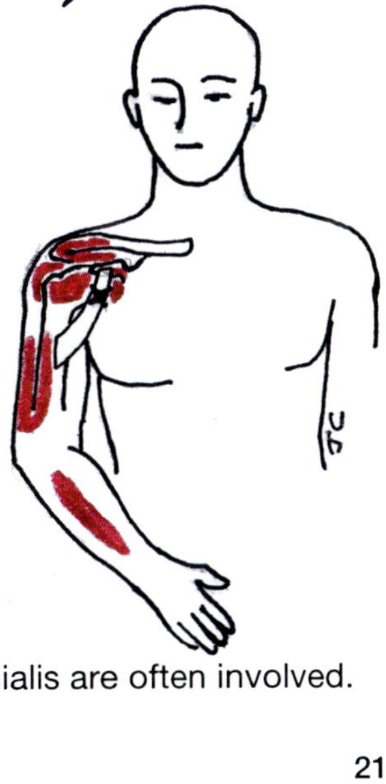

Figure 167: Coracobrachialis TrPs and their referred pain pattern

X = TrPs

Red area = the referred pain

NB. In shoulder pain syndromes, TrPs in the coracobrachialis are often involved.

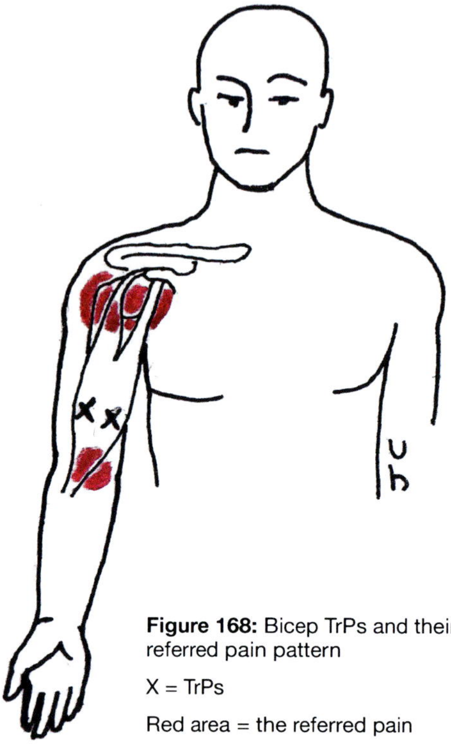

Figure 168: Bicep TrPs and their referred pain pattern

X = TrPs

Red area = the referred pain

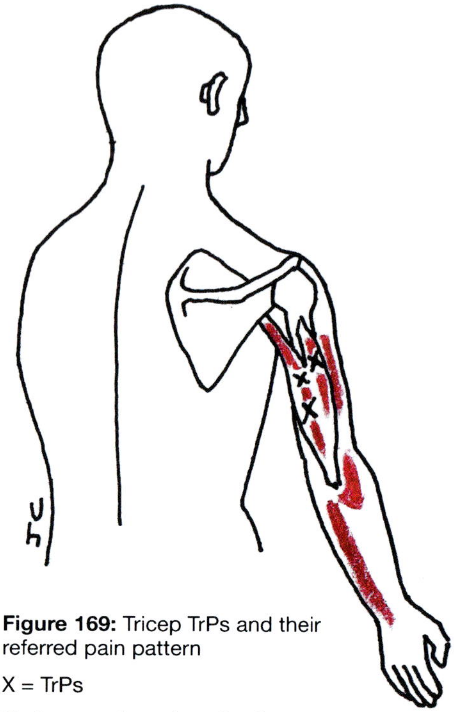

Figure 169: Tricep TrPs and their referred pain pattern

X = TrPs

Red area = the referred pain

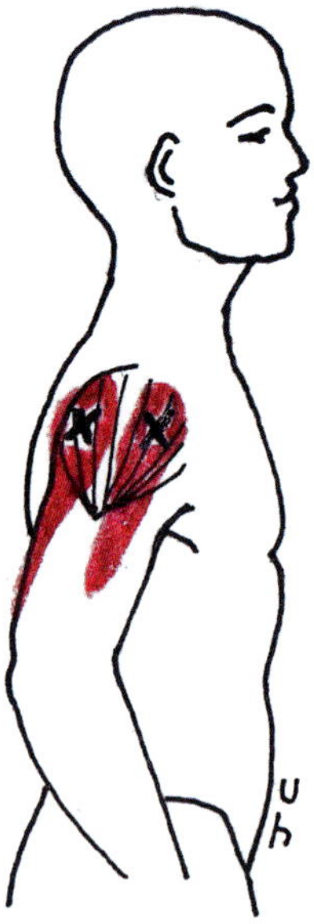

Figure 170: Deltoid TrPs and their referred pain pattern

X = TrPs

Red area = the referred pain

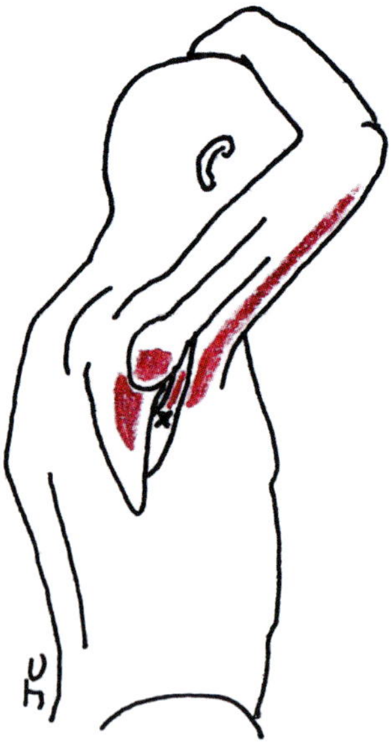

Figure 171: Subscapularis TrPs and their referred pain pattern

X = TrPs

Red area = the referred pain

A SUMMARY OF A PROPOSED APPROACH TO A PATIENT PRESENTING WITH SHOULDER OR HEAD AND NECK PAIN

1. Attempt to reach a diagnosis through a thorough history
2. Rule out any red-flag diagnosis
3. Examination targeted to confirm diagnosis and to exclude other possibilities
4. If appropriate, include palpation for trigger points (TrPs) around the shoulder and neck region. They may be part of, if not the main cause of, the pain. With practice, it will take a few minutes (see Fig. 172).
5. Order appropriate imaging or other investigations. Tests should not take precedence over, or replace, the above steps. Try not to order unnecessary tests that would not change the management plan. Tests often show multiple pathologies that are not the cause of the problem, thus, confusing the diagnostic process.
6. Plan treatment with the aim to cure or improve the condition, not just to treat the pain.

Finding trigger points and treating them successfully can

- **eradicate the pain completely (when the TrPs are the cause);**
- **improve some of the pain (as the TrPs cause some of the pain);**
- **exclude TrPs as the cause of the pain, and allow you to move on to consider other possible diagnoses; and**
- **often avoid expensive imaging or invasive treatments.**

NB. There are often many instances when a pain syndrome is wrongly diagnosed to be from a shoulder osteoarthritis or subacromial bursitis when the cause of pain is primarily from TrPs. However, just because significant TrPs are found in a patient, it doesn't always mean that is the diagnosis. The TrPs may be secondary to another condition. Often multiple conditions can coexist.

It is worth remembering that diagnoses are static entities, whereas a patient's condition changes and evolves with time. A patient with minor cervical nerve root impingement pain may evolve to have significant muscular TrP pain, overshadowing the original impingement pain. Someone with mainly TrP pain may evolve to develop a radiculopathy; or after eradicating the TrP pain in a patient, an underlying minor radiculopathy or OA pain may become more evident. As TrPs are very common and readily treatable, it is still worthwhile eradicating them first.

PALPATION FOR TRIGGER POINTS IN THE SHOULDER AND NECK REGION

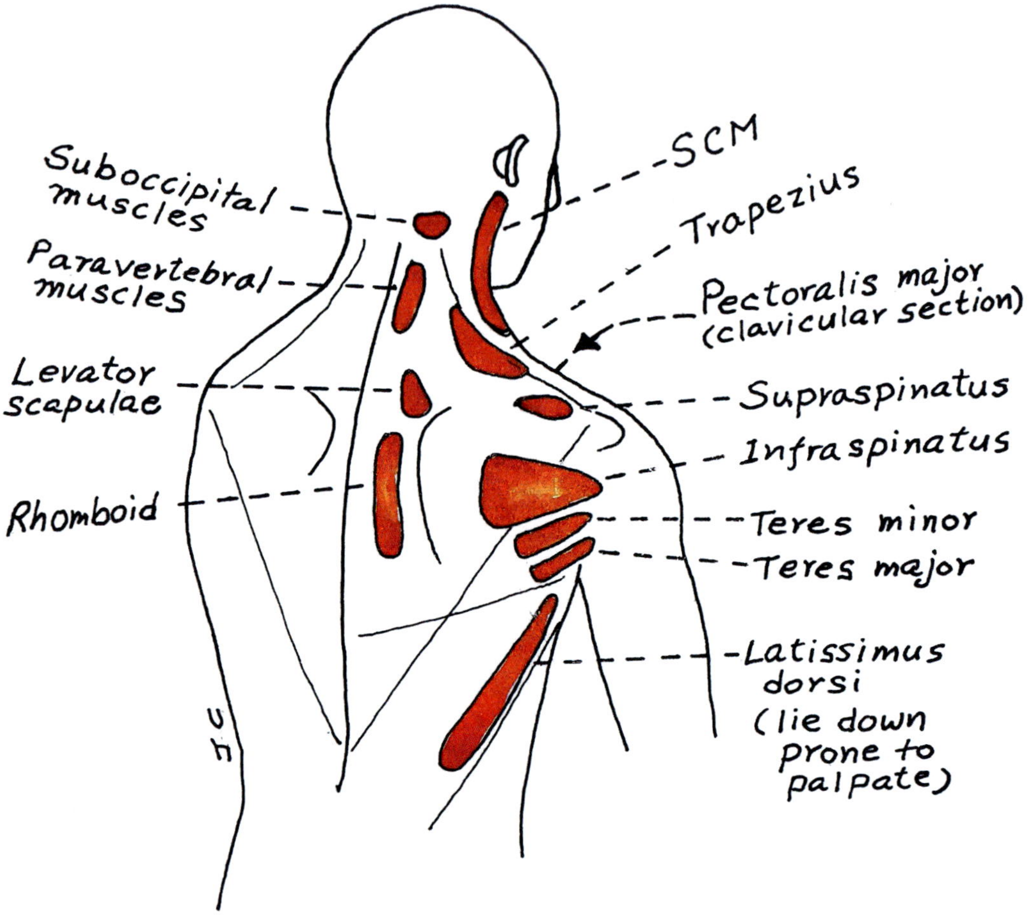

Figure 172: Palpation for TrPs in the shoulder, head and neck region

SOME GENTLE EXERCISES FOR PAINFUL SHOULDER CONDITIONS

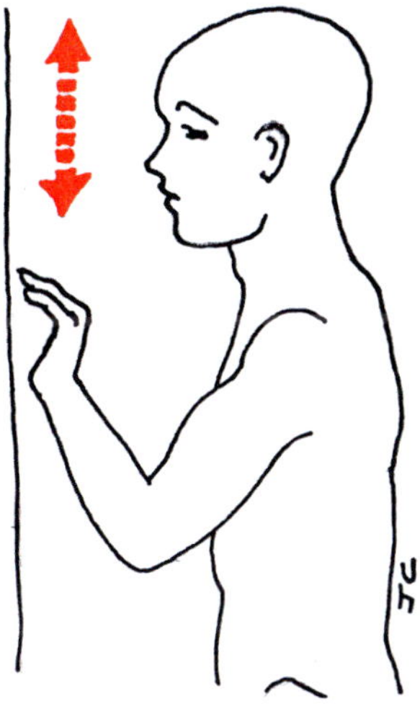

Crawling up and down the wall

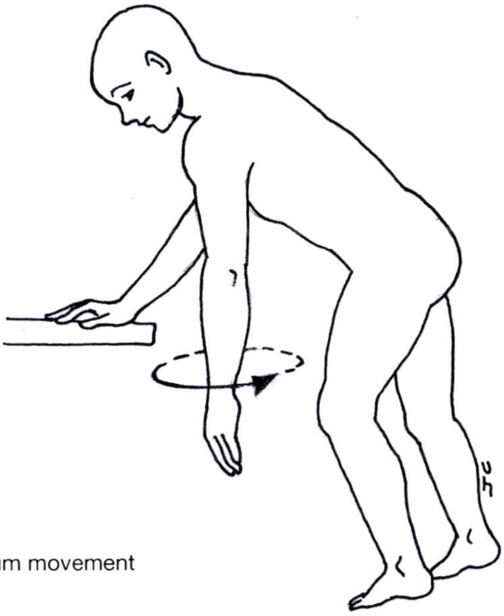

Pendulum movement

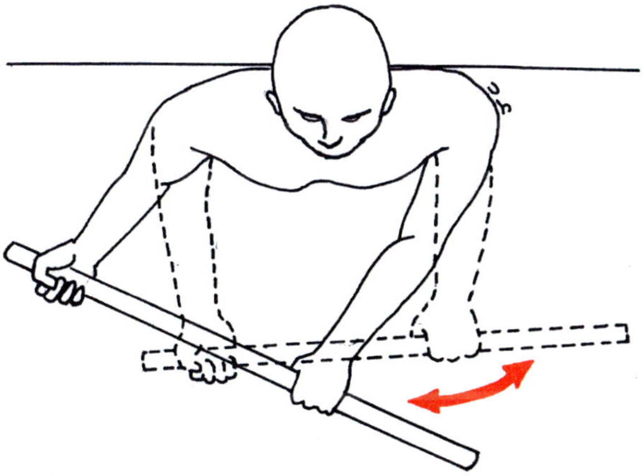

The unaffected arm helping the affected arm in external rotation

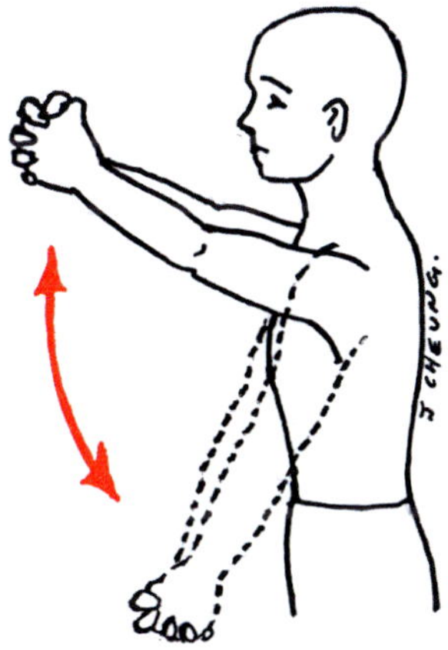

The unaffected arm lifting the affected arm upwards

Figure 173: Useful exercises for painful shoulder conditions

SOME SHOULDER STRETCHES

You need to feel the stretch in the designated muscles and relax all the adjacent muscles in order to target it. Maintain the stretch for eight breaths or 30 seconds and repeat if necessary. Be patient, do it every day.

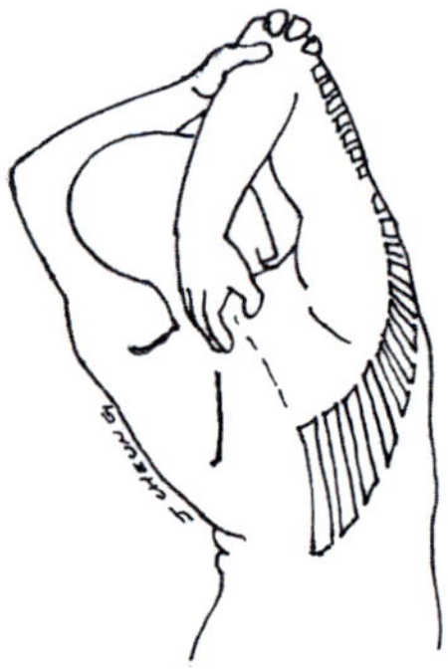

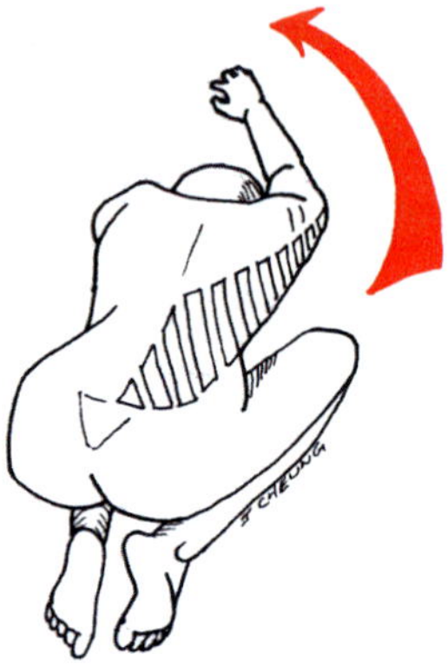

Triceps, Latissimus dorsi

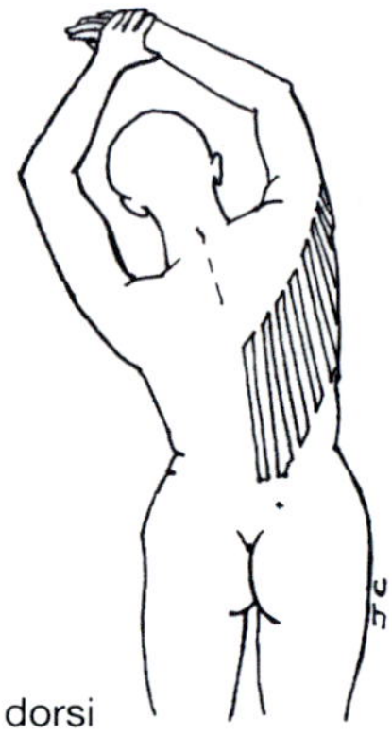

Latissimus dorsi

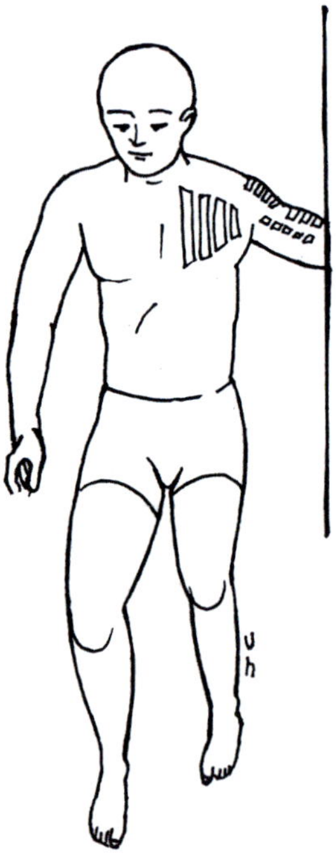

Pectoralis, Anterior Deltoid, Coracobrachialis, Biceps

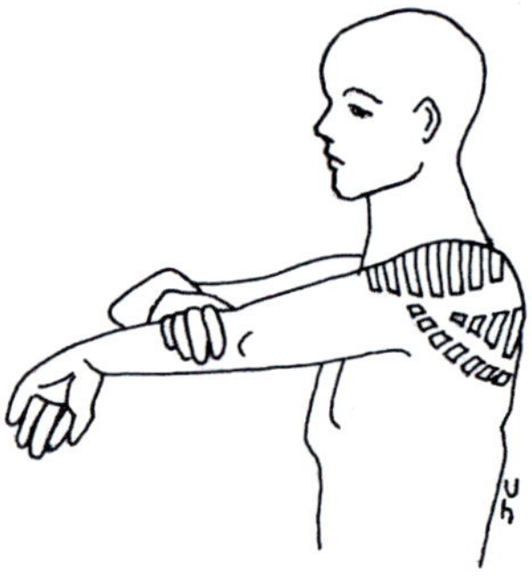

Posterior Deltoid, Infraspinatus, Teres minor

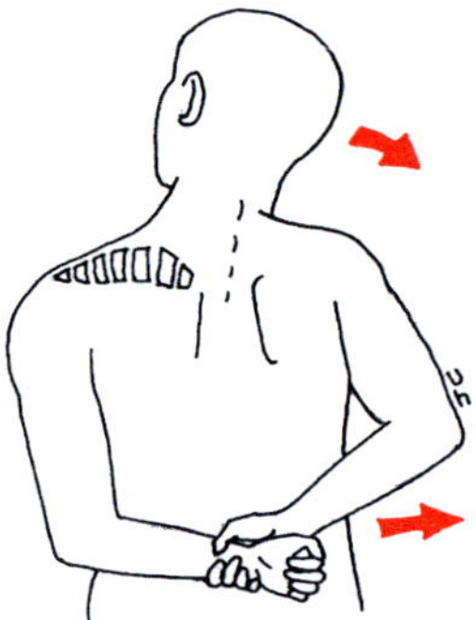

Supraspinatus

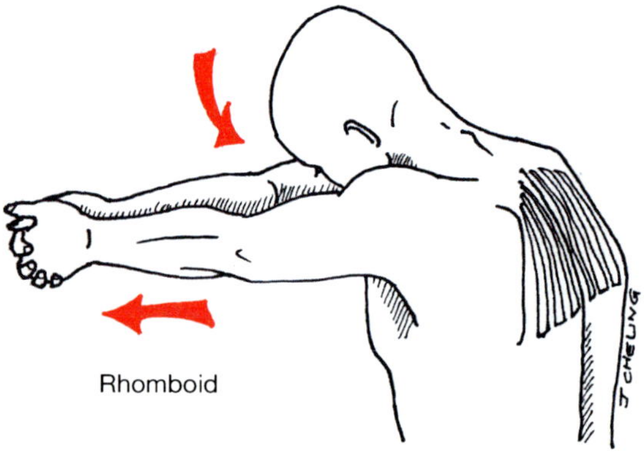

Rhomboid

Figure 174: Useful stretches for the shoulder

SOME STRENGTHENING EXERCISES FOR THE SHOULDER

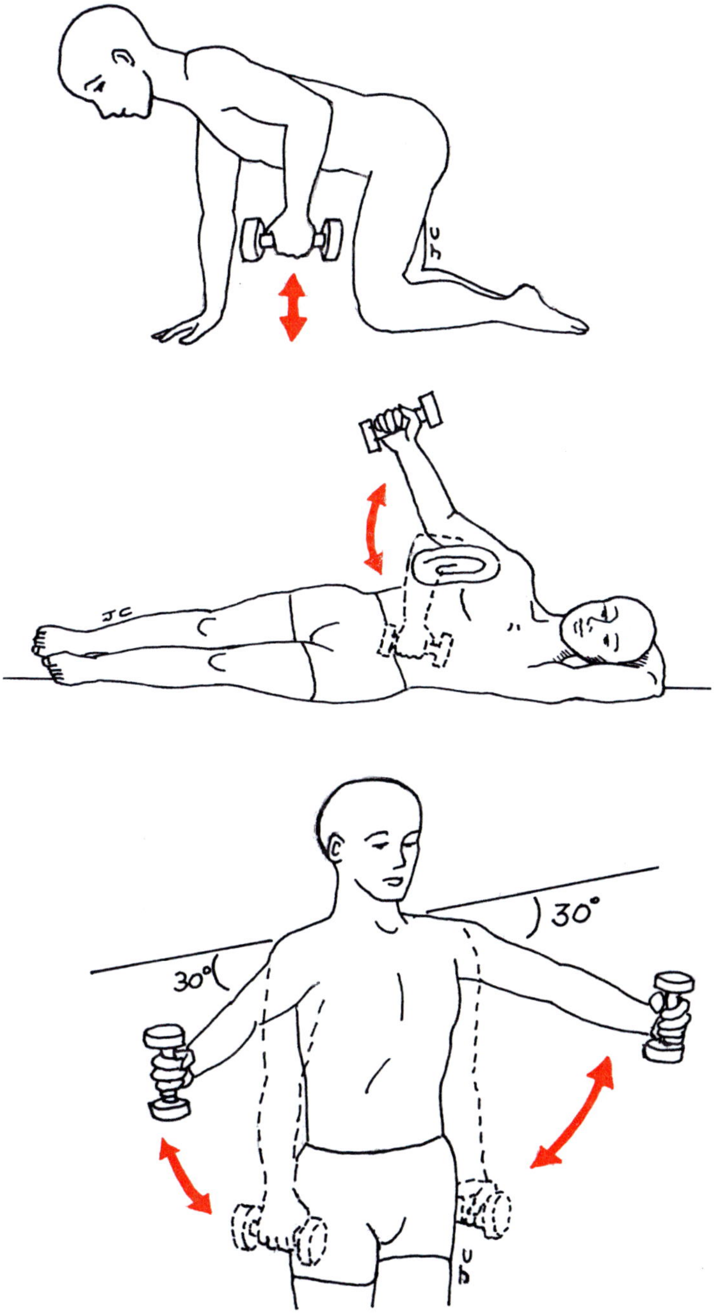

Figure 175: Useful strengthening exercises for the shoulder

SOME STRETCHES AND LOOSENING EXERCISES FOR THE NECK

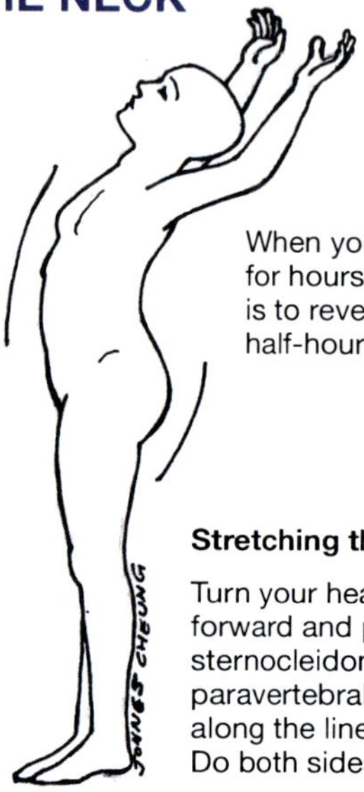

When you bend over a laptop for hours, the least you can do is to reverse the posture every half-hour.

Stretching the neck muscles

Turn your head 45° to one side (for the levator scapulae), face forward and pull the head to one side (for the trapezius and the sternocleidomastoid), face forward and pull the head down (for the paravertebral muscles); pull as shown until you can feel the stretch along the line, maintain the stretch for 30 seconds or eight breaths. Do both sides and repeat, if necessary, until muscles are relaxed.

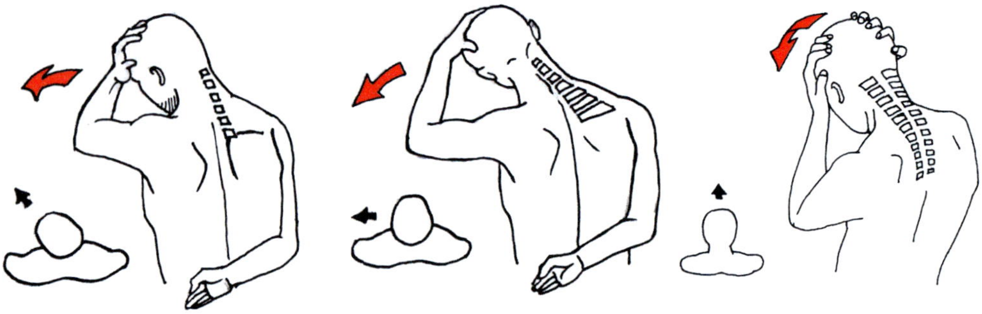

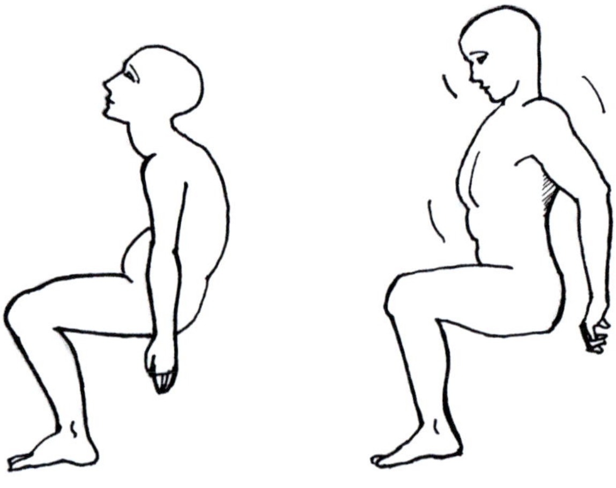

Slouching and straightening

Slouching is easy. To straighten, tuck in the chin, push the chest forwards and pull shoulder tips backwards. Alternate the two positions 20 times. It is as if you are giving yourself traction. When you are in the slouching position, think 'lethargic, lazy, unmotivated', then switch to thinking 'alert, happy, energetic' and let that feeling pull your posture to an upright position. Our mental state can help our posture and vice versa.

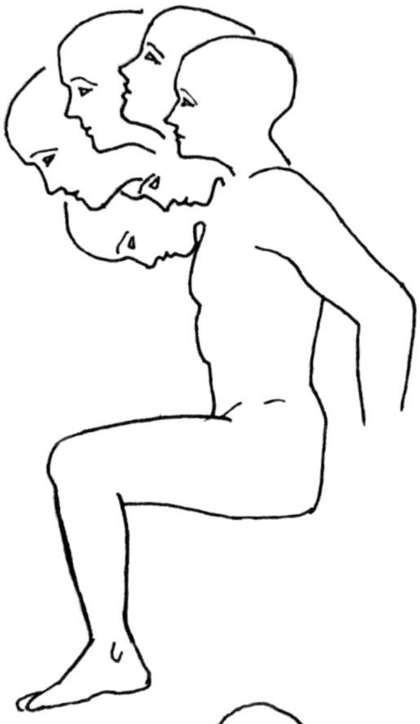

Do circles with your chin

Start with the neutral position, then draw a circle with your chin, moving it forwards until it is pressing on your lower chest. Then move your chin upwards along your chest until you reach the original neutral position. Repeat this 20 times. You should hear your neck joints clicking as you do this exercise.

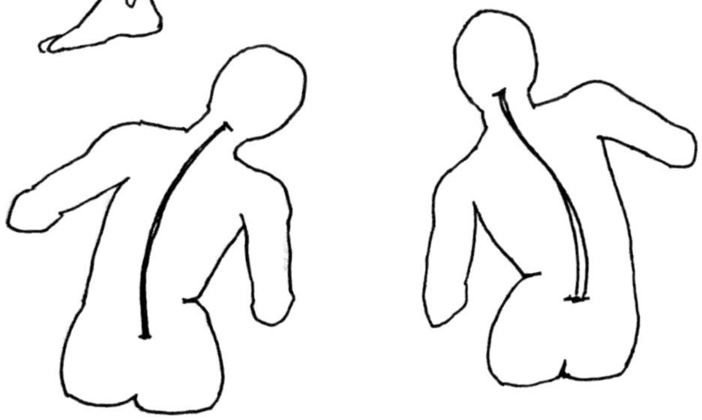

Chalk in the navel, do circles

Imagine you have a piece of chalk stuck in your navel and a blackboard right in front of your tummy. Try to draw a big circle clockwise 10 times and then anticlockwise 10 times. While you do the circles, let your head and neck relax and flop with the rhythmic movement – you are actually moving your neck sideways and loosening it indirectly as well.

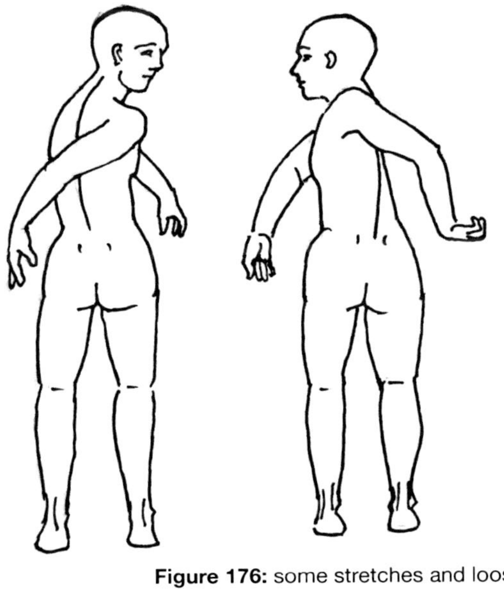

Spinning

With your feet slightly apart and toes gripping the floor, spin your whole trunk one way and then the other, using your arms to create the rotational momentum, thereby rotating your whole spine.

Figure 176: some stretches and loosening exercises for the neck

5. CONCLUSION

CHRONIC PAIN AND BEREAVEMENT

It is often said that at the very moment a patient makes an appointment to see us, the healing process has already begun, and hopefully we have the therapeutic skills to facilitate that process.

However, when it comes to chronic pain, more needs to be addressed than just the physical aspect of pain. For patients who have endured many years of pain, there is often a history of significant loss or bereavement that has not been grieved and processed in addition to the trauma of having suffered a long period of disability and pain. There may have been a relationship break-up, suicide of a close friend, a betrayal or an abandonment. It is not within the scope of this book to address these issues but it is important to be aware of these aspects and to allow the patient to verbalise and express any suppressed feelings. As their pain improves with our treatment, the patient may start to feel some hope and be more ready to let go of long suppressed feelings of grief, loneliness, despair and anger; and as the treating doctor, we must be ready to listen and facilitate these processes.

If the pain has been with the patient for a very long time, there may have been negative experiences towards other doctors and allied health colleagues previously. Negative feelings about these experiences may be transferred to us unknowingly. We should be aware of such possibilities, listen to any grievances with empathy and without judgement on either party. Emphasis should be directed gently towards possible future improvements and progress rather than the past.

It is also important to encourage and help the patient to rediscover their independence and to re-engage with the life they used to know. We should add on regular exercise regimes and encourage re-involvement in activities of daily life. To do all that, extra time must be allotted to allow for these processes. To be sure, it is a demanding challenge for the clinician but a worthwhile one.

THE QUESTION OF RESISTANCE AND COMPLIANCE

As clinicians, we often wonder why some patients follow our advice and management to the letter while others disregard even the simplest of instructions and argue with the most reasonable request. At times, patients may exhibit poor behaviour, irrational responses or unexplained anger. While such reactions can stem from external factors beyond our control, they can also arise from resistance we unintentionally create in our relationships with them.

It's important to consider where resistance might originate and how we can minimise it. Sometimes, it begins even before the patient sees us. For instance, a receptionist who is unhelpful, does not inquire about the urgency of the matter, or interacts abruptly can create resistance early on. This highlights the value of having a skilled and empathetic receptionist - if you have one, make every effort to retain them. Other factors might also contribute, such as difficulties finding parking near our practice or a poorly maintained, untidy, or unwelcoming clinic environment. These seemingly minor issues can leave a negative first impression, potentially influencing how patients engage with us.

In any relationship, being on time shows respect and running more than 20 minutes late starts to create resistance. (There are ways to avoid this, such as making longer appointments when appropriate, having catch-up time in our schedules, ringing patients when you are running an hour late, etc.) Do apologise if you are late.

When meeting patients, a warm greeting and a smile always helps. Once the consultation has started, drop all other concerns and concentrate purely on the patient. Break the ice, talk about something of mutual interest. A positive approach is always encouraging. Whenever there is a chance to say something to enhance a patient's self-esteem, it would be worthwhile to do so. For example, 'Well done! I am so impressed with you completing a degree while working full-time', 'You have done an amazing job as a parent', 'You look really healthy and vibrant today. I think losing some weight and your exercise regime are really working.'

Relate to your patients as equals and with respect; try to talk in accessible terms and limit the use of jargon. Ask for permission before examining the patient or doing a test, even though it is probably expected. For example, 'Can I listen to your chest?', 'Can I have a look at the mole on your back that you asked me about?', 'Can I do a cardiograph now?' Always explain before any test, palpation or procedure is undertaken. Do not assume that patients know what we intend to do. Explain and educate the patient on all topics – again, do not assume they know. When examining a patient, always cover exposed parts of the body that will not be examined.

Include the patients in making management and therapeutic decisions. Present your intended plan so that patients have a choice. For example, one might say, 'You have a very strong family history of heart disease, and your cholesterol is really quite high. I think it is very important that we lower it. Would you like to start some medications for it now, or would you like to try some dietary changes for another two months?' Or 'I think we can treat your lower back pain by different ways. I believe that acupuncture would work the best, but if you prefer, we can try physiotherapy instead. What do you think?'

Given that you know the medical procedures and pathways very well yourself, you should help guide the patient onto the easiest path, not just hand the forms or referral over and let the patient deal with them. For example, try to do the blood tests, ECGs, skin biopsies, lung function tests yourself in the rooms, thus, avoiding numerous appointments and waiting times for patients. Ring and expedite appointments with specialists or investigative tests yourself at appropriate times. When the patient rings, an appointment may only be available in four weeks' time, but if you ring and explain the urgency of the condition, it would be much earlier. Warn the patient of the costs of tests and specialist fees. Refer patients only to health professionals that you know well and share your view on what constitutes good 'bedside manner'. If you do this, your patient's appreciation would reduce resistance to treatment by miles and miles.

Giving patients time is also very important. It is always appreciated. Often when given time, patients will tell us what they REALLY came to see us for and, at times, the reason for the resistance they displayed. I remember a story about a very badly behaved palliative care patient who was extremely non-compliant and was abusing staff and patients. The doctor in charge was called in to deal with the situation. According to the story, he just sat with her patiently without judgement or expectations but with care and gave her unlimited time. She then voluntarily disclosed why she was behaving the way she did. It turned out that, years ago, she had a dispute with her brother and did not speak to him for years after that. Because of this, she was not able to talk to her brother before he died of cancer. After relating that to the doctor and weeping, she settled down. She became very apologetic, friendly and caring to her fellow patients and staff. She passed away at peace.

When faced with what appear to be insolvable obstacles and problems, stay with the patient and listen to them, allowing them time, to talk and feel. Opportunities and pathways may open up.

THE QUESTION OF SUCCESS, FAILURE AND HUMILITY

As doctors, being successful in our work is important for our patients, and deeply disheartening when we fail. In general practice, straightforward tasks are normally met with success. Whether it be controlling the blood pressure of a hypertensive patient, removing a simple skin lesion or cleaning an infected wound – all are relatively simple and we would feel quite in control of the expected outcome. However, other tasks may present far greater challenges and uncertainty, such as venepuncture in a six-year-old child, trying to motivate a diabetic patient to lose weight, treating someone with opioid use disorder, or treating someone with a chronic and complicated shoulder pain.

For more specialised procedures that are performed by our specialist colleagues, the sense of not being in control of the outcome is far more common. For example, carrying out a colonoscopy on a patient with known intra-abdominal adhesions and a previous endoscopic perforation, or trying to help a patient's chronic neck pain when two other specialists have failed. I always remember a time when I was assisting in an open repair of a leaking aortic aneurysm (in the days before percutaneous stenting) and the surgeon in charge tried for hours to stop the leakage from the grafted aorta. There have been heroic successes, but I have also seen colleagues who, burdened by the weight of a failed procedure or missed diagnosis, blamed themselves entirely and became disillusioned and despondent. On one occasion, one doctor became very depressed and never practised again.

If we are successful most of the time, some of us can become complacent and even boastful. I remember a patient recounting to me a consultation with a specialist surgeon who leaned across his desk towards the patient and said, 'You know, you are looking at the best.' I have also assisted a surgeon who could do a difficult operation twice as fast and better than most surgeons. He would remain very humble throughout his career.

Trying to own one's successes is often somewhat naïve. There have been times I thought that I was pretty good at treating lower back pains; and as soon as I thought that, I would fail the next few patients. It's a bit like 'writer's block' – after writing a wonderful bestseller, thinking that they will keep coming, only to find that for a protracted period of time, they are unable to write anything of note at all.

Related to success and failure is humility. In traditional Chinese culture, humility is a very desirable attribute. However, as soon as we see ourselves as humble, and claim that we are, we are already the opposite. It is a puzzling paradox.

A number of years ago, I came across a piece of writing that helped me to solve this riddle. One day, I picked up a somewhat neglected book from the bottom corner of my bookshelf, Plato's Apology. It told the story of his teacher, Socrates, and his quest for truth, which ultimately led to his execution. Socrates was named by the Oracle to be the wisest in the land. Being truly humble, Socrates did not consider himself to be wise at all, and in order to disprove it, he set out to find someone wiser than himself. According to what was written about him, Socrates was renowned for his honesty, logical mind and persistence at any given task. In essence, he went around ancient Athens, seeking out the wisest, the best of the poets and the best craftsmen and he would ask what made them the best in their field and wise, above all others, for he was truly mystified. At the end of his exhaustive search and questioning – which would have been very thorough, persistent and analytical – he concluded that none of them knew! Of course, the craftsmen practised their painting and sculpture, the orator debated all the time and had great tutors, but so had those who never reached their level of perfection. Socrates also found out that, amongst these great poets, the average bystanders would understand their poems better than the poets themselves. So where did their excellence and wisdom come from? They didn't know.

This helped me solve the puzzle. I believe we are the instrument of our arts, whether it is poetry, mathematics, swimming, music or medicine. We are all gifted with some excellence in something, in varying degrees. We are drawn to it and tend to become very good at it. These gifts come from whatever you believe in – genetics, a higher being, cosmic energy – but we are not the origin of these gifts. We don't own them. We are just the instrument of expression of that particular art. It comes through us; we are its messenger. I felt a sense of freedom after that realisation. When I approach any task, of course I will try to do my best and prepare for it the best I can. When I succeed, I am just being a good instrument for that art; I don't feel that I own nor do I claim the result, thereby achieving humility without even being aware of it – and I don't own that either. In the face of praise, I just smile and say thank you and, in my mind, say to myself, 'I have been a good instrument.' If I fail, I examine the instrument thoroughly and honestly. If I decide that I have done my best, I don't own the failure either.

If we try to own the result of a task and put ourselves on a pedestal, it can be quite hazardous. The ancient Taoist philosophers knew this and warned that we can only fall from a pedestal; the higher we are, the further we would fall, and fall we will. If we own a lot of precious gems and jewels, we will be always worry about losing them, and one day we probably will. But if we don't own any, we will not be worried about losing them.

Be grateful for your gifts, enjoy them, be a good instrument for them and be free.

REFERENCES

[1] Jordan, K.P., Kadam, U.T., Hayward, R., Porcheret, M., Young, C. and Croft, P., 2010. Annual consultation prevalence of regional musculoskeletal problems in primary care: an observational study. *BMC musculoskeletal disorders, 11*(1), pp.1–10.

[2] Minagawa, H., Yamamoto, N., Abe, H., Fukuda, M., Seki, N., Kikuchi, K., Kijima, H. and Itoi, E., 2013. Prevalence of symptomatic and asymptomatic rotator cuff tears in the general population: from mass-screening in one village. *Journal of orthopaedics, 10*(1), pp.8–12.

[3] Travell, J.G. and Simons, D.G., 1992. *Myofascial pain and dysfunction: the trigger point manual* (Vol. 1 and 2). Lippincott Williams & Wilkins.

[4] Ibid.

[5] Pavón, M. J. G., Redondo, I. C., Vizcaíno, V. M., Morales, A. F., García, P. L., and Bueno, C. Á., (2022). Comparative effectiveness of manual therapy interventions on pain and pressure pain threshold in patients with myofascial trigger points: A network meta-analysis. *The Clinical Journal of Pain, 38*(12), pp.749–760.

[6] Ganjaei, K.G., Ray, J.W., Waite, B. and Burnham, K.J., 2020. The fascial system in musculoskeletal function and myofascial pain. *Current Physical Medicine and Rehabilitation Reports, 8*(4), pp.364–372.

[7] Cao, Q.W., Peng, B.G., Wang, L., Huang, Y.Q., Jia, D.L., Jiang, H., Lv, Y., Liu, X.G., Liu, R.G., Li, Y. and Song, T., 2021. Expert consensus on the diagnosis and treatment of myofascial pain syndrome. *World journal of clinical cases, 9*(9), p.2077.

[8] Mazza, D. F., Boutin, R. D., and Chaudhari, A. J., (2021). Assessment of myofascial trigger points via imaging: a systematic review. *American journal of physical medicine & rehabilitation, 100*(10), pp.1003–1014.

[9] Pavón, M. J. G., Redondo, I. C., Vizcaíno, V. M., Morales, A. F., García, P. L., and Bueno, C. Á., (2022). Comparative effectiveness of manual therapy interventions on pain and pressure pain threshold in patients with myofascial trigger points: A network meta-analysis. *The Clinical Journal of Pain, 38*(12), pp.749–760.

[10] Gattie, E., Cleland, J. A., & Snodgrass, S., (2017). The effectiveness of trigger point dry needling for musculoskeletal conditions by physical therapists: a systematic review and meta-analysis. *Journal of orthopaedic & sports physical therapy, 47*(3), pp.133–149.

[11] Vickers, A.J., Vertosick, E.A., Lewith, G., MacPherson, H., Foster, N.E., Sherman, K.J., Irnich, D., Witt, C.M., Linde, K. and Acupuncture Trialists' Collaboration, 2018. Acupuncture for chronic pain: update of an individual patient data meta-analysis. *The Journal of Pain, 19*(5), pp.455–474.

[12] Liu, W., Fan, Y., Wu, Y., Hou, X., Xue, B., Li, P., Zhang, S. and Yue, Q., 2021. Efficacy of acupuncture-related therapy in the treatment of knee osteoarthritis: a network meta-analysis of randomized controlled trials. *Journal of Pain Research, 14*, p.2209.

[13] Lin, J.G., Kotha, P. and Chen, Y.H., 2022. Understandings of acupuncture application and mechanisms. *American journal of Translational Research, 14*(3), p.1469.

[14] Yamamoto, T., 1998. *Yamamoto New Scalp Acupuncture: YNSA.* "A." Springer Japan.

[15] Artioli, D.P., Azevedo, M.V.G.T. and Bertolini, G.R.F., 2018. Yamamoto new scalp acupuncture: its applications and results in painful conditions. Systematic review. *Brazilian Journal of Pain, 1*, pp.180–183.

[16] Schockert, T. (2011). Yamamoto New Scalp Acupuncture (YNSA): Development, Principles, Safety, Effectiveness and Clinical Applications. In *Acupuncture-Clinical Practice, Particular Techniques and Special Issues.*

[17] Ibid.

[18] Schockert, T., Schnitker, R., Boroojerdi, B., Smith, I. Q., Yamamoto, T., Vietzke, K., and Kastrau, F., (2010). Cortical activation by Yamamoto new scalp acupuncture in the treatment of patients with a stroke: a sham-controlled study using functional MRI. *Acupuncture in Medicine, 28*(4), pp.212–214.

[19] Molnár, I., Máté, A., Szoke, H., and Hegyi, G., (2018). Effects of permanent acupuncture of YNSA (Yamamoto new scalp acupuncture) on quality of life in patients suffering from post-stroke syndrome. *International Journal of Complementary & Alternative Medicine, 11*(3), 00356.

[20] Correia, L. M. F., Alberti, D., and Lopes, S. S., (2015). Evaluation of chronic head and neck myofascial pain control with Yamamoto New Scalp Acupuncture in eight weeks follow-up period. *Revista Dor, 16*, pp.81–85.

[21] Hasegawa, T. M., Baptista, A. S., de Souza, M. C., Yoshizumi, A. M., and Natour, J., (2014). Acupuncture for acute non-specific low back pain: a randomised, controlled, double-blind, placebo trial. *Acupuncture in Medicine, 32*(2), pp.109–115.

[22] Shaladi, A., Crestani, F., Tartari, S., and Trombella, T., (2010). Treatment of neck pain using Yamamoto new scalp acupuncture (YNSA). *Medical acupuncture, 22*(1), pp.41–44.

[23] Artioli, D. P., Azevedo, M. V. G. T., and Bertolini, G. R. F., (2018). Yamamoto new scalp acupuncture: its applications and results in painful conditions. Systematic review. *BrJP, 1*, pp.180–183.

[24] Teo, E., 2023. *Defining the Application of YNSA.*BA Printing and Publishing Services Pty Ltd.

[25] Yamamoto, T., 1998. *Yamamoto New Scalp Acupuncture: YNSA.* "A." Springer Japan.

[26] Konatalapalli, R.M., Lumezanu, E., Jelinek, J.S., Murphey, M.D., Wang, H. and Weinstein, A., 2012. Correlates of axial gout: a cross-sectional study. *The Journal of Rheumatology, 39*(7), pp.1445–1449.

[27] Konatalapalli, R.M., Demarco, P.J., Jelinek, J.S., Murphey, M., Gibson, M., Jennings, B. and Weinstein, A., 2009. Gout in the axial skeleton. *The Journal of rheumatology, 36*(3), pp.609–613.

[28] Jordan, K.P., Kadam, U.T., Hayward, R., Porcheret, M., Young, C. and Croft, P., 2010. Annual consultation prevalence of regional musculoskeletal problems in primary care: an observational study. *BMC musculoskeletal disorders, 11*(1), pp.1–10.

[29] Konatalapalli, R.M., Lumezanu, E., Jelinek, J.S., Murphey, M.D., Wang, H. and Weinstein, A., 2012. Correlates of axial gout: a cross-sectional study. *The Journal of Rheumatology, 39*(7), pp.1445–1449.

[30] Konatalapalli, R.M., Demarco, P.J., Jelinek, J.S., Murphey, M., Gibson, M., Jennings, B. and Weinstein, A., 2009. Gout in the axial skeleton. *The Journal of rheumatology, 36*(3), pp.609–613.

[31] Gaitonde, D.Y., Ericksen, A. and Robbins, R.C., 2019. Patellofemoral pain syndrome. *American family physician, 99*(2), pp.88–94.

[32] Nunes, G.S., Stapait, E.L., Kirsten, M.H., de Noronha, M. and Santos, G.M., 2013. Clinical test for diagnosis of patellofemoral pain syndrome: Systematic review with meta-analysis. *Physical Therapy in Sport, 14*(1), pp.54–59.

[33] Dong, C., Li, M., Hao, K., Zhao, C., Piao, K., Lin, W., Fan, C., Niu, Y. and Fei, W., 2021. Dose atrophy of vastus medialis obliquus and vastus lateralis exist in patients with patellofemoral pain syndrome. *Journal of Orthopaedic Surgery and Research, 16*(1), pp.1–6.

[34] de Marche Baldon, R., Nakagawa, T.H., Muniz, T.B., Amorim, C.F., Maciel, C.D. and Serrão, F.V., 2009. Eccentric hip muscle function in females with and without patellofemoral pain syndrome. *Journal of athletic training, 44*(5), pp.490–496

[35] Petersen, W., Ellermann, A., Gösele-Koppenburg, A., Best, R., Rembitzki, I.V., Brüggemann, G.P. and Liebau, C., 2014. Patellofemoral pain syndrome. *Knee surgery, sports traumatology, arthroscopy, 22*(10), pp.2264–2274.

[36] Lankhorst, N.E., Bierma-Zeinstra, S.M. and van Middelkoop, M., 2013. Factors associated with patellofemoral pain syndrome: a systematic review. *British journal of sports medicine, 47*(4), pp.193–206.

[37] Dillon, C.F., Rasch, E.K., Gu, Q. and Hirsch, R., 2006. Prevalence of knee osteoarthritis in the United States: arthritis data from the Third National Health and Nutrition Examination Survey 1991-94. *The Journal of rheumatology, 33*(11), pp.2271–2279.

[38] Cui, A., Li, H., Wang, D., Zhong, J., Chen, Y. and Lu, H., 2020. Global, regional prevalence, incidence and risk factors of knee osteoarthritis in population-based studies. *EClinicalMedicine, 29.*

[39] Litwic, A., Edwards, M.H., Dennison, E.M. and Cooper, C., 2013. Epidemiology and burden of osteoarthritis. *British medical bulletin, 105*(1), pp.185–199.

[40] Chen, L., Zheng, M., Chen, Z., Peng, Y., Jones, C., Graves, S., Chen, P., Ruan, R., Papadimitriou, J., Carey-Smith, R. and Leys, T., 2022. The burden of end-stage osteoarthritis in Australia: a population-based study on the incidence of total knee replacement attributable to overweight/obesity. *Osteoarthritis and Cartilage, 30*(9), pp.1254–1262.

[41] Jin, X., Gibson, A.A., Gale, J., Schneuer, F., Ding, D., March, L., Sainsbury, A. and Nassar, N., 2021. Does weight loss reduce the incidence of total knee and hip replacement for osteoarthritis? —A prospective cohort study among middle-aged and older adults with overweight or obesity. *International Journal of Obesity, 45*(8), pp.1696–1704.

[42] Chen, L., Zheng, M., Chen, Z., Peng, Y., Jones, C., Graves, S., Chen, P., Ruan, R., Papadimitriou, J., Carey-Smith, R. and Leys, T., 2022. The burden of end-stage osteoarthritis in Australia: a population-based study on the incidence of total knee replacement attributable to overweight/obesity. *Osteoarthritis and Cartilage, 30*(9), pp.1254–1262.

[43] Australian Medical Association. 2023. *Sugar tax, stronger focus on prevention and tackling health inequities key to reducing diabetes in Australia.*

[44] Wang, C., Schmid, C.H., Iversen, M.D., Harvey, W.F., Fielding, R.A., Driban, J.B., Price, L.L., Wong, J.B., Reid, K.F., Rones, R. and McAlindon, T., 2016. Comparative effectiveness of Tai Chi versus physical therapy for knee osteoarthritis: a randomized trial. *Annals of internal medicine, 165*(2), pp.77–86.

[45] da Costa, B.R., Pereira, T.V., Saadat, P., Rudnicki, M., Iskander, S.M., Bodmer, N.S., Bobos, P., Gao, L., Kiyomoto, H.D., Montezuma, T. and Almeida, M.O., 2021. Effectiveness and safety of non-steroidal anti-inflammatory drugs and opioid treatment for knee and hip osteoarthritis: network meta-analysis. *British Medical Journal, 375.*

[46] Bannuru, R.R., Osani, M.C., Vaysbrot, E.E., Arden, N.K., Bennell, K., Bierma-Zeinstra, S.M.A., Kraus, V.B., Lohmander, L.S., Abbott, J.H., Bhandari, M. and Blanco, F.J., 2019. OARSI guidelines for the non-surgical management of knee, hip, and polyarticular osteoarthritis. *Osteoarthritis and cartilage, 27*(11), pp.1578–1589.

[47] Wandel, S., Jüni, P., Tendal, B., Nüesch, E., Villiger, P.M., Welton, N.J., Reichenbach, S. and Trelle, S., 2010. Effects of glucosamine, chondroitin, or placebo in patients with osteoarthritis of hip or knee: network meta-analysis. *British Medical Journal, 341*.

[48] Belk, J.W., Keeling, L.E., Kraeutler, M.J., Snow, M.G., Mei-Dan, O., Scillia, A.J. and McCarty, E.C., 2021. Risk of infection in knee arthroscopy patients undergoing corticosteroid injections in the perioperative period. *Orthopaedic Journal of Sports Medicine, 9*(8).

[49] Burnett, R.A., Khalid, S., DeBenedetti, A., Terhune, E.B., Angotti, M.L. and Della Valle, C.J., 2022. Intra-articular corticosteroid injections are associated with a dose-dependent risk of total knee arthroplasty at 5 years. *Knee Surgery, Sports Traumatology, Arthroscopy, 31*(2), pp.426–431.

[50] Lewis, E., Merghani, K., Robertson, I., Mulford, J., Prentice, B., Mathew, R., Van Winden, P. and Ogden, K., 2022. The effectiveness of leucocyte-poor platelet-rich plasma injections on symptomatic early osteoarthritis of the knee: the PEAK randomized controlled trial. *The Bone & Joint Journal, 104*(6), pp.663–671.

[51] Price, A.J., Alvand, A., Troelsen, A., Katz, J.N., Hooper, G., Gray, A., Carr, A. and Beard, D., 2018. Knee replacement. *The Lancet, 392*(10158), pp.1672–1682

[52] Ibid.

[53] Zwerver, J., Bredeweg, S.W. and van den Akker-Scheek, I., 2011. Prevalence of Jumper's knee among nonelite athletes from different sports: a cross-sectional survey. *The American journal of sports medicine, 39*(9), pp.1984–1988.

[54] van Leeuwen, G. J., de Schepper, E. I., Rathleff, M. S., Bindels, P. J., Bierma-Zeinstra, S. M., & van Middelkoop, M., 2022. Incidence and management of Osgood–Schlatter disease in general practice: retrospective cohort study. *British Journal of General Practice, 72*(717), pp.301–306.

[55] Neuhaus, C., Appenzeller-Herzog, C. and Faude, O., 2021. A systematic review on conservative treatment options for OSGOOD-Schlatter disease. *Physical Therapy in Sport, 49*, pp.178–187.

[56] Eymard, F. and Chevalier, X., 2016. Inflammation of the infrapatellar fat pad. *Joint Bone Spine, 83*(4), pp.389–393.

[57] Lee, P.Y.F., Nixion, A., Chandratreya, A. and Murray, J.M., 2017. Synovial plica syndrome of the knee: a commonly overlooked cause of anterior knee pain. *The Surgery Journal, 3*(1), pp.9–16

[58] Ibid.

[59] Kessler, J. I., Nikizad, H., Shea, K. G., Jacobs Jr, J. C., Bebchuk, J. D., & Weiss, J. M., 2014. The demographics and epidemiology of osteochondritis dissecans of the knee in children and adolescents. *The American journal of sports medicine, 42*(2), pp.320–326.

[60] Sari, A., Günaydin, B. and Dinçel, Y.M., 2018. Meniscus Tears and Review of the Literature. *Meniscus of the Knee-Function, Pathology and Management*.

[61] Aprato, A., Sordo, L., Costantino, A., Sabatini, L., Barberis, L., Testa, D., & Massè, A., 2021. Outcomes at 20 years after meniscectomy in patients aged 50 to 70 years. Arthroscopy: *The Journal of Arthroscopic & Related Surgery, 37*(5), pp. 1547–1553.

[62] Sibilska, A., Góralczyk, A., Hermanowicz, K. and Malinowski, K., 2020. Spontaneous osteonecrosis of the knee: what do we know so far? A literature review. *International Orthopaedics, 44*(6), pp.1063–1069.

[63] Ibid.

[64] Ibid.

[65] Vosoughi, F., Dogahe, R.R., Nuri, A., Firoozabadi, M.A. and Mortazavi, J., 2021. Medial collateral ligament injury of the knee: a review on current concept and management. *Archives of Bone and Joint Surgery, 9*(3), p.255.

[66] Yamamoto, T., 1998. *Yamamoto New Scalp Acupuncture: YNSA*. "A." Springer Japan.

[67] Teo, E., 2023. Defining the application of YNSA. BA Printing and Publishing Services Pty Ltd, Australia.

[68] Litscher, G., 2020. History of laser acupuncture: A narrative review of scientific literature. *Medical Acupuncture, 32*(4), pp.201–208.

[69] Chon, T. Y., Mallory, M. J., Yang, J., Bublitz, S. E., Do, A. and Dorsher, P. T., 2019. Laser acupuncture: a concise review. *Medical acupuncture, 31*(3), pp.164–168.

[70] Litscher, G., and Opitz, G., 2012. Technical parameters for laser acupuncture to elicit peripheral and central effects: state-of-the-art and short guidelines based on results from the Medical University of Graz, the German Academy of Acupuncture, and the scientific literature. *Evidence-based Complementary and Alternative Medicine: eCAM, 2012.*

[71] Litwic, A., Edwards, M.H., Dennison, E.M. and Cooper, C., 2013. Epidemiology and burden of osteoarthritis. *British medical bulletin, 105*(1), pp.185–199.

[72] Menz, H.B., Thomas, M.J., Marshall, M., Rathod-Mistry, T., Hall, A., Chesterton, L.S., Peat, G.M. and Roddy, E., 2019. Coexistence of plantar calcaneal spurs and plantar fascial thickening in individuals with plantar heel pain. Rheumatology, 58(2), pp.237–245.

[73] Ibid.

[74] Ibid.

[75] Hoy, D., Brooks, P., Blyth, F. and Buchbinder, R., 2010. The epidemiology of low back pain. *Best practice & research Clinical rheumatology, 24*(6), pp.769–781.

[76] Jordan, K.P., Kadam, U.T., Hayward, R., Porcheret, M., Young, C. and Croft, P., 2010. Annual consultation prevalence of regional musculoskeletal problems in primary care: an observational study. *BMC musculoskeletal disorders, 11*(1), pp.1–10.

[77] Peng, T., Pérez, A., & Gabriel, K. P., 2018. The association among overweight, obesity, and low back pain in US adults: a cross-sectional study of the 2015 National Health Interview Survey. *Journal of manipulative and physiological therapeutics, 41*(4), pp.294–303.

[78] Alexander, C. E., Cascio, M. A., & Varacallo, M., 2023. Lumbosacral facet syndrome.

[79] Middleton, K. and Fish, D.E., 2009. Lumbar spondylosis: clinical presentation and treatment approaches. *Current Reviews in Musculoskeletal Medicine, 2*, pp.94–104.

[80] Will, J.S., Bury, D.C. and Miller, J.A., 2018. Mechanical low back pain. *American family physician, 98*(7), pp.421–428.

[81] Watts, J., Abimanyi-Ochom, J., Sanders, K., 2022. Osteoporosis costing all Australians. A new burden of disease analysis – 2012 to 2022. *Osteoporosis Australia.*

[82] Ma, Y., Wu, X., Xiao, X., Ma, Y., Feng, L., Yan, W., Chen, J. and Yang, D., 2020. Effects of teriparatide versus percutaneous vertebroplasty on pain relief, quality of life and cost-effectiveness in postmenopausal females with acute osteoporotic vertebral compression fracture: a prospective cohort study. *Bone, 131*, pp.115–154.

[83] Will, J.S., Bury, D.C. and Miller, J.A., 2018. Mechanical low back pain. *American family physician, 98*(7), pp.421–428.

[84] Mohile, N.V., Kuczmarski, A.S., Lee, D., Warburton, C., Rakoczy, K. and Butler, A.J., 2022. Spondylolysis and isthmic spondylolisthesis: a guide to diagnosis and management. *The Journal of the American Board of Family Medicine, 35*(6), pp.1204–1216.

[85] Peng, Z., Jia, Y., Li, J. and Wang, G., 2024. Diagnostic performance of SPECT in lumbar spondylolysis: a systematic review and meta-analysis. *Clinical Radiology, 79*(1), pp.137–146.

[86] Koslosky, E. and Gendelberg, D., 2020. Classification in brief: the Meyerding classification system of spondylolisthesis. *Clinical orthopaedics and related research, 478*(5), p.1125.

[87] Atalay, B., Gadjradj, P.S., Sommer, F.S., Wright, D., Rawanduzy, C., Ghogawala, Z. and Härtl, R., 2023. Natural history of degenerative spondylolisthesis. A systematic review and meta-analysis. *World Neurosurgery*.

[88] Robinson, P.C., 2020. Axial spondyloarthritis: what is it and how is it diagnosed and managed? *Medicine Today, 21*(2). pp.45–47.

[89] Ibid.

[90] Strand, V. and Singh, J.A., 2017. Evaluation and management of the patient with suspected inflammatory spine disease. In *Mayo Clinic Proceedings, 92*(4), pp.555–564.

[91] FitzGerald, O., Ogdie, A., Chandran, V., Coates, L.C., Kavanaugh, A., Tillett, W., Leung, Y.Y., deWit, M., Scher, J.U. and Mease, P.J., 2021. Psoriatic arthritis. *Nature reviews Disease primers, 7*(1), p.59.

[92] Ibid.

[93] Wendling, D., Prati, C., Chou, M., and Verhoeven, F., 2020. Reactive arthritis: treatment challenges and future perspectives. *Current rheumatology reports, 22*, pp.1–7.

[94] Jubber, A. and Moorthy, A., 2021. Reactive arthritis: a clinical review. *Journal of the Royal College of Physicians of Edinburgh, 51*(3), pp.288–297.

[95] Ibid.

[96] Konatalapalli, R.M., Lumezanu, E., Jelinek, J.S., Murphey, M.D., Wang, H. and Weinstein, A., 2012. Correlates of axial gout: a cross-sectional study. *The Journal of Rheumatology, 39*(7), pp.1445–1449.

[97] Konatalapalli, R.M., Demarco, P.J., Jelinek, J.S., Murphey, M., Gibson, M., Jennings, B. and Weinstein, A., 2009. Gout in the axial skeleton. *The Journal of rheumatology, 36*(3), pp.609–613.

[98] Kumar, N., Tan, W.L.B., Wei, W. and Vellayappan, B.A., 2020. An overview of the tumors affecting the spine—Inside to out. *Neuro-oncology practice, 7*(1), pp.10–17.

[99] Ibid.

[100] Ibid.

[101] Mekhail, N., Saweris, Y., Sue Mehanny, D., Makarova, N., Guirguis, M. and Costandi, S., 2021. Diagnosis of sacroiliac joint pain: predictive value of three diagnostic clinical tests. *Pain Practice, 21*(2), pp.204–214.

[102] Jung, M.W., Schellhas, K. and Johnson, B., 2020. Use of diagnostic injections to evaluate sacroiliac joint pain. *International Journal of Spine Surgery, 14*(1), pp.30–34.

[103] Parperis, K., Psarelis, S. and Nikiphorou, E., 2020. Osteitis condensans ilii: current knowledge and diagnostic approach. *Rheumatology international, 40*(7), pp.1013–1019.

[104] Ibid.

[105] Grimm, B.D., Blessinger, B.J., Darden, B.V., Brigham, C.D., Kneisl, J.S. and Laxer, E.B., 2015. Mimickers of lumbar radiculopathy. *JAAOS-Journal of the American Academy of Orthopaedic Surgeons, 23*(1), pp.7–17.

[106] Will, J.S., Bury, D.C. and Miller, J.A., 2018. Mechanical low back pain. *American family physician, 98*(7), pp.421–428.

[107] Berry, J.A., Elia, C., Saini, H.S. and Miulli, D.E., 2019. A review of lumbar radiculopathy, diagnosis, and treatment. *Cureus, 11*(10).

[108] van der Windt, D.A., Simons, E., Riphagen, I., Ammendolia, C., Verhagen, A.P., Laslett, M., Deville, W., Deyo, R.A., Boulter, L.M., de Vet, H.C. and Aertgeerts, B., 2010. Physical examination for lumbar radiculopathy due to disc herniation in patients with low back pain. *Cochrane Database Syst Rev,* (2).

[109] Lam, O.T., Strenger, D.M., Chan-Fee, M., Pham, P.T., Preuss, R.A. and Robbins, S.M., 2018. Effectiveness of the McKenzie method of mechanical diagnosis and therapy for treating low back pain: literature review with meta-analysis. *Journal of orthopaedic & sports physical therapy, 48*(6), pp.476–490.

[110] Halliday, M.H., Pappas, E., Hancock, M.J., Clare, H.A., Pinto, R.Z., Robertson, G. and Ferreira, P.H., 2016. A randomized controlled trial comparing the McKenzie method to motor control exercises in people with chronic low back pain and a directional preference. *Journal of Orthopaedic & Sports Physical Therapy, 46*(7), pp.514–522.

[111] Clark, R., Weber, R.P. and Kahwati, L., 2020. Surgical management of lumbar radiculopathy: a systematic review. *Journal of general internal medicine, 35*(3), pp.855–864.

[112] Wilson, H., Armstrong, F., & Thong, I., 2020. Opioid prescribing: what do the 2020 PBS changes mean for GPs? *Medicine Today, 21*(9), pp.21–28.

[113] Ibid.

[114] Katz, J.N., Zimmerman, Z.E., Mass, H. and Makhni, M.C., 2022. Diagnosis and management of lumbar spinal stenosis: a review. Journal of the *American Medical Association, 327*(17), pp.1688–1699.

[115] Ibid.

[116] Will, J.S., Bury, D.C. and Miller, J.A., 2018. Mechanical low back pain. *American family physician, 98*(7), pp.421–428.

[117] Cohen, S.P. and Raja, S.N., 2007. Pathogenesis, diagnosis, and treatment of lumbar zygapophysial (facet) joint pain. *The Journal of the American Society of Anaesthesiologists, 106*(3), pp.591–614.

[118] Will, J.S., Bury, D.C. and Miller, J.A., 2018. Mechanical low back pain. *American family physician, 98*(7), pp.421–428.

[119] Luesma, M.J., Galé, I. and Fernando, J., 2021. Diagnostic and therapeutic algorithm for pudendal nerve entrapment syndrome. *Medicina Clínica (English Edition), 157*(2), pp.71–78.

[120] Possover, M., Forman, A., 2012. Voiding Dysfunction Associated with Pudendal Nerve Entrapment. *Current Bladder Dysfunction Reports, 7*(4), pp.281–285.

[121] Board, T.N., Hughes, S.J. and Freemont, A.J., 2014. Trochanteric bursitis: the last great misnomer. *Hip international, 24*(6), pp.610–615.

[122] Klauser, A.S., Martinoli, C., Tagliafico, A., Bellmann-Weiler, R., Feuchtner, G.M., Wick, M. and Jaschke, W.R., 2013. Greater trochanteric pain syndrome. In *Seminars in musculoskeletal radiology, 17*(1), pp.43–48.

[123] Pianka, M.A., Serino, J., DeFroda, S.F., and Bodendorfer, B. M., 2021. Greater trochanteric pain syndrome: Evaluation and management of a wide spectrum of pathology. *SAGE Open Medicine, 9*.

[124] Tinetti, M.E., Speechley, M. and Ginter, S.F., 1988. Risk factors for falls among elderly persons living in the community. *New England journal of medicine, 319*(26), pp.1701–1707.

[125] Australian Bureau of Statistics. 2019. *Opioid-induced deaths in Australia*.

[126] Wilson, N., Kariisa, M., Seth, P., Smith IV, H. and Davis, N.L., 2020. Drug and opioid-involved overdose deaths—United States, 2017–2018. *Morbidity and Mortality Weekly Report, 69*(11), p.290.

[127] Wilson, H., Armstrong, F. and Thong, I., 2020. Opioid prescribing: what do the 2020 PBS changes mean for GPs? Medicine Today, 21(9), pp.21–28.

[128] Australian Bureau of Statistics. 2019. *Opioid-induced deaths in Australia*.

[129] Lintzeris, N., & Wilson, H., 2020. Take-home intranasal naloxone to prevent opioid overdose deaths. *Medicine Today, 21*(4), pp.45–49.

[130] Konatalapalli, R.M., Lumezanu, E., Jelinek, J.S., Murphey, M.D., Wang, H. and Weinstein, A., 2012. Correlates of axial gout: a cross-sectional study. *The Journal of Rheumatology, 39*(7), pp.1445–1449.

[131] Konatalapalli, R.M., Demarco, P.J., Jelinek, J.S., Murphey, M., Gibson, M., Jennings, B. and Weinstein, A., 2009. Gout in the axial skeleton. *The Journal of rheumatology, 36*(3), pp.609–613.

[132] Australian Orthopaedic Association National Joint Replacement Registry (AOANJRR). 2021. Lay Summary: Supplementary Report, in Hip, Knee & Shoulder Arthroplasty: Annual Report.

[133] Kara, M., and Alp, G., 2023. Can normal erythrocyte sedimentation rate and c-reactive protein level be a reason for diagnostic delay in polymyalgia rheumatica? *British Medical Journal, 82*(1), pp.1576–1577.

[134] Onks, C., Silvis, M., Loeffert, J., Tucker, J. and Gallo, R.A., 2021. Conservative or surgical management for that shoulder dislocation?. *The Journal of Family Practice, 70*(2).

[135] Ibid.

[136] Shanahan, E.M. and Buchbinder, R., 2010. The painful shoulder. *Medicine Today, 11*(9), pp.73–79.

[137] Jordan, K.P., Kadam, U.T., Hayward, R., Porcheret, M., Young, C. and Croft, P., 2010. Annual consultation prevalence of regional musculoskeletal problems in primary care: an observational study. *BMC musculoskeletal disorders, 11*(1), pp.1–10.

[138] Cross, T., 2006. Rotator cuff problems in sport. *Medicine Today,* 7(11), pp.75–79.

[139] Park, H.B., Yokota, A., Gill, H.S., El Rassi, G. and McFarland, E.G., 2005. Diagnostic accuracy of clinical tests for the different degrees of subacromial impingement syndrome. *Journal of Bone and Joint Surgery, 87*(7), pp.1446–1455.

[140] Hermans, J., Luime, J.J., Meuffels, D.E., Reijman, M., Simel, D.L. and Bierma-Zeinstra, S.M., 2013. Does this patient with shoulder pain have rotator cuff disease? The Rational Clinical Examination systematic review. *Journal of the American Medical Association, 310*(8), pp.837–847.

[141] Minagawa, H., Yamamoto, N., Abe, H., Fukuda, M., Seki, N., Kikuchi, K., Kijima, H., & Itoi, E., 2013. Prevalence of symptomatic and asymptomatic rotator cuff tears in the general

population: from mass-screening in one village. *Journal of orthopaedics, 10*(1), pp.8–12.

[142] Konatalapalli, R.M., Lumezanu, E., Jelinek, J.S., Murphey, M.D., Wang, H. and Weinstein, A., 2012. Correlates of axial gout: a cross-sectional study. *The Journal of Rheumatology, 39*(7), pp.1445–1449.

[143] Konatalapalli, R.M., Demarco, P.J., Jelinek, J.S., Murphey, M., Gibson, M., Jennings, B. and Weinstein, A., 2009. Gout in the axial skeleton. *The Journal of rheumatology, 36*(3), pp.609–613.

[144] Cohen, S.P., 2015. Epidemiology, diagnosis, and treatment of neck pain. In *Mayo Clinic Proceedings, 90*(2), pp.284–299.

[145] Peene, L., Cohen, S. P., Brouwer, B., James, R., Wolff, A., Van Boxem, K., & Van Zundert, J., 2023. 2. Cervical radicular pain. *Pain Practice, 23*(7), pp.800–817.

[146] Cohen, S.P., 2015. Epidemiology, diagnosis, and treatment of neck pain. In *Mayo Clinic Proceedings, 90*(2), pp.284–299.

[147] Kirpalani, D. and Mitra, R., 2008. Cervical facet joint dysfunction: a review. *Archives of physical medicine and rehabilitation, 89*(4), pp.770–774.

[148] Hurley, R.W., Adams, M.C., Barad, M., Bhaskar, A., Bhatia, A., Chadwick, A., Deer, T.R., Hah, J., Hooten, W.M., Kissoon, N.R. and Lee, D.W., 2021. Consensus practice guidelines on interventions for cervical spine (facet) joint pain from a multispecialty international working group. *Pain Medicine, 22*(11), pp.2443–2524.

[149] Suer, M., Wahezi, S.E., Abd-Elsayed, A. and Sehgal, N., 2022. Cervical Facet Joint Pain and Cervicogenic Headache Treated with Radiofrequency Ablation: A Systematic Review. *Pain Physician, 25*, pp.251–263.

[150] Hurley, R.W., Adams, M.C., Barad, M., Bhaskar, A., Bhatia, A., Chadwick, A., Deer, T.R., Hah, J., Hooten, W.M., Kissoon, N.R. and Lee, D.W., 2021. Consensus practice guidelines on interventions for cervical spine (facet) joint pain from a multispecialty international working group. *Pain Medicine, 22*(11), pp.2443–2524.

[151] Kirpalani, D. and Mitra, R., 2008. Cervical facet joint dysfunction: a review. *Archives of physical medicine and rehabilitation, 89*(4), pp.770–774.

[152] Dengler, N. F., Pedro, M. T., Kretschmer, T., Heinen, C., Rosahl, S. K., & Antoniadis, G., 2022. Neurogenic Thoracic Outlet Syndrome: Presentation, Diagnosis, and Treatment. *Deutsches Ärzteblatt International, 119*(43), pp.735–743.

[153] Jones, M.R., Prabhakar, A., Viswanath, O., Urits, I., Green, J.B., Kendrick, J.B., Brunk, A.J., Eng, M.R., Orhurhu, V., Cornett, E.M. and Kaye, A.D., 2019. Thoracic outlet syndrome: a comprehensive review of pathophysiology, diagnosis, and treatment. *Pain and therapy, 8*(1), pp.5–18.

[154] Illig, K.A., Rodriguez-Zoppi, E., Bland, T., Muftah, M. and Jospitre, E., 2021. The incidence of thoracic outlet syndrome. *Annals of Vascular Surgery, 70*, pp.263–272.

[155] Jones, M.R., Prabhakar, A., Viswanath, O., Urits, I., Green, J.B., Kendrick, J.B., Brunk, A.J., Eng, M.R., Orhurhu, V., Cornett, E.M. and Kaye, A.D., 2019. Thoracic outlet syndrome: a comprehensive review of pathophysiology, diagnosis, and treatment. *Pain and therapy, 8*(1), pp.5–18.

[156] Ibid.

[157] Gibson, J., Nouri, A., Krueger, B., Lakomkin, N., Nasser, R., Gimbel, D. and Cheng, J., 2018. Focus: sensory biology and pain: degenerative cervical myelopathy: a clinical review. *The Yale Journal of Biology and Medicine, 91*(1), p.43.

[158] Ibid.

[159] Cohen, S.P., 2015. Epidemiology, diagnosis, and treatment of neck pain. In *Mayo Clinic Proceedings, 90*(2), pp.284–299.

[160] Kazeminasab, S., Nejadghaderi, S.A., Amiri, P., Pourfathi, H., Araj-Khodaei, M., Sullman, M.J., Kolahi, A.A. and Safiri, S., 2022. Neck pain: global epidemiology, trends and risk factors. *BMC musculoskeletal disorders, 23*(1), pp.1–13.

[161] Konatalapalli, R.M., Lumezanu, E., Jelinek, J.S., Murphey, M.D., Wang, H. and Weinstein, A., 2012. Correlates of axial gout: a cross-sectional study. *The Journal of Rheumatology, 39*(7), pp.1445–1449.

[162] Konatalapalli, R.M., Demarco, P.J., Jelinek, J.S., Murphey, M., Gibson, M., Jennings, B. and Weinstein, A., 2009. Gout in the axial skeleton. *The Journal of rheumatology, 36*(3), pp.609–613.

[163] Ibid.

[164] Do, T. P., Remmers, A., Schytz, H. W., Schankin, C., Nelson, S. E., Obermann, M., ... & Schoonman, G. G., 2019. Red and orange flags for secondary headaches in clinical practice: SNNOOP10 list. *Neurology, 92*(3), pp.134–144.

[165] Liebert, A., Rebbeck, T., Elias, S., Hawkins, D. and Adams, R., 2013. Musculoskeletal physiotherapists' perceptions of non-responsiveness to treatment for cervicogenic headache. *Physiotherapy theory and practice, 29*(8), pp.616–629.

[166] Ray, J.C., Hutton, E.J., Cheng, S., Zhang, L. and Stark, R.J., 2021. New horizons in migraine therapy CGRP monoclonal antibodies. *Medicine Today, 22*(6), pp.61–64.

Made in United States
North Haven, CT
04 November 2026

21730342R00137